Special aspects
of psychopharmacology

Proceedings of the symposium on special aspects of psychopharmacology, Sainte-Maxime, France, April 25-30, 1982

Possible clinical significance
of recent biochemical and pharmacological findings
with ortho-methoxybenzamides

Chairman : N. Matussek, Munich

Co-Chairmen : H. Dufour, Marseille
K. Fuxe, Stockholm
P. Grof, Hamilton
J. Mendlewicz, Brussels
G. Sedvall, Stockholm

Technical : Sesif/Delagrange, Paris

Organization : Schürholz Arzneimittel GmbH, Munich

Expansion Scientifique Française
15, rue St-Benoît - Paris 6e

ISBN : 2-7046-1134-3

© Expansion Scientifique Française, 1983
15, rue St-Benoît, 75278 PARIS CEDEX 06

Contents

Contributors

Prof. Manfred Ackenheil, M.D.
Psychiatric Clinic
University of Munich
Nussbaumstrasse 7
8000 Munich 2 (Federal Republic of Germany)

Prof. Guiseppe Bartholini, M.D.
Research Department
Synthélabo — LERS
58, rue de la Glacière
75013 Paris (France)

Guy Chazot, M.D.
Neurometabolism Department
Neurologic Hospital
59, Bd Pinel
69394 Lyons Cedex 3 (France)

Prof. Giovanni U. Corsini, M.D.
Clinical Pharmacology
University of Cagliari
Via Porcell 4
09100 Cagliari (Italy)

Brenda Costall, M.D.
Postgraduate School of Studies in
Pharmacology
University of Bradford
Bradford, BD7 1DP (United Kingdom)

Prof. Christian Eggers, M.D.
Child Psychiatric Unit
University of Essen
Hufelandstrasse 55
4300 Essen 1 (Federal Republic of Germany)

William H. Fennell, M.D.
Section of Cardiology
Department of Internal Medicine
Baylor College of Medicine
Houston, Texas 77030 (USA)

Prof. Kjell Fuxe, M.D.
Department of Histology
Karolinska Institute
P.O. Box 60400
104 01 Stockholm (Sweden)

Prof. Carlo Gennari, M.D.
Institute of Medical Semeiotics
University of Siena
P. zza Duomo 2
53100 Siena (Italy)

Prof. Menek Goldstein, Ph. D.
Department of Psychiatry
New York University Medical Center
550 First Avenue
New York, 10016 (USA)

Prof. Paul Grof, M.D., Ph.D.
Department of Psychiatry
McMaster University Medical Center
1200 Main Street West
Hamilton, Ontario L8N3Z5 (Canada)

Gerhard Gross, M.D.
Institute of Pharmacology
University of Essen
Hufelandstrasse 55
4300 Essen 1 (Federal Republic of Germany)

Claus Hagen, M.D.
Department of Endocrinology
Hvidovre University Hospital
2650 Hvidovre (Denmark)

Peter Jenner, M.D.
University Department of Neurology
Institute of Psychiatry
& King's College Hospital Medical School
Denmark Hill
London SE5 (United Kingdom)

Gösta Jonsson, M.D.
Department of Histology
Karolinska Institute
P.O.Box 60400
104 01 Stockholm (Sweden)

Jin-Soo Kim, M.D.
Department of Neurology
University of Ulm
7959 Schwendi 1
(Federal Republic of Germany)

Salomon Z. Langer, M.D.
Biology Department
Synthélabo — LERS
58, rue de la Glacière
75013 Paris (France)

Yves Lecrubier, M.D.
Department of Psychiatry
University Hospital Pitié-Salpêtrière
47, Bd de l'Hôpital
75651 Paris Cedex 13 (France)

Prof. Brian E. Leonard, Ph.D., D.Sc.
Pharmacology Department
University College
Galway (Republic of Ireland)

Prof. Norbert Matussek, M.D.
Psychiatric Clinic
University of Munich
Nussbaumstrasse 7
8000 Munich 2 (Federal Republic of Germany)

Prof. Julien Mendlewicz, M.D., Ph.D.
Department of Psychiatry
Erasme Hospital/Free University of Brussels
808, route de Lennick
Brussels 1070 (Belgium)

Charles Oliver, M.D.
Department of Endocrinology and Metabolic
Disorders
Hospital of the Conception
144, rue Saint-Pierre
13385 Marseille Cedex 5 (France)

Robert M. Post, M.D.
Biological Psychiatry Branch
National Institute of Mental Health
Bethesda, Maryland 20205 (USA)

Annick Pouplard, M.D.
Unit Neuroimmunology
University Hospital
49040 Angers Cedex (France)

Prof. Philippe Protais, Ph.D.
Laboratory of Pharmacodynamics and
Physiology
Medicine & Pharmacy University of Rouen
Avenue de l'Université
76800 Saint Etienne du Rouvray (France)

Alain J. Puech, M.D.
Department of Pharmacology
University Hospital Pitié-Salpêtrière
91, Bd de l'Hôpital
75634 Paris Cedex 13 (France)

Prof. Göran Sedvall, M.D.
Department of Psychiatry and Psychology
Karolinska Institute
104 01 Stockholm (Sweden)

Pierre Sokoloff, M.D.
Research Unit of Neurobiology (U 109)
Paul Broca Center
2ter, rue d'Alésia
75014 Paris (France)

Prof. Bernard Testa, Ph.D.
School of Pharmacy
University of Lausanne
Place du Château 3
1005 Lausanne (Switzerland)

Prof. Paul Trouillas, M.D.
Neurology Unit
Antiquaille Hospital
1, rue de l'Antiquaille
69005 Lyons (France)

Marc Valli, M.D.
Department of Clinical Pharmacology
University Hospital La Timone
Bd Jean Moulin
13385 Marseille Cedex 5 (France)

Prof. Wolfgang Vogel, Ph.D.
Department of Pharmacology
Jefferson Alumni Hall, Room 326
Thomas Jefferson University
1020 Locust Street
Philadelphia, Pennsylvania 19107 (USA)

Foreword

The development of psychopharmacology is due to two factors, firstly and empirically due to the careful, clinical observations of patients who have been treated with a certain substance and secondly, due to the precise work of the neurobiological basic researchers with regard to the mode of action of such drugs. Thus, the clinicians and theoricians have participated equally in the progress of psychopharmacology over the decades. In spite of this, at many congresses and symposia there is still a lack of dialogue between both these groups and for this reason it should be greatly appreciated that at this symposium both theoricians and clinicians had an opportunity to present their results and opinions on psychopharmacology and biological psychiatry and to discuss them. The main point of these discussions was the ortho-methoxy-benzamides, a substance class with a special mode of action which has already found a wide spectrum of application both in the clinic and pratice, although it has only come to the notice of the basic researchers in the past few years and has since been increasingly studied. This volume summarizes the present clinical and neurobiological state of development of these interesting substances and, furthermore, deals with modern biological aspects of specific psychiatric and neurological syndromes. The editors and the participants are grateful to the companies Sesif/Delagrange, Paris, and Schürholz, Munich, especially to Dr. Herrmann, Mrs. Heim, Dr. Fischer, and Mr. Meyran, Dr. Fabregou, for the splendid organization of this symposium and we hope that interested clinicians and basic researchers will profit from this publication.

M. Ackenheil and N. Matussek

1

Structural studies of orthopramides and topographical elements of the dopamine receptor

B. Testa, H. van de Waterbeemd and L. Anker

School of Pharmacy, University of Lausanne, Switzerland

Summary : The conformational behavior of orthopramides has been studied by means of a quantum mechanical method. Four classes of derivatives were investigated, which differ in the nature of their basic side chain. In all four classes (aminoethyl, 2-pyrrolidyl, 3-pyrrolidyl, and 4-piperidyl derivatives), extended conformers are either energetically possible, or the only permitted ones. These conformational properties control one of the key structural features of the molecules, namely the distance between the cationic head and the aromatic moiety. Topographical comparison between dopamine and orthopramides leads to the recognition of a virtual cycle of high electron density and delocalization. These results define a possible mode of binding of the orthopramides on the dopamine receptor and suggest additional topographical elements of this receptor.

Introduction

Substituded *o*-methoxybenzamide drugs (substituted *o*-anisamides, orthopramides) are a group of dopamine (DA) receptor antagonists which belong to four main chemical classes, as summarized in Table 1. The mechanism of action of these compounds is not fully understood, but it is generally thought that they act selectively as DA antagonists on populations of DA receptors not linked to adenylate cyclase (Jenner and Marsden, 1979 ; Kebabian and Calne, 1979 ; Kebabian and Cote, 1981 ; Laduron, 1980 ; Sokoloff et al., 1980). Recent findings, however, indicate that the more lipophilic orthopramides are also moderate inhibitors of DA-sensitive adenylate cyclase (Fleminger et al., in press ; Usuda et al., 1981 ; Woodruff et al., 1980).

Table 1 - *The four main classes of orthopramide derivatives*

Structure	Class of derivatives	Example	R^a	R^b	R^c	R^d
I	Aminoethyl	Metoclopramide	Cl	NH_2	Et	—
		Tiapride	SO_2CH_3	H	Et	—
II	2-Pyrrolidyl	Sulpiride	SO_2NH_2	H	Et	—
		Sultopride	SO_2Et	H	Et	—
		Flubepride	SO_2NH_2	H	$CH_2C_6H_4$-p-F	—
III	3-Pyrrolidyl	YM-08050	Cl	MeNH	$CH_2C_6H_5$	H
		YM-09151-2	Cl	MeNH	$CH_2C_6H_5$	Me
IV	4-Piperidyl	Clebopride	Cl	NH_2	$CH_2C_6H_5$	—

3

These effects of orthopramides on dopamine receptor(s) must be accounted for by structural properties of the molecules including physicochemical properties and stereochemical features. According to this working hypothesis, topographical and conformational features of orthopramides are of considerable interest for an understanding of their receptor selectivity and its rational improvement. Stereoselective activity has been observed for (-)-sulpiride and (-)-sultopride (Jenner et al., 1980).

Theoretical conformational studies of orthopramides

We have investigated the conformational behavior of the four classes of orthopramides using the all-valence-electron semi-empirical PCILO procedure (Diner et al., 1969). One model molecule (Table 1, $R^a = R^b = R^d = H$; $R^c = Me$) was used for each of the four classes. From 360 MHz ^{1}H-NMR spectroscopy, we have observed that the aromatic substituents other than the o-methoxy group, have no discernible influence on the side-chain conformation of orthopramides, as seen in the identical CH_2-CH_2 H-H coupling constants of metoclopramide and its corresponding model o-anisamide (Anker et al., to be published). Standard bond lengths and bond angles (Sutton, 1965) were used, and the molecules were taken in their protonated form which is predominant under physiological conditions. The o-methoxybenzamide moiety was fixed in a planar conformation, which corresponds to its energy minimum (Pannatier et al., 1981). In particular, a strong intramolecular H-bond exists between the amide hydrogen atom and the methoxy oxygen atom.

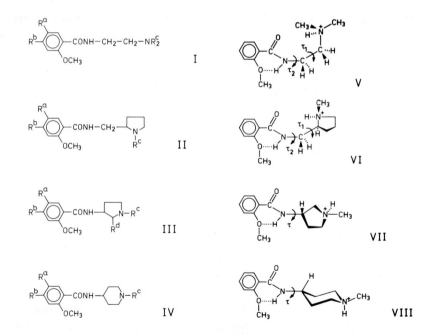

The model of metoclopramide, N-(2-dimethylaminoethyl)-o-anisamide is shown in diagram V with the two torsions angles $\tau_1 = \tau_2 = 0$. The conformational map displayed in Figure 1 was obtained for this molecule (Pannatier et al., 1981). A

4

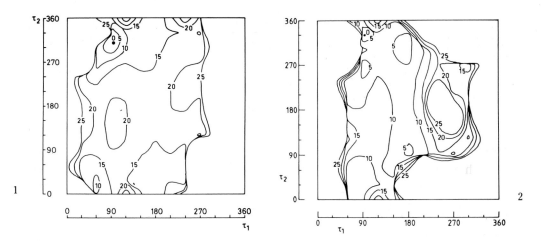

Fig. 1 — Conformational energy map of N-(2-dimethylaminoethyl)-*o*-anisamide. For a definition of torsion angles see diagram V. The isoenergy contours are in kcal/mol.

Fig. 2 — Conformational energy map of N-(1-methyl-2-pyrrolidylmethyl)-*o*-anisamide. For a definition of torsion angles see diagram VI. The isoenergy contours are in kcal/mol.

global energy minimum is observed for $\tau_1 = 90^0$, $\tau_2 = 305^0$, corresponding to a folded conformation. No other energy minimum is seen, but Figure 1 shows that extended conformers in the range $\tau_1 = 150\text{-}240^0$, $\tau_2 = 20\text{-}90^0$ are 10-15 kcal/mol less stable than the preferred conformer. The topographical features corresponding to the preferred, folded conformer, as well as to extended conformers are given in Table 2.

Table 2 - *Topographical features of N-(2-dimethylaminoethyl)-o-anisamide (V) and N-(1-methyl-2-pyrrolidylmethyl)-o-anisamide (VI)*

Compound	τ_1	τ_2	Energy (kcal/mol)	Distances in Å N+/aro. center	N+/molec. plane	N+/O=
V	90°	305°	0.0	5.95	0.75	2.46
	150-240°	20-90°	10-15	6.9.-7.2	0.0-2.2	3.8-4.8
VI	90°	330°	0.0	6.16	0.03	2.56
	90°	270°	1.96	6.29	2.13	3.45
	180°	315°	2.79	7.12	1.32	4.00
	180°	100°	4.21	7.24	1.75	4.69

The model molecule N-(1-methyl-2-pyrrolidylmethyl)-*o*-anisamide (VI) was used for the class of 2-pyrrolidyl derivatives. The conformational map is displayed in Figure 2 (van de Waterbeemd and Testa, 1981), showing a global minimum for the folded conformer defined by $\tau_1 = 90^0$; $\tau_2 = 330^0$. Local energy minima are also apparent, in particular two extended conformers ($\tau_1 \sim 180^0$) which are just a few kcal/mol less stable than the preferred one. The conformers corresponding to energy minima, as well as their topographical features, are listed in Table 2.

When 3-pyrrolidyl (III) and 4-piperidyl (IV) derivatives are considered, the conformational problem becomes more complex than with 2-pyrrolidyl derivatives. Indeed, the flexibility of the saturated heterocycle can no longer be neglected, since

5

Table 3 - *Topographical features of N-(1-methyl-3-pyrrolidyl)-o-anisamide (VII)*

Pyrrolidine conformation*	τ	Energy (kcal/mol)	Distances in Å N+/aro. center	N+/molec. plane	N+/O=
1	0°	9.67	5.80	1.61	2.73
	75°	4.89	5.76	1.18	2.45
2	60°	6.13	6.92	0.74	3.66
3	30°	3.29	5.98	0.62	2.48
4	45°	15.7	6.53	0.23	3.07
5	0°	6.03	7.07	0.62	3.86
	45°	5.39	7.06	0.40	3.81
6	45°	1.00	6.25	0.18	2.72
7	30°	0.58	5.75	0.64	2.24
	60°	0.00	5.75	0.57	2.22
8	60°	16.2	6.39	0.72	3.78

* The conformations of the pyrrolidine ring are :
1 : envelope C_2 up ; 2 : env. N_1 up ; 3 : env. C_4 up ; 4 : planar ; 5 : env. C_3 up ; 6 : env. N_1 down ; 7 : env. C_3 down ; 8 : half-chair C_3 up C_4 down.

the torsion angle τ_1 is included in the heterocycle. As a first step, we (van de Waterbeemd and Testa, in press) have calculated the full geometry of several conformers of pyrrolidine and piperidine using a force-field method (Allinger, 1975, 1976). These conformers were then used to construct the complete molecules VII and VIII, N-(1-methyl-3-pyrrolidyl)-o-anisamide and N-(1-methyl-4-piperidyl)-o-anisamide, respectively. For N-(1-methyl-3-pyrrolidyl)-o-anisamide, 8 curves of potential energy versus torsion angle were calculated by the PCILO method, all of which yield an energy minimum for values of τ between 30° and 90°. The pyrrolidine conformations 6 and 7, which correspond to folded conformers of molecule VII, lead to the lowest energy. It should be noted that the pyrrolidine conformation 5, which corresponds to extended conformers of molecule VII, leads to an energy minimum which is only a few kcal/mol above the global minimum.

Some remarkable topographical features of molecule VII are presented in Table 3. The global minimum corresponds to the shortest distance between N+ and the center of the aromatic ring, with the N+/O= distance implying a strong intramolecular H-bond. Other folded conformers are just a few kcal/mol less stable. Table 3 also shows that extended conformers exhibiting a N+/aromatic center distance of ca 7Å are less stable by only 5-6 kcal/mol.

For N-(1-methyl-4-piperidyl)-o-anisamide, the above mentioned two-step approach was used. First, the geometry of several conformations of piperidine was calculated by a force-field method. The complete molecule was constructed from these conformations. For example, diagram VIII shows this molecule with the piperidine ring in a chair conformation and the anisamidyl substituent in an equatorial position. Six curves of potential energy versus torsion angle were calculated by the PCILO method. The three forms with the equatorial anisamidyl moiety are of the lowest energy, the chair form being the preferred one. All three forms display an energy minimum at $\tau = 180°$, with only a limited variation in energy as a function of τ. The three forms with an axial anisamidyl moiety are of much higher energy. Two local energy minima are seen, namely for $\tau = 90-120°$ and $\tau = 240-270°$.

Table 4 - *Topographical features of N-(1-methyl-4-piperidyl)-o-anisamide (VIII)*

No.	Piperidine geometry* Piperidine conformation	Anisamidyl position	τ	Energy (kcal/mol)	Distances in Å N+/aro. center	N+/molec. plane	N+/O=
1	chair	eq	0°	6.55	7.88	0.02	5.59
			180°	0.0	7.63	0.02	4.32
2	chair	ax	90°	30.88	6.15	2.91	4.14
			270°	36.71	6.18	2.91	4.24
3	boat	eq	180°	10.58	7.67	0.07	4.67
4	boat	ax	120°	28.76	5.14	2.28	2.74
			240°	28.76	5.14	2.28	2.74
5	twist-boat	eq	180°	8.64	7.70	0.02	4.66
6	twist-boat	ax	120°	29.47	5.25	2.28	2.75

* The l-methyl substituent is in equatorial position

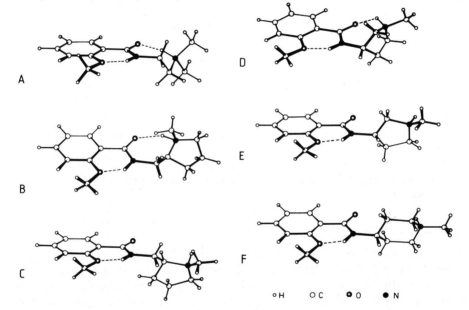

Fig. 3 — Representations, based on computer-generated drawings, of : A : N-(2-dimethylaminoethyl)-o-anisamide in its preferred, folded conformation ($\tau_1 = 90^0$, $\tau_2 = 305^0$) ; B and C : N-(1-methyl-2-pyrrolidylmethyl)-o-anisamide in a folded conformation ($\tau_1 = 90^0$, $\tau_2 = 330^0$) and in an extended conformation ($\tau_1 = 180^0$, $\tau_2 = 315^0$), respectively ; D and E : N-(1-methyl-3-pyrrolidyl)-o-anisamide, conformation 7, $\tau = 60^0$, and conformation 5, $\tau = 45^0$, respectively ; F : N-(1-methyl-4-piperidyl)-o-anisamide in its preferred, extended conformation (chair, $\tau = 180^0$).

Some remarkable topographical features of compounds VIII are presented in Table 4, showing that the preferred conformations are the extended ones (distance from N+ to aromatic center larger than 7.5 Å). The folded conformations with an intramolecular H-bond are less stable by ca 30 kcal/mol. Clearly compound VIII, and hence clebopride, can only exist as an extended conformer under normal condition.

In Figure 3, some conformers of compounds V-VIII are presented in perspective drawing.

Experimental conformational study of metoclopramide using ^{1}H-NMR

Using 360 MHz ^{1}H-NMR spectroscopy, we have investigated the conformational behavior of N-(2-dimethylaminoethyl)-*o*-anisamide (V) and metoclopramide as hydrochlorides in $CDCl_3$ and D_2O (Anker et al., to be published). Of special relevance here is the $-CH_2-CH_2-$ portion of the molecules, which in all four cases appears as an apparently perfect A_2B_2 system with $J_{AB} = J'_{AB} = 6.1$ Hz (Fig. 4). This implies that in all four cases the trans conformer has an energy level identical to that of the two gauche conformers. Hence metoclopramide HCl·HCl in $CDCl_3$ and D_2O exists as a gauche (folded) population of 2/3 and a trans (extended) population of 1/3.

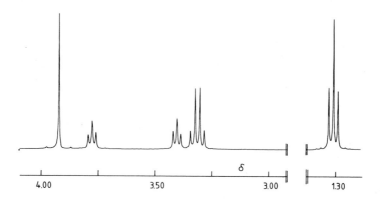

δ

4.00   3.50   3.00   1.30

Fig. 4 — Part of the 360 MHz ^{1}H-NMR spectrum of metoclopramide HCl·HCl in D_2O.

Discussion

Our theoretical investigations indicate that the four main classes of orthopramides have different conformational behaviors. The aminoethyl derivatives, such as metoclopramide, display a 10-15 kcal/mol preference for folded conformers over extended forms. In 2- and 3-pyrrolidyl derivatives (e.g., sulpiride and YM-08050, respectively), the same preference exists, but the energy differences are reduced to 3-5 kcal/mol. In contrast, 4-piperidyl derivatives, such as clebopride, favor extended over folded conformations by a forbiddingly large difference of 30 kcal/mol. These conformational differences, particularly between metoclopramide and clebopride, are so large and incompatible that they suggest different pharmacophores.

It must be remembered that the above results apply only to molecules in the vacuum, that is without any interaction with the environment. A large body of evidence indicates that molecules with a cationic side-chain, when dissolved in water, tend to favor extended forms due to hydration factors. Our NMR investigations confirm that this is also true for orthopramides. As assessed by quantum mechanical calculations, in vacuum the intramolecular H-bond between C=O and N+-H is the main conformational determinant. In water or chloroform solution, this intramolecular H-bond is in competition with intermolecular H-bonds (solvation). A comparison of our results for metoclopramide shows that solvation effects increase the stability of extended conformers by 10-15 kcal/mol.

If this stabilizing effect is assumed to be approximately constant for all orthopramides, then protonated 2-pyrrolidyl, 3-pyrrolidyl, and 4-piperidyl derivatives must all exist predominantly or exclusively as extended conformers in solution. In contrast, as shown above by NMR, metoclopramide exists in a 2/1 folded/extended mixture. We, therefore, hypothesize that the pharmacologically active conformation of orthopramides is an extended one, with an N+/aromatic center distance in the range of 7.1-7.6 Å.

From a study of some rigid neuroleptics such as butaclamol, Humber et al. (Humber et al., 1979 ; Philipp et al., 1979) have derived the topographical features of a dopamine receptor. Of relevance in the present context is the presence, in this model, of two phenyl binding sites, an α- and β-region, located at a distance of 5.1 Å and 6.4 Å, respectively, of the nitrogen binding site (Philipp et al., 1979).

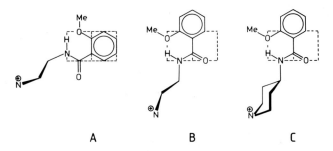

A   B   C

Fig. 5 — Possible modes of interaction of benzamide drugs with the topographical model of the dopamine receptor (Humber et al., 1979 ; Philipp et al., 1979). A and B : two possible modes ; C : interaction of clebopride-like compounds.

Clearly all neuroleptic orthopramides cannot exist with their basic nitrogen only 5.1 Å away form the center of the aromatic ring, as discussed above. However, all these compounds exhibit a virtual six-membered ring, stabilized by the strong intramolecular H-bond which exists between the amide N-H group and the methoxy-O atom (Pannatier et al., 1981). We speculate that this virtual cycle binds to the α-region of the topographical dopamine receptor. This mode of binding leaves the binding site of the phenyl ring undefined. The latter can indeed be conceived to interact with the β-region (Fig. 5 A) or with another, as yet unrecognized, region above the α- and β-region (Fig. 5 B). This latter mode of binding seems more probable, since it is the only one compatible with the conformational behavior of clebopride (Fig. 5 C). Furthermore, as originally derived, the β-region binds to a phenyl ring devoid of electrodonating substituents, whereas such substituents are necessary for the activity of orthopramides.

We believe that the mode of binding of orthopramides to the topographical dopamine receptor is that shown in Figure 5 C. If this assumption turns out to be correct, the topographical dopamine receptor will have to be completed by an additional aromatic binding site.

Acknowledgements
The authors are indebted to the Swiss National Science Foundation for research grants 3.448-0.79 and 3.013-0.81.

REFERENCES

Allinger, N.L. *1975* — Molecular Mechanics MMI/MMPI, QCPE Program No. 318.

Allinger, N.L. *1976* — Calculation of molecular structure and energy by force-field methods. *Adv. Phys. Org. Chem,* 13 : 1.

Anker, L., Testa, B. and Lauterwein, J. (*to be published*).

Diner, S., Malrieu, J.P., Jordan, F. and Gilbert, M. *1969* — Localized bond orbitals and the correlation problem. *Theor. Chim. Acta,* 15 : 100, and ref. therein.

Fleminger, S., van de Waterbeemd, H., Rupniak, N.M.J., Reavill, C., Testa, B., Jenner, P., and Marsden, C.D. — *J. Pharm. Pharmacol.* (in press).

Humber, L.G., Bruderlein, F.T., Philipp, A.H., Götz, M. and Voith, K. *1979* — Mapping the dopamine receptor. 1. Features derived from modifications in ring E of the neuroleptic butaclamol. *J. Med. Chem,* 22 : 761.

Jenner, P., Clow, A., Reavill, C., Theodorou, A. and Marsden, C.D. *1980* — Stereoselective actions of substituted benzamide drugs on cerebral dopamine mechanisms; *J. Pharm. Pharmacol,* 32 : 39.

Jenner, P. and Marsden, C.D. *1979* — Substituted benzamides — Novel class of dopamine antagonists. *Life Sci,* 25 : 479.

Kebabian, J.W. and Calne, D.B. *1979* — Multiple receptors for dopamine. *Nature,* 277 : 93.

Kebabian, J.W. and Cote, T.E. *1981* — Dopamine receptors and cyclic AMP : a decade of progress. *Trends Pharmacol. Sci,* 2 : 69.

Laduron, P. *1980* — Dopamine receptor : from an in vivo concept towards a molecular characterization. *Trends Pharmacol. Sci,* 1 : 471.

Pannatier, A., Anker, L., Testa, B. and Carrupt, P.A. *1981* — A theoretical conformational stydy of substituted ortho-anisamides as models of a class of dopamine antagonists. *J. Pharm. Pharmacol,* 33 : 145.

Philipp, A.H., Humber, L.G. and Voith, K. *1979* — Mapping the dopamine receptor. 2. Features derived from modifications in the rings A/B region of the neuroleptic butaclamol. *J. Med. Chem,* 22 : 768.

Sokoloff, P., Martres, M.P. and Schwarz, J.C. *1980* — Three classes of dopamine receptors (D-2, D-3, D-4) identified by binding studies with ^{3}H-apomorphine and ^{3}H-domperidone, *N. S. Arch. Pharmacol.* 315 : 89.

Sutton, L.E. *1965* — *Tables of interatomic distances and configuration in molecules and ions,* London, The Chemical Society.

Usuda, S., Nishikori, K., Noshiro, O. and Maeno, H. *1981* — Neuroleptic properties of cis-N-(1-benzyl-2-methylpyrrolidin-3-yl)-5-chloro-2-methoxy-4-methylaminobenzamide (YM-09151-2) with selective antidopaminergic activity. *Psychopharmacology,* 73 : 103.

van de Waterbeemd, H. and Testa, B. *1981* — PCILO and CD conformational study of sulpiride, a dopamine antagonist. *Helv. Chim. Acta,* 64 : 2183.

van de Waterbeemd, H. and Testa, B., *1983* — *J. Med. Chem.*

Woodruff, G.N., Freedman, S.B. and Poat, J.A. *1980* — Why does sulpiride not block the effect of dopamine on the dopamine-sensitive adenylate cyclase ? *J. Pharm. Pharmacol,* 32 : 802.

DISCUSSION

M. Ackenheil
It is known that the isomers of some benzamides, e.g. of sulpiride, act differentially on dopamine receptors. What is known about their conformations ?

B. Testa
In principle, two enantiomers have identical energy levels and conformation behavior. In my presentation, I considered only the conformational aspects of benzamides and not the configurational selectivity of the dopamine receptor.

M. Ackenheil
But in your opinion, why do they act differentially on the receptors?

B. Testa
The model of Humber et al. in its present state of development does not incorporate comprehensive enantio-selectivity. In order to do so the model will have to be enlarged. Presumably, the protein environment conditions the enantio-selectivity by providing additional binding or hindering groups, for example, close to the binding site of the nitrogen atom. Our goal is a global topographical view of the dopamine receptor(s) incorporating all steric aspects, of which conformational and configurational selectivity are a part.

G. Bartholini
Concerning the optimal receptor conformation of benzamides, as for the distance between the N-atom and the center of the aromatic ring, do you find it in the region of the 5-6 Å as in the non-benzamide neuroleptics?

B. Testa
That is a very interesting question, but you will have to wait for the presentation of Dr. Jenner to get the answer, because as I mentioned, we are co-ordinated and he will be discussing the biological relevance.

Analysis of transmitter-identified neurons by morphometry and quantitative microfluorimetry. Evaluation of the actions of psychoactive drugs, especially sulpiride

K. Fuxe, L.F. Agnati, K. Andersson, L. Calza, F. Benfenati, I. Zini, N. Battistini, C. Köhler, S.-O. Ögren and T. Hökfelt

Department of Histology, Karolinska Institute, Stockholm, Sweden,
Departments of Human Physiology and Endocrinology, University of Modena, Modena, Italy
Astra Research Laboratories, Södertälje, Sweden.

Summary : Methods have been developed for the morphometric characterization of transmitter-identified nerve cell bodies, dendrites and terminals of central neurons. Different quantitative approaches have also been developed for the determination of the entity of the coexistence of transmitters in neurons. Recently, it has also been possible to develop a methodology for the quantitation of immunofluorescence, using indirect fluorescence methods according to Coons et al. These methods are complementary to those known to quantitate catecholamine fluorescence in sections, making it possible to determine catecholamines in absolute amounts in nerve cells of the central nervous system. All these methods are of paramount importance for the analysis of the mechanism of action of psychoactive drugs in view of their ability to reveal changes in discrete nerve terminals and cell body systems in the brain.
This methodology is applied to the analysis of the actions of antidepressant drugs, such as desipramine and zimelidine and of antipsychotic drugs, such as haloperidol and sulpiride on various types of catecholamine and 5-hydroxytryptamine nerve cells of the rat brain.

Introduction

Morphofunctional studies have become increasingly important in analyzing the actions of psychoactive drugs on the central nervous system in view of the marked heterogeneities present in the various types of transmitter-identified neurons of the brain. The present paper summarizes the recent methodological developments in this area with particular attention on the various central catecholamine (CA) neurons. This article also reports the quantitative microfluorimetrical results obtained by analyzing the action of the two substituted benzamides, sulpiride and tiapride, on the various dopamine (DA) systems both at the cell body and nerve terminal levels. Sulpiride is at present considered a D_2 receptor blocking agent with antipsychotic activity (Spano et al., 1980). Using quantitative microfluorimetrical measurements of DA fluorescence in coronal sections of rat brains, Fuxe et al. (1977 a, b) have demonstrated that dl-sulpiride preferentially increases DA turnover in the tuberculum olfactorium and particularly in the entorhinal cortex.

Morphometrical procedures used to analyze transmitter-identified cell bodies and nerve terminal systems

Cell body level

In a recent paper (Agnati et al., 1982a,b) we have outlined the principles for the morphometrical characterization of transmitter-identified nerve cell groups and for the determination of possible subpopulations within such groups. Cartesian axes are superimposed on the photomontage of the transmitter-identified cell groups under study. Usually the X-axis and the Y-axis are chosen according to neuroanatomical landmarks, for example the midline and the tangent to the inferior border of the brain. Thus, each cell body has its own XY co-ordinates. The next step is the assessment of the number of cells per unit area. A unit area is a square with sides 10 times the size of the mean cell body radius. The density of cell bodies per square, as well as the cell body parameters (mean diameter, mean perimeter, mean area, shape factor) and cell group parameters (number of cells, mean free distance between cells, volume fraction, gravity center, major axis slope with respect to the midline) are obtained by using a semi-automatic image analyzer (MOP Zeiss 02 Kontron) connected to an Apple II computer. This procedure is illustrated in Figures 1 and 2, which show the morphometric description of the 5HT and Substance P (SP) cell groups in nucleus raphe pallidus (B2) obscurus (B2), using as markers 5HT and SP antibodies. Using this type of analysis, it will be possible to detect, for example, whether a chronic neuroleptic treatment increases the degeneration rate of certain types of DA nerve cells in the midbrain.

In addition, we have proposed two approaches which make it possible to objectively determine the possible existence of subgroups within a cell group of transmitter-identified neurons. The first approach involves an analysis of cell body densities within the cell group. The second one detects changes, especially in the shape of the cell group, which can be assumed to result from the partial fusion of two cell clusters. The assessment of subgroups could be important, since it might thus be possible to decide whether, for example, a neuroleptic compound affects preferentially the DA turnover within a special DA cell body subgroup.

Nerve terminal level

Recently we have also proposed a new approach to quantitate the density and antigen contents of transmitter-identified nerve terminals (Agnati et al., 1982). Here again a semi-automatic image analyzer connected to an Apple II computer was used, together with suitable computer programs. A densitometric method has been applied on the original photographs followed by a systematic sampling carried out by means of a grating of circles. This procedure makes it possible to study quantitatively the density and intensity of all types of transmitter-identified nerve terminals. As described above, the procedure involves, first, the selection of the X- and Y-axes, then the division of the area under study into squares in which the number of positive circles (filled by terminals) is calculated. Furthermore, the uniformity of the density of distribution of the nerve terminals per square can be analyzed by Lorenz curves from which a concentration index, the s.c. Gini's index, can be calculated. This index gives an estimation of the degree of unevenness in the distribution of the nerve terminals in the area analyzed. Thus, an overall quan-

14

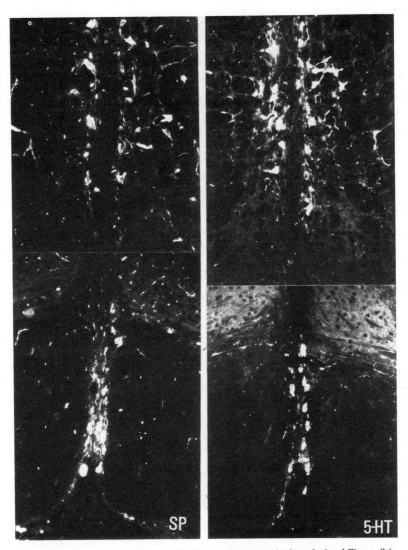

Fig. 1. The two photographs, on which the morphometrical analysis of Figure 2 is based. The cell groups are shown and in agreement with the morphometric analysis there seems to be more 5HT cell bodies than SP cell bodies in the B2 group (Magnification × 120).

titative evaluation of the degree of concentration of various types of nerve terminals in a certain region can be obtained (Agnati et al., 1982c,d). This procedure is illustrated by studying the dorsal-caudal midline area of the medulla oblongata containing mainly the nucleus tractus solitarius, but also the nucleus dorsalis motorius nerve vagi, the nucleus commisuralis and the area postrema. Thus, by means of the present procedure the density distribution of various types of transmitter-identified

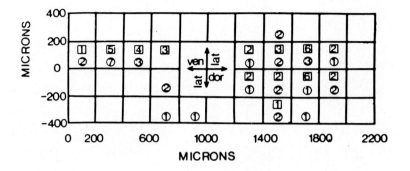

MORPHOMETRICAL EVALUATION OF THE CELL GROUP

PARAMETERS	5HT POSITIVE PROFILES (■)	SP POSITIVE PROFILES (●)
CELL BODY PARAMETERS		
Profile number	39	34
Ferret diameter		
- along the X-axis	34.2	30.6
- along the Y-axis	23.2	21.4
Mean profile perimeter	93	83
Mean profile area	513	395
Shape factor	.73	.71
CELL GROUP PARAMETERS		
Volume fraction	.60	.02
Meann free distance	580	630
Gravity center		
- along the X-axis	977	810
- along the Y- axis	-41	-63

Fig. 2. Density distribution of 5HT and SP immunoreactive nerve cell bodies in the B1 and B2 cell groups of the medulla oblongata of the male rat. The rostrocaudal level is indicated. Two adjacent sections containing 5HT and SP immunoreactive nerve cell bodies were analyzed. Indirect immunofluorescence procedures have been used to analyze coronal cryostat sections of the medulla oblongata of the male rat. The procedure of Agnati, Fuxe et al. (1982a) has been used for this analysis. In brief, a Cartesian plan has been used so that both photographs have common X- and Y-axes. The X-axis has been made coincident with the midline, and the tangent to the ventral surface of the medulla oblongata has been considered as the Y-axis. Each square had a side approximately 10 times greater than the mean diameter of the 5HT and SP nerve cell bodies. The number of cells in each square is shown in the Figure. The morphometrical evaluation of the two cell groups is given in the table below the Figure. The higher number of 5HT nerve cell bodies in group B2 should be noticed.

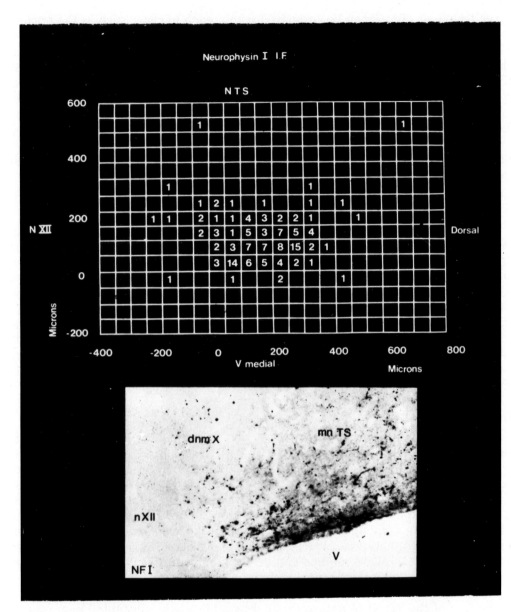

Fig. 3. Morphometrical evaluation of the density of neurophysin I immunoreactive nerve terminals in nucleus tractus solitarius of the normal male rat. An indirect immunofluorescence procedure has been used to demonstrate the neurophysin I immunoreactivity in a coronal section of the medulla oblongata (level -6.2 mm). (Magnification × 300). The procedure is based on the method of Agnati, Fuxe et al. (1982d) to evaluate the distribution density of immunoreactive nerve terminals. A systematic sampling of the area analyzed has been carried out using a suitable grid. The number of positive terminals were counted in each square, with a size of 40 μm. The periventricular border was used to determine the X-axis and the Y-axis was perpendicular to the X-axis, passing through an arbitrary origin.

17

nerve terminals (Fig. 3) can be compared within each nucleus, such as the nucleus of the tractus solitarius. It is thus possible to assess objectively whether or not and to which extent interactions may take place between different types of transmitter-identified nerve terminals. A preferential innervation of a part of a nucleus can also be discovered in this manner. By analyzing adjacent sections showing, for example, PNMT-like immunoreactivity and oxytocin-like immunoreactivity, it is possible to carry out a correlation analysis to evaluate whether a significant co-distribution of the two types of nerve terminal networks takes place.

Histochemical analysis of central CA cell bodies and nerve terminal networks by quantitative microfluorimetrical measurements of CA fluorescence

Cell body level

The CA levels and turnover can be evaluated in Falck-Hillarp preparations, using the tyrosine hydroxylase inhibition model, by the densitometric method of Agnati et al. (1978). This method makes it possible to obtain a rapid evaluation of the overall CA levels and turnover within CA nerve cell groups. Thus, using a photographic method, which involves the use of high contrast Kodalith plates and different exposure times, it is possible to separate the various tones in the negative and, from the areas of the various tones to obtain an overall evaluation of the fluorescence intensity in that area. By this procedure it was possible to demonstrate that a subgroup of A10, located in the medial part, had a considerably higher turnover rate than the DA cell bodies of the substantia nigra (Group A9) (Agnati et al., 1980a).

Nerve terminal level

The quantitative microfluorimetrical determinations of CA fluorescence in various CA nerve terminal populations make it possible to study very discrete CA nerve terminal systems and to discover heterogeneities in the responses, for example to psychoactive drugs administered either for a short time or chronically (Löfström et al., 1976). By demonstrating that the fluorescence yield is the same in the section and in the standard included in the section, it is also possible to determine the absolute amounts (nmol/g) of CA present in the individual DA nerve terminal networks (Agnati et al., 1979). Thus, absolute quantitation of the CA fluorescence by the Falck-Hillarp method can be obtained, and this illustrates once more the usefulness of this histochemical technique.

Evaluation of the action of antipsychotic drugs, especially substituted benzamides, on the DA nerve terminal systems

Evaluation of the dl-, l- and d-sulpiride action

As mentioned in the introduction, we had previously demonstrated that dl-sulpiride preferentially increases DA turnover in the tuberculum olfactorium and in cortical areas, for example the ventral entorhinal cortex (Fuxe et al., 1977a,b ; 1980 ; Agnati et al., 1980a,b). This study has now been continued by analyzing the action of l-sulpiride, which is the active isomer, and d-sulpiride, on the DA turnover

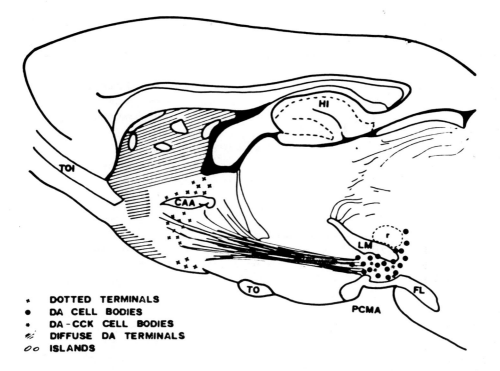

DOTTED TERMINALS
DA CELL BODIES
DA - CCK CELL BODIES
DIFFUSE DA TERMINALS
ISLANDS

Fig. 4. Schematic illustration of the dotted and diffuse types of DA nerve terminal systems in the forebrain, shown in a sagittal plane. The ascending DA pathways are also shown together with the DA-CCK positive and the DA-CCK negative cell bodies.

in the various dotted (CCK-positive) and diffuse (CCK-negative) types of DA nerve terminal systems of the forebrain (Fuxe et al., 1979a ; Hökfelt et al., 1980). The dotted types of DA nerve terminals are in minority and are found in special parts of the nucleus accumbens, tuberculum olfactorium and neostriatum (Fig. 4). They have a lower DA turnover than the diffuse systems and seem to possess CCK-like immunoreactivity. The CCK immunoreactive DA nerve terminals seem to originate mainly from the lateral A10 and medial A9 group. The results with l-sulpiride are summarized in Figure 5. From the dose response curves obtained in the various DA nerve terminal populations it can be shown that, unlike the dl-sulpiride, l-sulpiride does not have any preferential action on the tuberculum olfactorium or the nucleus accumbens compared with the nucleus caudatus. As a matter of fact, the diffuse types of DA nerve terminal systems found in the medial and lateral caudatus appear to be preferentially sensitive to l-sulpiride, since these two areas are the only ones to show a significant enhancement of the H 44/68- induced depletion of DA at a dose of 25 mg/kg. The dotted types of DA nerve terminals in the marginal zone of the nucleus caudatus and within the nucleus accumbens appear to be less sensitive to l-sulpiride, since the enhancement of DA turnover was not significant even at a dose of 100 mg/kg. The results obtained with the inactive form d-sulpiride on DA turnover in various DA nerve terminal populations are summarized in Figure 6. It should be noticed that d-sulpiride can selectively reduce DA turnover in

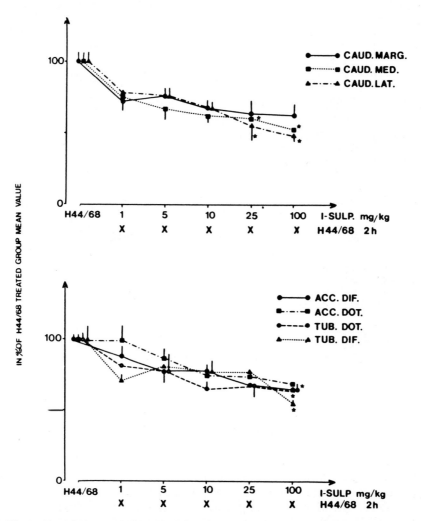

Fig. 5. Effects of l-sulpiride on the H 44/68 (250 mg/kg, i. p., 2 h) induced DA fluoresensce disappearance in various forebrain regions of the male rat. The l-sulpiride was given in various doses at the same time as the H 44/68. The fluorescence value (Y-axis) is given as percent of the mean value of the respective H 44/68 treated group. Each group consisted of 3-4 animals. The statistical analysis was carried out according to the Wilcoxon test : treatment vs controls. *= p<0.05 ; **= p<0.01. 100 % of the DA fluorescence value for the various regions of the control group represents the following absolute concentrations of DA, expressed in nmol/g tissue. Means ± S.E.M. CAUD marg. = marginal zone of the nucleus caudatus : 91 ± 4 ; CAUD med. = medial part of the nucleus caudatus : 96 ± 5 ; CAUD cent. = central part of the nucleus caudatus : 82 ± 3 ; ACC dif. = diffuse type of DA nerve terminals of the anterior nucleus accumbens : 82 ± 3 ; ACC dot. = dotted type of DA nerve terminals of the posterior nucleus accumbens : 165 ± 5 TUB dot. = dotted type of DA nerve terminals of the medial — posterior part of the tuberculum olfactorium : 159 ± 6 ; TUB dif. = diffuse type of DA nerve terminals of the lateral — posterior part of the tuberculum olfactorium : 82 ± 3.

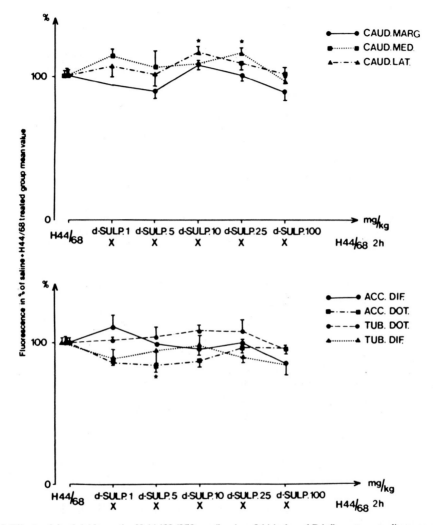

Fig. 6. Effects of d-sulpiride on the H 44/68 (250 mg/kg, i. p. 2 h) induced DA fluorescence disappearance in various forebrain regions of the male rat. The d-sulpiride was given at the same time as the H 44/68 the fluorescence value is given as percent of the mean value of the respective H 44/68 treated group. Each group consisted of 3-4 animals. Statistical analysis was carried out according to the Wilcoxon test : treatment vs controls. * = $p < 0.05$; ** = $p < 0.01$. CAUD marg. = 96 ± 6 ; CAUD med. = 114 ± 7 ; CAUD cent. = 83 ± 6 ; ACC dif. = 79 ± 2 ; ACC dot. = 178 ± 6 ; TUB dot. = 184 ± 8 ; TUB dif. = 79 ± 7. For further details, see text of previous figure.

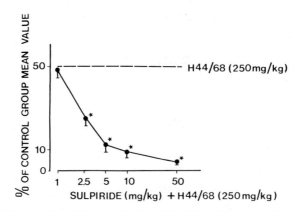

Fig. 7. Effects of dl-sulpiride on the H 44/68 (250 mg/kg, i. p., 2 h) induced DA fluorescence disappearance in DA islands of the ventral entorhinal cortex of the male rat. The dl-sulpiride was given in various doses at the same time as the H 44/68. The Falck-Hillarp procedure was carried out on vibrotome sections (Fuxe et al. , 1977b). The fluorescence value (Y-axis) is given as per cent of the mean value of the control group. Statistical analysis was carried out according to the test for multiple comparisons : treatment vs controls, non parametrical procedures.

the lateral and medial part of the nucleus caudatus at doses of 10 and 25 mg/kg, respectively. Furthermore, d-sulpiride, at a dose of 5 mg/kg, can increase DA turnover in the dotted type DA terminals in the nucleus accumbens. These results can, to some extent, explain the preferential effects of dl-sulpiride on DA turnover in the tuberculum olfactorium and especially in the entorhinal cortex (Fig. 7) in comparison with the nucleus caudatus, (Fuxe et al., 1977a,b) since d-sulpiride can reduce DA turnover in the lower dose range in the diffuse types of DA nerve terminal systems of the nucleus caudatus. Thus, it seems possible that d-sulpiride may exert some DA agonistic activity on pre-synaptic and/or post-synaptic D_2 receptors in the diffuse types of striatal DA nerve terminal systems. In the same experiment, the actions of l- and d-sulpiride were also analyzed using biochemical measurements of DA and NA in the anteromedial frontal cortex. As shown in Figure 8, l-sulpiride at a dose of 25, but not of 10 mg/kg, produced an enhancement of the H 44/68 induced DA depletion. Thus, this area is not as sensitive as the entorhinal cortex to the action of dl-sulpiride. However, it seems as if, within the anteromedial frontal cortex, l-sulpiride might preferentially increase DA turnover compared with its effects on the subcortical limbic areas and in the various areas of the nucleus caudatus. Previous studies have shown that dl-sulpiride can preferentially block apomorphine-induced hyperactivity (ID_{50} value, 15 mg/kg) compared with apomorphine-induced stereotypies (ID_{50} value = 103 mg/kg) (Fuxe et al., 1977 ; Köhler et al., 1979). In view of the present results on DA turnover with l- and d-sulpiride, it seems possible that these behavioral findings could, in part, be produced by a possible agonistic activity of dl-sulpiride at post-synaptic DA receptors of the D_2 types, belonging to the diffuse types of DA nerve terminal populations of the nucleus caudatus, since apomorphine- induced hyperactivity and locomotion are probably mostly dependent on the activation of DA receptors in the nucleus accum-

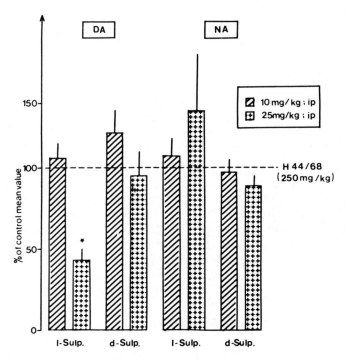

Fig. 8. Effects of d- and l-sulpiride on the H 44/68 (250 mg/kb, i. p., 2 h) induced DA and NA disappearance in the anteromedial frontal cortex of the male rat. The doses used were 10 and 25 mg/kg given at the same time as H 44/68. The DA levels (Y-axis) are expressed as percent of the mean value of the H 44/68. Each group consisted of 4 rats. The statistical analysis was carried out by comparing each treated group with its respective control group using the Student's t-test. * = $p < 0.05$. Means ± S.E.M. are shown. The DA levels in the H 44/68 treated group were 42 ± 6 ng/g, and the NA levels 388 ± 42 ng/g.

bens. Such an agonistic activity of d-sulpiride (Benfenati et al., 1981) could explain, to some extent, the lack of extrapyramidal side effects of dl-sulpiride in the clinic, where it is used as an antipsychotic drug (Jenner and Marsden, 1979 ; Spano et al., 1980). This activity may also contribute to explain why sulpiride produces only weak catalepsy, in contrast to the classical antipsychotic drugs chlorpromazine and haloperidol. The capacity of dl-sulpiride as well as l-sulpiride to increase preferentially cortical DA turnover could be related to a selective *in vivo* distribution of sulpiride in the cortical areas, rather than to differences in DA receptor populations in cortical vs noncortical areas, since *in vitro* sulpiride has not been shown to displace preferentially 3H- spiperone from its binding sites in limbic vs striatal areas (Ögren et al., 1978). In agreement with this proposal, Fuxe et al. (1980b) have found that chronic treatment with l-sulpiride and haloperidol, using the ID$_{50}$ doses to block apomorphine-induced hyperactivity, results in an enhancement of the ability of

23

apomorphine to induce both hyperactivity and stereotypies. This finding shows that, after chronic sulpiride and haloperidol treatment, a DA receptor hypersensitivity is developed both to apomorphine-induced hyperactivity and to apomorphine-induced stereotypies.

Finally, one may also think that a relative lack of DA autoreceptors in the mesocortical DA systems can contribute to the preferential effects observed on cortical DA turnover after dl-sulpiride, since d-sulpiride can also exert pre-synaptic DA agonistic effects in the striatal regions. However, l-sulpiride preferentially increases also DA turnover in the prefrontal cortex, indicating that l-sulpiride may actually be preferentially distributed to some cortical areas.

In vivo binding studies with l-sulpiride

It has been demonstrated that sulpiride cannot block DA sensitive adenylate cyclase activity in any brain area studied *in vitro* or *in vivo* (Spano et al., 1975 ; Scatton et al., 1977 ; Jenner and Mardsen, 1979). Therefore, it has been suggested that sulpiride and other substituted benzamides represent a novel class of DA antagonists, which can only block those DA receptors which are not linked to an activation of the adenylate cyclase, and which have been called D_2 receptors (Kebabian and Calne, 1979). *In vitro*, sulpiride and related substituted benzamide drugs displace ^{3}H-spiroperidol with a lower affinity than other types of neuroleptic compounds (Elliot et al., 1977) and, in contrast to other neuroleptic drugs, with a low Hill coefficient (Fuxe et al., 1979b). The finding of a low Hill coefficient may indicate either a negative co-operativity or a multiplicity of neuroleptic binding sites. Studies on the regional displacement of ^{3}H-spiperone binding *in vivo* by sulpiride show that, in contrast with other neuroleptic drugs such as haloperidol and spiperone, sulpiride can only displace about 40 % of the ^{3}H-spiperone binding sites in any of the regions studied (caudatus, tuberculum) even at high doses (Köhler et al., 1979, Fig. 9B). Köhler et al. (1979) also found that a dose of 10 mg/kg of dl-sulpiride acts preferentially on limbic and nigral DA receptors rather than striatal receptors. These *in vivo* findings on ^{3}H-spiperone binding sites and dl-sulpiride are in good agreement with our DA turnover findings, which show preferential increases of DA turnover in the tuberculum olfactorium and in the ventral entorhinal cortex (Fig. 7), where Köhler et al. (1979) also demonstrated marked effects of dl-sulpiride at low doses. Finally it should be noticed that the affinity of substituted benzamides for ^{3}H-spiperone or ^{3}H-haloperidol binding sites is not correlated with their potency as antipsychotics (Jenner et al., 1978). Therefore, we have also analyzed the action of l-sulpiride on DA agonist sites, using ^{3}H-N-propylnorapomorphine (^{3}H-NPA) as a radioligand. As shown in this and in a previous paper, l-sulpiride displaces ^{3}H-NPA from practically all (91 %) of its binding sites in the striatum and tuberculum olfactorium (Köhler et al., 1981, and Fig. 9). A trend for a preferential action on the tuberculum olfactorium can be observed, as compared with the striatum. It should be noticed, however, that *in vivo* binding experiments show that already after a dose of about 5 mg/kg of l-sulpiride, more than 50 % of the ^{3}H-NPA binding sites are affected by l-sulpiride both in the tuberculum olfactorium and in the striatum, (Fig. 9), while at this low dose the ^{3}H-spiperone binding sites in the striatum and in the nucleus accumbens remain unaffected (Köhler et al., 1979). Only 39 % of the striatal ^{3}H-spiperone binding sites can be maximally displaced *in vivo* by dl-sulpiride, and

24

A

I-Sulpiride displacement of ^{3}H-NPA

B

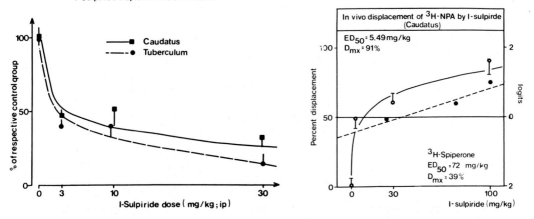

Fig. 9. Effects of l-sulpiride on *in vivo* ^{3}H-NPA in the striatum and tuberculum olfactorium of mice. The l-sulpiride was given 10 min. after the injection of ^{3}H-NPA (5 μCu). The animals were killed 45 min. after the injection of the isotope. The procedure used was that of Köhler et al. (1981). The various doses of l-sulpiride are plotted on the X-axis. On the Y-axis are plotted the remaining specific ^{3}H-NPA binding in the striatum and in the tuberculum olfactorium, expressed as percent of the total specific binding as means ± S.E.M. n=5. A slight preferential action of l-sulpiride can be observed in the tuberculum olfactorium in comparison with the striatum, although it is not significant. The percent displacement by l-sulpiride in the striatum is shown in B, and it is possible to calculate the ED_{50} values by logits transformation. In the lower right corner, the results of the same analysis are shown for the actions of dl-sulpiride on *in vivo* ^{3}H-spiperone binding in the striatum. ^{3}H-spiperone (4μCi) was injected i.v. 90 min. before killing, and the sulpiride was given 30 min. earlier (Köhler et al., 1979).

the ED_{50} value for dl-sulpiride in the striatum is of 72 mg/kg (Fig. 9B). It seems possible, therefore, that some of the behavioral effects and possibly also the antipsychotic activity of sulpiride are related to its ability to block receptors labelled *in vivo* with ^{3}H-NPA, but not with ^{3}H-spiperone. *In vivo* probably only the high affinity type ^{3}H-agonist sites are labelled, focusing the interest on this type of D_2 receptor. The neuroleptic receptors may represent regulatory sites at the DA receptor. This hypothesis may partially explain why sulpiride, as various DA agonists, can displace only about 40 % of the ^{3}H-spiperone bound. The failure of sulpiride and other substituted benzamides to block D_1 receptors may be due to differences in the topography of the neuroleptic binding sites at the level of the D_1 and D_2 receptors, so that sulpiride can only interact with the D_2 receptor, especially the high affinity type D_2 receptor labelled *in vivo* by ^{3}H-NPA. The latter possibility is supported by the fact that the ^{3}H-sulpiride and ^{3}H-spiperone binding sites probably represent different entities (Spano et al., 1980 ; Jenner, this symposium) in view, *inter alia*, of the absolute sodium ion dependency of the ^{3}H-sulpiride binding.

Evaluation of tiapride action

Tiapride is a substituted benzamide of special interest, since it can inhibit dyskinesias induced by DA receptor agonists in laboratory animals (Costall et al., 1978, 1979), and it diminishes dyskinesias caused by L-dopa in Parkinsonian pa-

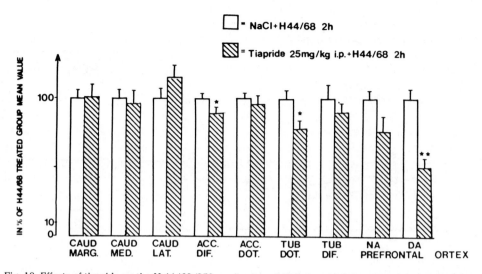

Fig. 10. Effects of tiapride on the H 44/68 (250 mg/kg, i. p., 2 h) induced DA fluorescence disappearance in various forebrain regions of the male rat. Tiapride (25 mg/kg, i.p.), was given at the same time as H44/68. The fluorescence value (Y-axis) is given as percent of the mean value of the respective H 44/68 treated groups. Each group consisted of 5 animals. The statistical analysis was carried out according to the Mann Whitney U-test. $* = p < 0.05$; $** = p < 0.01$. For further details, absolute amounts and abbreviations, see text of Figure 5. The results obtained in the prefrontal cortex (anteromedial frontal cortex) were obtained by means of biochemical measurements using HPLC in combination with electrochemical detection.

tients. Tiapride may also have the ability to block more effectively supersensitive DA receptors than normal DA receptors, as indicated by behavioral studies using the DA receptor agonist apomorphine (Costall et al., 1979). Like sulpiride, tiapride displaces *in vitro* ^{3}H-spiperone or ^{3}H-Cis(z)-flupentixol only when administered at high doses (Jenner et al., 1978 ; Hyttel, 1980). Potent displacers of ^{3}H-l-sulpiride binding from its striatal binding sites are DA, DA receptor agonists and substituted benzamide, while classical neuroleptic drugs can only compete weakly with the ^{3}H-l-sulpiride binding sites (Spano et al., 1980). These results (see also previous section) indicate that substituted benzamides, such as l-sulpiride, can act by exerting an antagonistic activity at the ^{3}H-NPA binding sites, which may label the DA receptors as such and not through actions on the neuroleptic receptors.

The possibility that tiapride, at a low dose of 25 mg/kg, which almost completely inhibits apomorphine- induced hyperactivity with little influence on apomorphine induced sterotypies (Fuxe et al., 1977a, 1980 ; Costall et al., 1977), could differentially influence the diffuse and dotted DA nerve terminal systems of the striatum and limbic forebrain including the anteromedial frontal cortex, has been tested. As seen in Figure 10, the drug produces a selective increase in DA turnover in the limbic areas, especially in the anteromedial frontal cortex where a marked enhancement of the H 44/68- induced DA depletion is obtained (Fuxe et al., 1979c). An increase in DA turnover is also observed in the dotted- type DA terminals of the tuberculum olfactorium and the diffuse type DA terminals of the nucleus accumbens. The striatal DA systems remained unaffected at this dose of tiapride. It seems, therefore, likely that the behavioral effects of tiapride involve actions on DA receptors in subcortical and cortical limbic areas. It remains unclear whether these selective changes are related to a selective *in vivo* distribution of tiapride to the cortical and subcortical limbic areas, or due to differences in D_2 receptor characteristics in striatal and limbic areas. Due to the selectivity of its action on certain types of DA receptors *in vivo*, tiapride may possess, like sulpiride, unique properties which can explain its activity in behavioral syndromes and special clinical cases. It should be noticed, however, that in spite of its ability to increase limbic DA turnover, tiapride is not an antipsychotic drug, which illustrates the problem of correlating antipsychotic activity with DA turnover changes. The antidyskinetic properties of tiapride appear only at higher doses and the mechanisms for this activity are unknown (Costall, this symposium).

Novel approaches to the morphofunctional analysis of transmitter-identified neurons

Quantitative immunocytochemistry

Through immunofluorescence histochemistry it is now possible to locate 5HT and neuropeptide transmitters, as well as co-modulators in central neurons. In order to understand the functional role of, for example, the neuropeptide neurons of the brain, it is necessary to develop a method to quantitate immunofluorescence in sections, in order to discover changes in peptide content in discrete cell body and nerve terminal populations. We have, therefore, developed a new methodology to satisfy this need. The procedure is shown on 5HT nerve cell bodies of the medulla oblongata, which can be demonstrated by a specific anti-5HT antibody (Steinbusch et al., 1978). The 5HT immunoreactivity in nerve cell bodies and terminals were measured with a Zeiss microscopy fluorimeter (03) equipped with a standard FITC interference filter set. The transmittance range was from 450 to 490 nm with a steep cut- off (LP 520). The 5HT immunoreactivity was determined in different sections, using various dilutions of the specific 5HT antibody. The intensity of the specific immunofluorescence was obtained by subtracting the background fluorescence from the value obtained in the area under study. The reaction of the antibody with the antigen is based on the law of mass action. Therefore, it should be possible to obtain a relative value of the antigen content in 5HT nerve cell bodies and terminals by using the saturation analysis indicated above, followed by Scatchard plots, which, in the presence of only one type of recognition site and in the absence of co-operativity, should give a straight line. Two different 5HT antibodies have been used on pairs of subsequent sections of medulla oblongata and, as shown in Figure 11, they both give the same B_{max} values (same intercept with the X-axis), but different K_D values (different slopes). The same B_{max} values obtained with the two antibodies indicate that, as expected, the two procedures result in a similar relative value of the 5HT content in the cell bodies, while the different slope values show, as expected, that the antibodies used have different affinities for the antigen 5HT. By this procedure, it will now be possible to perform a quantitative immunocytochemical analysis of structures demonstrated by indirect immunofluorescence technique. This new procedure opens up a new field in the area of brain research. Using this procedure we have recently been able to demonstrate

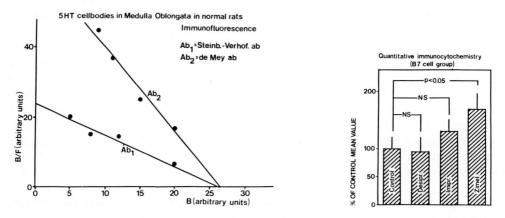

Fig. 11. Quantitative immunocytochemical evaluation of the 5HT immunoreactivity in 5HT nerve cell bodies of the medulla oblongata (nucleus raphe obscurus). Two types of antibodies obtained from Drs. Steinbusch and Verhofstad and from Dr. De Mey, respectively, have been used to detect 5HT immunoreactivity. The 5HT immunoreactivity was evaluated in two corresponding set of sections, each set having been incubated with one type of antibody. An indirect immunofluorescence procedure was used, with an FITC-labelled second antibody. The antisera were diluted 1 : 100 - 1 : 1 000. The 5HT immunofluorescence was measured in 5HT nerve cell bodies quantitative microfluorimetry, using an optimal filter combination for FITC fluorescence. The specific 5HT fluorescence was obtained by subtracting the background fluorescence. A saturation curve of 5HT immunofluorescence was obtained by performing the measurements with different dilutions of the antibodies. The Scatchard plots of the saturation curves are shown in the figure. The two antibodies produce the same B_{max} values, but different K_D values as can be seen from the different slopes. In both cases the Scatchard plot has, as a best fit line, a straight line. It should also be noticed that the same B_{max} value was obtained with the two 5HT antibodies making it possible to obtain comparable results with different types of antibodies upon a quantitative basis.

Fig. 12. Effects of chronic treatment with desipramine, imipramine and zimelidine ($2 \times 10 \mu$ mol/kg per day for 2 weeks) on the 5HT immunoreactive content of the 5HT nerve cell bodies of the nucleus raphe dorsalis (B7). The rats were killed 24 h following the last oral treatment of the three antidepressants. Means ± S.E.M. out of 4 rats. Eight sections were studied for each animal. On the Y-axis the 5HT immunofluorescence values are expressed as per cent of the mean value of the control group. For each animal, the 5HT immunofluorescence value was obtained from the B_{max} value of the respective Scatchard plot. The statistical analysis was made according to the test for multiple comparisons : treatment vs controls, non parametrical procedures.

that chronic treatment with zimelidine, a new antidepressant drug, results in an increase in 5HT immunoreactivity in the nucleus raphe dorsalis of the midbrain (Fig. 12).

Quantitative evaluation of the coexistence of transmitters

During recent years it has become of importance to understand the functional significance of the coexistence of monoamines and peptides, or of two types of neuropeptides, in the same neuron (Agnati et al., 1982e). Therefore, it has become necessary to develop methods for the quantitative evaluation of the coexistence in various physiological and experimental states. One method is based on the use of a semi-automatic image analyzer to study the nerve cell bodies in a Cartesian plan.

When profiles show at least a 30 % overlap in the same or adjacent sections, it is possible to state that they coexist in the same nerve cell body. This procedure can be used after different staining techniques employed to demonstrate different transmitters in the nerve cell bodies. With the present set up the sensitivity of the procedure is 0.1 mm and the nerve cell body has a size of 3.5 mm (Agnati et al., 1982e). By this morphometric procedure it becomes thus possible to define, on objective grounds and in a quantitative fashion, the extent of coexistence of various substances in the same cell (Agnati et al., 1982e). Another procedure, which we have developed, is based on a statistical approach, which involves the analysis of three adjacent sections, randomly stained with antisera against neuromodulator I, neuromodulator II or against both neuromodulators I and II. The coexistence can then be shown by subtracting from the sum of the immunoreactive profiles obtained with the first and second antibodies (against neuromodulators I et II, respectively), the number of immunoreactive profiles obtained with the combined antibodies (against both types of neuromodulators) (Agnati et al., 1982f). This analysis can also be supplemented with another morphometric procedure to collect additional information on the extent of coexistence. The gravity centers of the two cell groups in question are calculated in adjacent sections, that is ACTH- and β-endorphin immunoreactive nerve cell groups. If, at various brain levels, the distances between the two gravity centers of the two, ACTH- and β-endorphin positive cell groups are significantly different it indicates that the coexistence is not of 100 %. The first procedure mentioned above has been further improved by the use of a grid of squares, which can be superimposed on photographs of adjacent sections having common X- and Y-axes. This grid was then analyzed by a mask consisting of circles (11 μm in diameter) arranged in a square pattern and with an intercenter distance of 40 μm. The sides of the squares were of 40 μm. By means of a semi-automatic image analyzer coupled with an Apple II computer and with suitable computer programs only the circles completely filled with fluorescence were counted (Agnati et al., 1982d ; Fuxe et al., 1982). When analyzing nerve cell body populations with a mean diameter of 21 μm one nerve cell body can only fill one circle and a 26 % overlap is required for a positive result. Therefore, when corresponding circles in the two photographs are positive, there exists an area of coexistence. The computer was programmed to plot such squares as black squares. The last method represents the simplest way to obtain a relative quantitation of the coexistence of substances in nerve cell bodies. With these various approaches it is possible to determine whether a chronic treatment with antidepressants or neuroleptic drugs of various types can modulate the coexistence in, for example the various monoamine pathways of the brain and spinal cord. Such information is quite important for the understanding of the mechanism of action of such drugs.

Receptor autoradiography

Due to the work of Kuhar, Young, Palacios et al. (Palacios et al., 1981 ; Young and Kuhar, 1979) it is possible to perform morphofunctional studies at the postsynaptic level of transmitter-identified neurons. The results obtained on turnover in discrete nerve terminal populations can then be correlated with possible changes occuring in the receptors belonging to those nerve terminal networks. Furthermore, with the recent development of autoradiography with tritium-sensitive

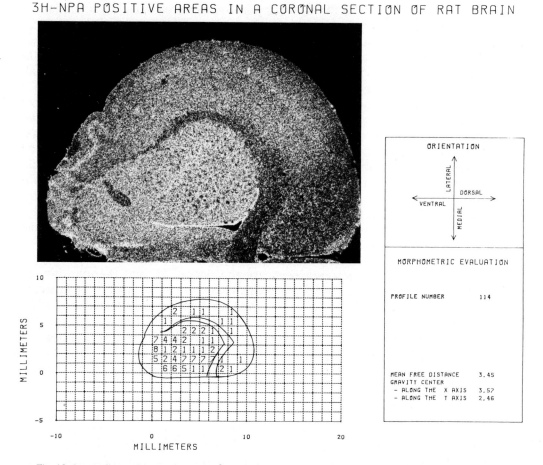

Fig. 13. Autoradiographic distribution of ^{3}H-NPA binding sites in a coronal section of rat brain at the level of A 8620. The procedure was that of Palacios et al. (1981). Sections were prepared and incubated with 1 nM of ^{3}H-NPA (60 Cu/mmol, New England Nuclear Corporation, Boston, Maryland, U.S.A.). Sheets of ^{3}H-Ultrofilm (LKB) were used and the exposure time was of 3 weeks at —20° C. A morphometrical approach to evaluate the radioligand positive areas in the autoradiogram is shown. A quantitation of the most positive areas was obtained by a grid of squares (1mm[2] per square) using a mask of circles (100 μm in diameter ; 10 circles per square).

film, it is possible to quantitate in a simple way the distribution of receptors in sections by means of computerized densitometry and morphometrical evaluation of the size and distribution of the radioligand positive areas after incubation (Agnati and Fuxe, 1982). This procedure is illustrated in Figure 13, which shows the localization of ^{3}H-NPA binding sites by autoradiograhy using a tritium sensitive film (^{3}H-Ultrofilm LKB). It has been discovered that there exists a high density of ^{3}H-NPA binding sites in certain types of DA nerve terminal networks in the nucleus accumbens and tuberculum olfactorium and in the marginal zone of nucleus caudatus.

Acknowledgements
This work has been supported by grants from the Swedish Medical Research Council (04X-715), Magnus Bergwalls Stiftelse, Knut & Alice Wallenberg's Foundation, NIH, U.S.A. (MH25504), and a CNR international grant. Dr. L. Calza is the recipient of a « Legato Dino Ferrari », Dr. F. Benfenati is the recipient of a « Villa Rusconi grant ». We are grateful to Mrs. Ulla Altimimi, Ms. Berith Hagman, Ms. Birgitta Johansson, Ms. Catharina Nilsson and Ms. Barbro Tinner for excellent technical assistance and to Ms. Elisabeth Sandqvist for her excellent secretarial assistance.

REFERENCES

Agnati, L. F., Fuxe, K. *1982* - A morphometrical method to measure the size and distribution of radioligand positive areas in autoradiography. *Neurosci. Lett.*, submitted.

Agnati, L. F., Benfenati, F., Cortelli, P., D'Alessandro, R. *1978* - A new method to quantify catecholamine stores visualized by means of the Falck-Hillarp technique. *Neurosci. Lett., 10* : 11-17.

Agnati, L. F., Anderson, K., Wiesel, F., Fuxe K. *1979* - A method to determine dopamine levels and turnover rate in discrete dopamine nerve terminal systems by quantitative use of dopamine fluorescence obtained by Falck-Hillarp methodology. *J. Neurosci. Meth., 1* : 365.

Agnati, L. F., Fuxe, K., Andersson, K., Benfenati, F., Cortelli, P., D'Alessandro, R. *1980a* - The mesolimbic dopamine system. Evidence for a high amine turnover and for a heterogeneity of the dopamine neuron population. *Neurosci. Lett., 18* : 45-52.

Agnati, L. F., Andersson, K., Fuxe, K., Benfenati, F., Cortelli, P., D'Alessandro, R., Ögren S.-O. *1980b* - Effects of chronic treatment with 1-sulpiride and haloperidol on central dopamine turnover evaluated in dopamine cell body and nerve terminal-rich areas. *In : Long-term Effects of Neuroleptics,* F. Cattabeni et al. (ed.) pp. 75-80, New York, Raven Press.

Agnati, L. F., Fuxe, K., Zini, I., Benfenati, F., Hökfelt, T., De Mey, J. *1982a* - Principles for the morphological characterization of transmitter-identified nerve cell groups. *J. Neurosci. Meth., 6 :* 157-167.

Agnati. L. F., Fuxe, K., Hökfelt, T., Benfenati, F., Calza, L., Johansson, O., De Mey, J. *1982b* - Morphometric characterization of transmitter-identified nerve cell groups : Analysis of mesencephalic 5HT nerve cell bodies. *Brain Res. Bull., 9 :* 45-51.

Agnati, L. F., Fuxe, K., Calza, L., Hökfelt, T., Johansson, O., Benfenati, F., Goldstein, M. *1982c* - A morphometrical analysis of transmitter-identified dendrites and nerve terminals. *Brain Res. Bull., 9 :* 53-60.

Agnati, L. F., Fuxe, K., Hökfelt, T., Calza, L., Benfenati, F., Zini, I., Zoli, M., Goldstein, M. *1982d* - A new approach to quantitative the density and antigen contents of high densities of transmitter-identified terminals. Immunocytochemical studies on different types of tyrosine hydroxylase immunoreactive nerve terminals in nucleus caudatus putamen of the rat. *Neurosci. Lett., 32* : 253-258.

Agnati, L. F, Fuxe, K., Andersson, K., Hökfelt, T., Skirboll, L., Benfenati, F., Battistini, N., Calza, L. *1982e* - Possible functional meaning of the coexistence of monoamines and peptides in the same neurons. A study on the interactions between cholecystokinin-8 and dopamine in the brain. *Proc. of the 2nd Eur. Neurosci. Meeting in Capoboj,* (G.V. Corsini, ed.), Pergamon Press, in press.

Agnati, L.F., Fuxe, K., Locatelli, V., Benfenati, F., Panerai, A. E., El Etreby, M. F., Hökfelt, T., Zini, I. *1982f* - Neuroanatomical methods for the quantitative evaluation of coexistence of transmitters in nerve cells. Analysis of the ACTH and β-endorphin immunoreactive nerve cell bodies of the mediobasal hypothalamus of the rat. *J. Neurosci. Meth., 5* : 203-214.

Benfenati, F., Bernardi, P., Cortelli, P., Copelli, M., Adami, C., Calza, L., Agnati, L. F. *1981* - Possible mixed agonist-antagonist activity of d-sulpiride at dopamine receptor level in man. *Neurosci. Lett., 26* : 289-293.

Costall, B., Naylor, R. J., Cannon, J. G., Lee, T. *1977* - Differentiation of the dopamine mechanism mediating sterotyped behaviour and hyperactivity in the nucleus accumbens and caudate putamen. *J. Pharm. Pharmacol., 29* : 337-342.

Costall, B., Fortune, D. H., Naylor, R. J. *1978* - Tiapride : A benzamide derivative having a unique activity spectrum. *7th International Congress of Pharmacology*, Abstract 2185, p. 928.

Costall, B., Fortune, D. H., Naylor, R., Nohria, V. *1979* - A study of drug action on normal and denervated striatal mechanisms. *Eur. J. Pharmacol., 56* : 207-216.

Elliot, P.N.C., Jenner, P., Huizing, G., Marsden, C. D., Miller, R. *1977* - Substitutive benzamides as cerebral dopamine antagonists in rodents. *Neuropharmacol., 16* : 333-342.

31

Fuxe, K., Ögren, S.-O., Fredholm, B., Agnati, L. F., Hökfelt, T., Perez de la Mora, M. *1977a* - Possibilities of a differential blockade of central monoamine receptor. *In : Rhinencéphale, neurotransmetteurs et psychoses*, J. de Ajuriaguerra and R. Tissot (eds), Symposium Bel-Air V. pp. 253-289 Genève, Georg & Cie.

Fuxe, K., Hökfelt, T., Agnati, L. F., Johansson, O., Ljungdahl, A., Perez de la Mora, M. *1977b* - Regulation of the mesocortical dopamine neurons. *Adv. Biochem. Psychopharmacol.*, tome : 47-55.

Fuxe, K., Andersson, K., Schwarcz, R., Agnati, L. F., Perez de la Mora, M., Hökfelt, T., Goldstein, M., Ferland, L., Possani, Tapia, R. *1979a* - Studies on different types of dopamine nerve terminals in the forebrain and their possible interaction with hormones and with neurons containing GABA, glutamate and opiod peptides. *Adv. Neurol.*, 24 : 199-215.

Fuxe, K., Schwarcz, R., Agnati, L. F., Fredholm, B., Ögren, S.-O., Köhler, C., Gustafsson, J.-Å. *1979b* - Actions of ergot derivatives at dopamine synapses. *In : Dopaminergic ergot derivatives and motor function*, K. Fuxe, D. B. Calne (eds), Oxford and New York, Pergamon Press.

Fuxe, K., Andersson, K., Agnati, L. F., Ögren, S.-O, *1979c* - The effects of d- and l-sulpiride and tiapride on central dopamine mechanisms in the normal male rat. III Eur. Neurosci. Metting, Rome, Italy, Sept.11-14, 1979. *Neurosci. Lett., suppl. 3*, p. 237.

Fuxe, K., Ögren, S.-O, Hall, H., Agnati, L. F., Anderson, K., Köhler, C., Schwarcz, R. *1980* - Effects of chronic treatment with l-sulpiride and haloperidol on central monoaminergic mechanisms. *In : Long-term effects of neuroleptics*, F. Cattabeni et al. (eds) pp. 193-206 New York, Raven Press.

Fuxe, K., Agnati, L. F., Ganten, D., Lang, R. E., Poulsen, K., Hökfelt, T., Calza, L., Infantellina, F. *1982* - A morphometrical method for the quantitation of the entity of cœxistence of substances in nerve cell bodies. Analysis of renin-like and oxytocin-like immunoreactivity in nerve cells of the paraventricular hypothalamic nucleus. *Neurosci, Lett., 33 :* 19-24.

Hökfelt, T., Skirboll, L., Rehfeld, J. F., Goldstein, M., Makrey, K., Dann, O. *1980* - A subpopulation of mesencephalic dopamine neurons projecting to limbic areas contains a cholecystokinin-like peptide : Evidence from immunohistochemistry combined with retrograde tracing. *Neurosci, 5 :* 2093-2124.

Hyttel, J. *1980* - No evidence for increased dopamine receptor binding in superresponsive mice after a single dose of neuroleptics. *In : Long-term effects of neuroleptics*, F. Cattabeni et al. (eds), pp. 167-173 New York, Raven Press.

Jenner, P., Clow, A., Rcavill, C., Theodorou, A. and Marsden, C. C. *1978* - A behavioural and biochemical comparison of dopamine receptor blockade produced by haloperidol with that produced by substituted benzamides drugs. *Life Sci., 23 :* 545-550.

Jenner, P., Marsden, C. D. *1979-* The substituted benzamides - a novel class of dopamine antagonists. *Life Sci.*, 25 : 479-486.

Johansson, O., Hökfelt, T., Pernow, B., Jeffcoate, S. L., White, N., Steinbusch, H.W.M., Verhofstad, A.J.J., Emson, P. C., Spindel, E. *1981* - Immunohistochemical support for three putative transmitters in one neuron : Coexistence of 5-hydroxytryptamine, substance P- and thyrotrophin releasing hormone-like immunoreactivity in medullary neurons projecting to the spinal cord. *Neurosci., 6 :* 1857-1881.

Köhler, C., Ögren, S.-O., Haglund, L., Ängeby, T. *1979* - Regional displacement by sulpiride of (^{3}H) spiperone binding in vivo. Biochemical and behavioural evidence for a preferential action on limbic and nigral dopamine receptors. *Neurosci. Lett., 13 :* 51-56.

Köhler, C., Fuxe, K., Roos, S. B. *1981* - Regional in vivo binding of (^{3}H)N-propylnorapomorphine in the mouse brain. Evidence for labelling of central dopamine receptors. *Eur. J. Pharmacol., 72 :* 397-402.

Löfström, A., Jonsson, G., Wiesel, F.-A., Fuxe, K. *1976* - Microfluorimetric quantitation of catecholamine fluorescence in rat median eminence. II : turnover changes in hormonal states. *J. Histochem. Cytochem., 24 :* 430-442.

Ögren, S-O., Hall, H., Köhler, C. *1972* - Studies on the stereoselective dopamine receptor blockade in the rat brain by rigid spiroamines. *Life Sci., 23 :* 1969-1774.

Palacios J., Niehoff, D., Kuhar, M. *1981* - Receptor autoradiography with tritum-sensitive film. Potential for computerized densitometry. *Neurosci. Lett., 25 :* 101-105.

Scatton, B., Bischoff, S., Dedek, J., Korf, I. *1977* - Regional effects of neuroleptics on doapmine metabolism and dopamine sensitive adenylate cyclase. *Eur. J. Pharmacol., 44 :* 287-292.

Spano, P. F., Memo, M., Stefanini, E., Fresisa, P., Trabucchi, M. *1980* - Detection of multiple receptors for dopamine. *In : Receptors for neurotransmitters and peptide,* G. Pepeu, M.-J. Kuhar and S.-J. Enna (eds) pp 243-251, New York, Raven Press.

Steinbusch, H.W.M., Verhofstad, A. A., Joosten, H.W.J. *1978* - Localization of serotonin in the central nervous system by immunohistochemistry : description of a specific and sensitive technique and some applications. *Neurosci., 3 :* 811-819.

Young, W.S., Kuhar, M. J. *1979* - A new method for receptor autoradiography ^{3}H-opiod receptor labelling in mounted tissue sections. *Brain Res. :* 179-255.

32

DISCUSSION

Ch. Eggers
I am astonished at your findings, which seem to indicate that tiapride does not only act on the nigro-striatal system, but also on the limbic level. How could you explain that, since clinically tiapride has no antipsychotic activities ?

K. Fuxe
I must say that we have not studied the mechanism of action for tiapride very carefully, but obviously there are changes in dopamine turnover. One could speculate that maybe there could be a pre-synaptic dopamine blocking action in those areas. A pre-synaptic dopamine receptor could therefore mainly be involved in producing these dopamine turnover changes with tiapride, explaining the absence of antipsychotic acting. On the other hand, it could well be that the dopamine turnover change is not related to actions on the dopamine receptors of the limbic dopamine systems. Therefore, the dopamine turnover change is a complex phenomenon. Obviously, in these types of studies we do not have any way of knowing what the integrated output is from the nerve cells controlled by the dopamine terminals affected by tiapride. Therefore, it is just a study of the dopamine turnover change. We have no idea what the final net action is on the neuronal network with regard to enhancement or reduction of activity.

G. Bartholini
If I understood correctly, you found a similar displacement of NPA by sulpiride in caudate and tuberculum olfactorium ?

K. Fuxe
That is correct. I could say that the ED_{50} value was somewhat lower in the tuberculum.

G. Bartholini
We might discuss this further tomorrow, as we find a much greater displacement in limbic regions with the racemic sulpiride.

K. Fuxe
This is in perfect agreement with Köhler's data in 1979 on ^{3}H-spiperone binding *in-vivo*. He obtained data with dl-sulpiride which agreed excellently with my turnover data from 1977 with dl-sulpiride, which I presented at the Bel-Air conference in Geneva. It sounds as though your data are also in agreement. There is certainly a trend for preferential activity with l-sulpiride, but it is not nearly as clear-cut as with the dl.

M. Goldstein
Perhaps this means that the l-enantiomer does not penetrate into the striatum to the same extent as the d. Therefore, there are vast differences between dl versus l.

K. Fuxe
Yes, this is one possibility. Interestingly, d-sulpiride may also have partial dopamine agonistic activity in the striatal regions. Thus, it reduced dopamine turnover in some striatal dopamine terminal populations. Agnati and colleagues also have evidence from analysis of cardiovascular parameters, that d-sulpiride has a partial agonistic activity at dopamine receptors.

The use of substituted benzamides and domperidone in the identification of the location and hemodynamic significance of peripheral dopamine receptors in dogs and man

W. H. Fennell, A. A. Taylor, and J. R. Mitchell.

Sections of Cardiology, Hypertension and Clinical Pharmacology/Toxicology, Department of Internal Medicine, Baylor College of Medicine, Houston.

Summary : Study of the hemodynamic significance of dopamine receptors has been hampered by the lack of specific agonists and antagonists. Recently a small number of n-dialkyl dopamine analogues (including n-dipropyl dopamine and n-propyl butyl dopamine (PBDA)) have been demonstrated to have dopaminergic properties without alpha or beta adrenergic effects.
Simultaneously, metoclopramide and sulpiride have been documented in isolated systems to be specific antagonists of the dopamine renal (DA1) and neurogenic pre-synaptic (DA2) receptors. PBDA decreased blood pressure and increased renal blood flow without a reflex tachycardia in anesthetized and conscious dogs and patients with congestive heart failure and hypertension. The reduction in blood pressure was inhibited by S-sulpiride (0.1 mg/kg), a specific DA2 antagonist, in conscious dogs, by domperidone (0.5 mg/kg) and metoclopramide (8 μg/kg) in anesthetized dogs and by metoclopramide (8 μg/kg) in patients with hypertension. The increase in renal blood flow was inhibited only by metoclopramide (145 μg/kg) in anesthetized dogs and also in hypertensive patients. These data suggest that the reduction in blood pressure is due to activation of peripheral pre-synaptic DA2 receptors and the increase in renal blood flow at post-synaptic DA1 receptors. Low dose metoclopramide appears to be a specific antagonist of peripheral pre-synaptic DA2 receptors and in high doses of post synaptic DA1 receptors in dogs and man.

Introduction

Dopamine (DA), the third endogenous catecholamine is of interest to physiologists, pharmacologists and clinicians. As a neurotransmitter within and outside the central nervous system, it is of great interest to physiologists. In the last two decades, the presence of dopamine receptors has been confirmed by pharmacologists. Agonists and antagonists for these receptors have been developed to increase our understanding of the physiological role of dopamine in many systems and have also become important agents useful in the diagnosis and therapy of many disease states (Goldberg, 1974). Despite the widespread clinical applications for many dopamine antagonists, the study of the hemodynamic roles for dopamine receptors *in vivo* has been hampered by the lack of specific agonists and antagonists for these receptors. In particular, the structural requirements for dopamine-induced vasodilation have been demonstrated to be extraordinarily restricted (Volkman et al., 1977). All the earlier dopamine antagonists, phenothiazines and butyrophenones, were nonspeci-

35

fic and with concomitant alpha-adrenergic antagonist activity. The demonstration of the specificity of the substituted benzamides, metoclopramide and sulpiride, to antagonise dopamine-induced renal vasodilation, has been an important step in the quest to characterise the hemodynamic significance of dopamine receptors (Kohli et al., 1978a). The subsequent demonstration of the specificity of the enantiomers of sulpiride, S(−) and R(+) for the pre- (DA$_2$) and post- (DA$_1$) synaptic dopamine receptors respectively has also helped to characterise better the difference between pre- and post-synaptic receptors (Goldberg et al. 1979).

In 1975, Enero and Langer described the inhibition by dopamine of noradrenaline release elicited by nerve stimulation in the cat nictitating membrane (Enero and Langer, 1975). This pointed to a location and role for pre-synaptic dopamine receptors. Another important landmark in the bid to characterise dopamine receptors was the finding that n-dialkyl substitution on the dopamine molecule produced analogs of dopamine without alpha or beta adrenergic effects (Ginos et al., 1978). Such analogs permitted the relative potencies at dopamine receptors to be quantitated using the most specific antagonists.

Our studies have attempted 1) to characterise the hemodynamic profiles in dogs and man of these n-dialkyl dopamine analogs, 2) to define their relative potency at the putative dopamine receptors within the central nervous system and periphery, and 3) to examine the similarities and differences in the hemodynamic importance of dopamine receptors in the dog and man.

Methods

We have studied the hemodynamic responses to the n-dialkyl dopamine analogs n-n-dipropyldopamine (DPDA), n-propyl-n-butyl dopamine (PBDA), n-ethyl-n-butyl dopamine (EBDA), and n-propyl-n-pentyl dopamine (PPDA) in conscious chronically instrumented dogs and acutely instrumented anesthetised dogs. The details for the methods of anesthesia, surgical techniques and instrumentation have previously been described (Fennell et al., 1980a ; Pinsky et al., 1979). The following hemodynamic parameters were recorded : left ventricular systolic and end diastolic pressures (mm Hg), dp-dt in mm Hg/sec, aortic pressure (phasic and mean), heart rate and renal blood flow using pulsed Doppler flow probes placed on the renal artery. A linear relationship between flow and frequency shift for ultrasonic crystals of this type has been established previously *in vivo* (Hartley et al., 1974).

Results

Kohli et al. described the properties of n-dipropyl dopamine (DPDA), an analog of dopamine with ability to activate pre-(DA$_2$) and post-(DA$_1$) synaptic dopamine receptors without activation of alpha or beta adrenergic receptors (Kohli et al., 1978b). Excited by the availability of a « pure » dopamine analog, we studied the hemodynamic effects of DPDA in anesthetised dogs (Fennell et al., 1980a). DPDA at 20, 40 and 80 μg/kg/min caused a rapid (within 2 minutes) fall in mean arterial pressure and renal vascular resistance (not dose-related) but there was a dose-related reduction in heart rate. At 20 μg/kg/min, the predominant effect appeared to be iliac vasodilation while renal blood flow increased with each dosage increment, the iliac blood flow decreased with each dosage increment. All the hemodynamic effects of DPDA were partially prevented by pretreatment with hexamethonium, 10 mg/kg and totally prevented by sulpiride, 0.5 mg/kg. Sodium nitroprusside was infused to cause a similar fall in mean aortic pressure but was not antagonised by either hexamethonium or sulpiride. These results confirmed the exciting potential of a « pure » dopamine analog and strongly suggested that the hypotensive-renal vasodilator properties were due to a combination of pre-synaptic (neurogenic) and post-synaptic (vascular) effects.

We then studied DPDA in conscious chronically instrumented dogs. However, there was a prohibitive incidence of vomiting in these animals at 20 μg/kg/min (the lowest effective dose in anesthetised dogs). We then studied the hemodynamic properties of three other n-dialkyl dopamine analogs, n-propyl-n-butyl dopamine (PBDA), n-ethyl-n-butyl dopamine (EBDA), and n-propyl-n-pentyl dopamine (PBDA) in conscious dogs (Fennell et al., 1980b). PBDA had a similar hemodynamic profile as DPDA but with significantly less vomiting, reducing mean arterial pressure without reflex tachycardia while increasing renal blood flow. In anesthetised dogs, the effects were similar except for a dose-related decrease in heart rate. The resting heart rate in anesthetised dogs was substantially greater (>50 b/min). At a dosage of 40 μg/kg/min, PBDA caused significant vomiting in conscious dogs. Pretreatment with S-sulpiride, 0.0125 mg/kg prevented vomiting while S-sulpiride, 0.1 mg/kg prevented the blood pressure lowering effect without attenuating the renal vasodilator effect. Pretreatment with R$^{(+)}$ sulpiride (0.0125 to 0.1 mg/kg) was less potent in preventing vomiting and did not attenuate the hypotensive effects of PBDA. These results supported the role of pre-synaptic DA_2 receptor activation in the hypotensive effect. However, as sulpiride penetrates the central nervous system, it was not possible to distinguish if the pre-synaptic DA_2 receptors being activated were predominantly central or peripheral. We subsequently gave PBDA following pretreatment with the peripherally active DA antagonist, domperidone, 0.5 mg/kg i.v. to anesthetised dogs (Fennell et al., 1981a). Again, the hypotensive and bradycardic effects were antagonised but not the renal vasodilation. These findings strongly suggested a peripheral location for the DA_2 receptors responsible for the hypotensive effect of PBDA. In preparation for human studies, PBDA was also administered following metoclopramide, 40 μg/kg in anesthetised dogs and again, the hypotensive and bradycardic effects were antagonised, but not the renal vasodilator effects. Higher doses of metoclopramide >145 μg/kg only antagonised the renal vasodilator effect of PBDA, supporting the earlier findings that relatively high doses of metoclopramide are required to antagonise the renal dopamine receptors (Fig. 1).

We subsequently extended our studies to healthy volunteers and patients with congestive heart failure. PBDA did not reduce the blood pressure in volunteers but did cause a substantial increase in renal plasma flow as measured by the clearance of para-amino-hippurate (Taylor et al., 1981). This effect was antagonised by pretreatment with metoclopramide, (20 mg i.v.). In the patients with heart failure PBDA caused a dose-related reduction in systemic vascular resistance and left ventricular end diastolic pressure without a reflex tachycardia (Fennell et al., 1981b). The onset of effect was prompt and loss of effect was complete within 10 minutes of discontinuation of infusion. There was no vomiting in man at doses from 5 to 20 μg/kg/min.

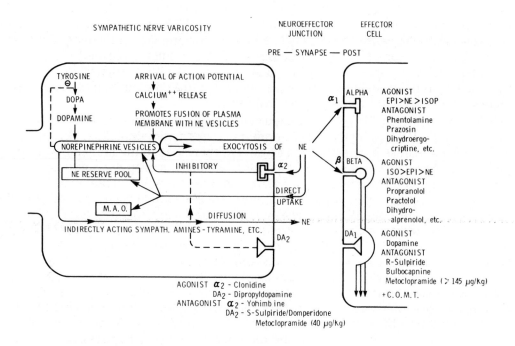

Fig. 1 - The use of substituted benzamides and domperidone in the identification of the location and significance of peripheral dopamine receptors in dogs and man.

The similarity of hemodynamic effects in dog and man of PBDA strongly suggests that in both species the effect is occurring by similar mechanisms. It is probable that the afterload or blood pressure lowering effect is at pre-synaptic DA_2 receptors located in the periphery, while the renal vasodilation is occurring at post-synaptic DA_1 receptors. Preliminary studies in hypertensive patients suggest similar important dual effects as found in the healthy volunteers and heart failure patients (Taylor et al., 1981). The finding of differential sensitivity of metoclopramide for pre- and post-synaptic DA receptors in the dog also opens possible means to characterise the importance of pre- and post-synaptic DA receptor activation in patients with hypertension using DA agonists such as PBDA.

Acknowledgements

This work was supported in part by the National Institutes of Health, Grant Number HL-17269, and a grant from the American Heart Association, Texas Affiliate. The domperidone hydrochloride used in these studies was generously provided by Janssen Pharmaceuticals, New Brunswick, New Jersey. RS-sulpiride and S-sulpiride hydrochloride were gifts from Laboratoires Delagrange, Paris, France.
The authors wish to acknowledge the help and patience of Mrs. Linda Adams in the preparation of this manuscript.

REFERENCES

Enero, M.A., Langer, S.Z. *1975* - Inhibition by dopamine of 3H-noradrenaline release elicited by nerve stimulation in the isolated cat's nictitating membrane. *Arch. Pharmacol., 289* : 179-203.

Fennell, W.H., Kohli, J.D., Goldberg, L.I. *1980a* - Hypotensive effects of N-N-di-n-propyl dopamine in the anesthetized dog : Comparison with sodium nitroprusside. *J. Cardiovasc. Pharmacol., 2* : 247-256.

Fennell, W.H., Taylor, A.A., Brandon, T.A., Goldberg, L.I., Mitchell, J.R., Miller, R.R. *1980b* - Dopamine analogs to reduce afterload. *Clin. Res., 28* : 469A.

Fennell, W.H., Taylor, A.A., Ginos, J.Z., Mitchell, J.R. *1981a* - Selective activation of peripheral dopamine presynaptic receptors decreases blood pressure and heart rate in dogs. *Clin. Res., 29* : 819A.

Fennell, W.H., Taylor, A.A., Young, J.B., Farmer, J.A., Ginos, J.Z., Goldberg, L.I., Mitchell, J.R., Miller, R.R. *1981b* - Activation of presynaptic dopamine receptors in man : A new mechanism for afterload reduction. *Clin. Res., 29* : 271A.

Ginos, J.Z., Kohli, J.D., Goldberg, L.I. *1978* - Cardiovascular actions of N-substituted dopamine analogs in the dog. *Fed. Proc. 37* : 683.

Goldberg, L.I. *1974* - Dopamine - clinical uses of an endogenous catecholamine. *N. Engl. J. Med., 291* : 707-710.

Goldberg, L.I., Kohli, J.D., Listinsky, J.J., McDermed, J.D. *1979* - Structure activity relationships of pre- and post-synaptic dopamine receptors mediating vasodilation. *In : Catecholamines : Basic and Clinical Frontiers.* E. Usdin, I.J. Kopin, and J. Barchas, (eds) pp. 447-449. New York, Pergamon Press.

Hartley, C.J., Cole, J.S. *1974* - An ultrasonic pulsed Doppler system for measuring blood flow in small vessels. *J. Appl. Physiol., 37* : 626-629.

Kohli, J.D., Volkman, P.H., Glock, D., Goldberg, L.I. *1978a* - Metoclopramide and sulpiride : antagonists of the vascular dopamine receptor. *Fed. Proc. 57* : 792.

Kohli, J.D., Goldberg, L.I., Volkman, P.H., Cannon, J.G. *1978b* - N-N-di-n-propyl dopamine : A qualitatively different dopamine vascular agonist. *J. Pharmacol. Exp. Ther., 207* : 16-22.

Pinsky, W.W., Lewis, R.M., Hartley, C.J., Entman, M.L. *1979* - Permanent changes of ventricular contractility and compliance in chronic volume overload. *Am. J. Physiol. : Heart Cir. Physiol., 6 (5)* : H575-583.

Taylor, A.A., Fennell, W.H., Mitchell, J.R. *1981* - Propylbutyl dopamine increases renal blood flow and decreases blood pressure in man by activation of specific DA_1 and DA_2 dopamine receptors. *Clin. Res. 29* : 859A.

Volkman, P.H., Kohli, J.D. Goldberg, L.I., Cannon, J.G., Lee, T. *1977* - Conformational requirements for dopamine-induced vasodilation. *Proc. Natl. Acad. Sci. USA, 74* : 3602-3606.

DISCUSSION

S.-Z. Langer

In the experiments where you used the 40 µg/kg infusion of PBDA, did you have any incidents of nausea or vomiting, or can you go that high for humans without any effects at this level ?

W.-H. Fennell

We went to 40 µg/kg per minute in 3 patients and in 3 volunteers. In the volunteers the infusion was for more than 10 minutes. The average length of each dosage infusion in the patients with heart failure and in man was 10 to 15 minutes. At 40 µg, 2 of the 3 volunteers and one patient vomited. That brings the therapeutic-toxic-ratio quite close. I think, however, the fact that we were able to block the vomiting and the blood pressure effect with widely different doses of S-sulpiride suggests that these effects are separable.

S.-Z. Langer

You also reported a very pronounced bradycardia in an animal experiment, particularly in the anaesthetized animal, yet in the other experimental conditions, particularly in man in the congestive heart failure experiments you show that there is no bradycardia in spite of the fact that you observed hypotension. Could you expand on this result ?

W.-H. Fennell

There is a difference in the effect on heart rate in anaesthetized and conscious dogs. In anaesthetized dogs the average heart rate is approximately 150, in conscious dogs it is between 70 and 90. So, I think there is a far higher sympathetic tone in anaesthetized dogs and in my opinion, whether pre-synaptic receptor activation has an effect, may depend on the high sympathetic tone. In heart failure patients, we did not get a reflex tachycardia, we can only speculate that this is may be due to altered kinetics of catecholamines as a result of heart failure.

S.-Z. Langer

You have elegantly shown with domperidone, that these effects are very likely to be located in the periphery and one question, which arises with dopamine agonists acting pre-synaptically to reduce blood pressure and heart rate, is whether these effects are likely to develop tolerance on chronic administration. I would also like to ask, whether in addition to your acute experiments you have tried if such dopamine agonists such as anti-hypertensives retain their effectiveness under sub-acute or chronic administration ?

W.-H. Fennell

We just gave a sub-acute administration, as our permission for man is limited by the Food & Drug Administration Authorities and is at present allowed up to one hour with continuous administration. We were impressed that in the hypertensive patient in contrast to normal volunteers the blood pressure lowering effect is quite strong and in those patients with repeated on and off administration the blood pressure effect still persisted.

P. Herrmann

You mentioned that domperidone would be an exclusively peripherally acting agent and that supposes that it would not pass the blood-brain barrier. On what experience do you base this statement, as we have learned that it is more or less a question of blood concentration of such a compound whether it passes through the blood-brain barrier or not ?

W.-H. Fennell

I am only able to quote from the literature. I know that it enters the brain in isolated systems and that some cases of dystonic reactions have been reported in man.

The substituted benzamides :
Selective dopamine receptor blockade

B. Costall and R.J. Naylor

Postgraduate School of Studies in Pharmacology,
University of Bradford, Bradford, England.

Summary : The proven clinical value of substituted benzamides, especially in the fields of psychiatry and gastroenterology, has been attributed to their ability to cause dopamine blockade. The uniqueness of the benzamide action emerges from the selectivity of this dopamine blockade, for their effectiveness cannot be correlated with actions via other major neurotransmitter mechanisms, cholinergic, adrenergic or serotonergic. The corollary to such a selectivity of action is a consideration that the pharmacological or clinical differences between the substituted benzamides may reflect differential affinities for dopamine receptor mechanisms which, in turn, is suggestive of different types of dopamine receptors. This is an important concept, for the introduction of further substituted benzamides is critically dependent on the demonstration of differences in site and mode of action of existing agents. In the present study we take tiapride as an example and discuss its ability to inhibit the abnormal involuntary facial-lingual movements induced by dopamine and dopamine agonists in the rodent. We review the evidence that, amongst the substituted benzamides, tiapride has a unique antidyskinetic action, and finally give careful consideration to the different types of dyskinesias that can be induced and antagonised by drugs with the view to clarifying the appreciation and distinction of « antidyskinetic action ».

Since the introduction of the substituted benzamides into pharmacology and medicine (Justin-Besançon and Laville, 1964), the accumulative experience of nearly two decades of intensive investigation has been the consistent demonstration of a selectivity of action for dopamine receptors (Puech et al., 1978 ; Jenner and Marsden, 1979). The evidence has derived essentially from animal studies where, for example, the substituted benzamides have a general ability to block the dopamine receptors in the area postrema mediating emesis, the dopamine receptors in the hypothalamo-hypophysial system moderating a variety of endocrinological changes, and the dopamine receptors in the mesolimbic and striatal systems regulating psychomotor activity. Within the brain systems the ability of the substituted benzamides to modify dopamine turnover (Jenner et al., 1978) and to bind to "dopamine-neuroleptic" receptors (Fortune et al., 1980 ; Jenner and Marsden, 1981 ; Freedman et al., 1981) supports an action on cerebral dopamine systems. Within the peripheral systems the substituted benzamides have been extensively used to identify "dopamine" responses, although an ability of (+) and (—) sultopride and (+) sulpiride to antagonise at an α_2-type adrenoceptor in a stomach circular smooth muscle preparation is very unusual, and cannot be immediately correlated to any "dopamine" receptor antagonism (Sahyoun et al., 1982).

41

Accepting that the substituted benzamides have a very high selectivity for dopamine receptors, particularly those in the central nervous system, it has become of major interest that these agents do not exert identical spectra of pharmacological and clinical activities. For example, notwithstanding that metoclopramide has incisive dopamine antagonist actions in many behavioral and biochemical tests for neuroleptic action, in some tests its dopamine antagonist action is weak, a notable situation being in the assessment of ability to inhibit a raised mesolimbic dopamine function (Costall et al., 1978). A direct clinical corollary of these observations is the difficulty of demonstrating an antipsychotic action for metoclopramide without the use of large doses and anticholinergic cover to prevent the development of the more easily attainable extrapyramidal side effects (Stanley et al., 1979). This directly contrasts with the pharmacological and clinical activities of sulpiride. That different substituted benzamides may have differential affinities for dopamine receptor mechanisms is an important concept, not least because the successful clinical introduction of further agents will be critically dependent on the demonstration of differences in site and/or mode of action from existing agents.

Whilst the substituted benzamides, particularly sulpiride, have a proven usefulness in psychiatry, the treatment of many neurological disease states has continued to provide a major challenge to drug design. With respect to the therapy of abnormal involuntary movement disorders, it has been appreciated for some years that neuroleptic agents appear to offer virtually the only effective treatment, even though the appearance of "side effects" may severely reduce all other aspects of motor performance, and notwithstanding the ability of neuroleptic drugs to induce motor dysfunction per se, particularly on chronic administration (Marsden et al., 1975 ; Baldessarini and Tarsy, 1978). A major impetus to an understanding of abnormal movement development in terms of a dopaminergic involvement also undoubtedly derived from the introduction of 1-dopa and other dopamine agonists for the treatment of Parkinson's disease, and the rapid realisation that a limiting side effect of such therapy was dyskinesia development. The dyskinetic responses obtained to neuroleptic agents and dopamine agonists indicate the basic clinical antidyskinetic challenge, the restoration of normal motor behavior without a further imposition of other forms of motor impairment. The two most urgent problems in « the seventies » were to find ways of limiting the acute dyskinesias caused by dopamine agonist treatment and to alleviate the dyskinesias occuring late in persistent neuroleptic therapy (i.e. tardive dyskinesias).

In our attempts to design a simple animal model for the detection of "antidyskinetic activity", we considered that a significant component of the dyskinesias induced both by the dopamine agonists and neuroleptics was the development of the orobuccolingual-facial dyskinesias. The simplest animal model, derived from the most logical approach, was to induce such abnormal movements by direct striatal dopamine stimulation, achieved by a stereotaxic approach to intracerebral injection. Initial studies showed the guinea-pig to be most sensitive to this approach, and this species was appropriate for use in large numbers for an anticipated usefulness of the model as a screening procedure for "antidyskinetic agents". The guinea-pig was found to respond to intrastriatal dopamine with intense orobuccolingual movements, often associated with other types of abnormal movement and, particularly important, a locomotor hyperactivity (Costall and Naylor, 1975). The use of this model has allowed the detection of drug action to antagonise abnormal movements (particularly orobuccolingual movements) with a concomitant assessment of the potential of the same drugs to reduce overall motor responding (shown as a reduction in locomotor hyperactivity). Many neuroleptic and potential neuroleptic agents from many different chemical series were "screened" using this model, and it soon became evident that an antidyskinetic action was exceptionally difficult to distinguish. In contrast, most neuroleptic agents from all chemical series could be shown to have potential to inhibit the dopamine mechanisms of locomotor hyperactivity to cause akinesia. This directly correlates with the spectrum of activity shown by the neuroleptics in the clinic. However, two agents were detected which could successfully antagonise the dopamine-induced dyskinesias. The first of these was oxiperomide (Costall and Naylor, 1975) which exerted an incisive inhibition of the dyskinesias, although locomotor hyperactivity was inhibited at similar doses. The importance of this first observation was its extension to the clinic where oxiperomide was shown to inhibit dyskinesias in man (Bédard et al., 1978 ; Casey and Gerlach, 1980), although a careful titration of dosage was necessary to avoid undue motor depression. Thus the value of the "dopamine dyskinesia model" using the guinea-pig was established and its application continued with the detection of a substituted benzamide having antidyskinetic activity, tiapride. Tiapride was shown in the guinea-pig to antagonise the orobuccolingual dyskinesias with less effect to inhibit the locomotor hyperactivity (Costall and Naylor, 1977). In man, tiapride antagonises dyskinesias (Lhermitte et al., 1977 ; Price et al., 1978 ; Lees et al. 1979), although again a careful titration of dose is necessary to avoid undue motor depression. The specificity of tiapride's action, amongst the substituted benzamides, to inhibit dopamine-induced dyskinesias in the guinea-pig is shown in Table 1.

Table 1. — *Neuroleptic antagonism of the orobuccolingual dyskinesias induced by intrastriatal dopamine in the guinea-pig*

Drug	Dose mg/kg	No. of animals inhibited
Haloperidol	16	0/8
Oxiperomide	0.5	0/8
	1	6/6
Tiapride	40	0/8˙
	80	6/8
	160	6/6
Metoclopramide	40	0/8
(—) Sulpiride	80	0/4
(+) Sulpiride	80	0/4
(—) Sultopride	80	0/4
(+) Sultopride	80	0/4
Clebopride	40	0/4
Bromopride	40	0/4

Neuroleptic agents were administered i.p. 2 h after intrastriatal dopamine (100 μg 2 h after pretreatment with nialamide, 75 mg/kg i.p.).

The development of a second animal model for the assessment of antidyskinetic activity allowed further analyses of the specificity of tiapride's action as an antidyskinetic agent. This second model was a logical extension of the first in which a potent dopamine agonist (2-di-n-propylamino-5,6-dihydroxytetralin) was used instead of dopamine to induce the dyskinesias because of the inherent disadvantages associated with the necessity of using a monoamine oxidase inhibitor pretreatment to allow the effect of dopamine. Secondly, the model was based on a knowledge of the topography of dyskinesia and hyperactivity "sites" in the striatum, and was designed to allow both the agonist inducing the dyskinesias and the potential antagonist to be administered intracerebrally into a carefully selected striatal site (Costall et al., 1980). The orobuccolingual movements and locomotor hyperactivity induced by the tetralin compound can be antagonised by neuroleptic agents. However, tiapride is again shown to be more effective against the dyskinesias with a typical neuroleptic such as fluphenazine or α-flupenthixol being more effective against the locomotor hyperactivity. Other substituted benzamides tested are similarly more effective as antagonists of the locomotor hyperactivity (Table 2).

Table 2. — *Selectivity and specificity of action of tiapride to antagonise the orobuccolingual dyskinesias induced by intrastriatal tetralin.*

Drug	Intrastriatal Dose µg	% Inhibition Dyskinesia	% Inihibition Hyperactivity
Tiapride	12.5	17	0
	25	60	8
	50	100	34
	100	100	91
Fluphenazine	12.5	0	25
	25	0	57
	50	8	100
	100	4	100
α-flupenthixol	50	0	84
	100	5	100
(±) sulpiride	50	0	68
	100	17	100
Metoclopramide	50	0	58
	100	25	78

Potential antagonists were administered bilaterally into the striatum 15 min. before tetralin (2-di-n-propylamino-5, 6-dihydroxytetralin, 12.5 µg bilateral) (Costall et al., 1980).

Of the substituted benzamides, tiapride is indicated as having a specific action to antagonise dyskinesias. It would be of clear advantage to determine if analogues of tiapride could even further dissociate an antidyskinetic activity from a potential to cause a general motor inhibition.

These results from simple experimental models of "dyskinesias" and the preliminary clinical data have stimulated further use of oxiperomide and tiapride in primate models. Both the acute and long-term treatment of primates with neuroleptic agents can elicit dyskinetic syndromes, and the diverse spectrum of such movements is remarkable (Gunne and Bárány, 1976 ; Weiss et al., 1977 ; Meldrum et al., 1977 ; Liebman et al., 1978 ; Bárány and Gunne, 1979 ; Neale et al., 1981 ;

Porsolt and Jalfre, 1981). Gunne and Bárány (1976) were the first to report their findings in terms of two distinct syndromes, an acute dyskinetic response which they considered to be a "dystonic phase" and a second delayed phase or tardive dyskinesia, the two phases showing respectively the essential sensitivity and resistance to anticholinergic treatment, directly analogous to human dyskinetic movements induced by neuroleptic agents. The dystonic reactions can be induced in a number of primates not only by classical neuroleptic agents such as haloperidol but also by the substituted benzamides, for example, sulpiride, metoclopramide and tiapride, and by oxiperomide (see references above). The dystonic response, idiosyncratic or other, may appear to occur to the administration of any dopamine receptor antagonist, a modified dopamine-cholinergic interaction causing the motor deficit. This interpretation is supported by the potent ability of anticholinergic agents to rapidly reverse dystonic reactions and/or these reactions to very rarely occur to the administration of neuroleptic agents having concomitant anticholinergic potential, for example, thioridazine, clozapine. The dystonic reactions, readily susceptible to anticholinergic treatment, should be distinguished from the tardive dyskinesias which are resistant to such treatment, and which are the concern of the present paper. It would be of obvious interest to determine the activity of oxiperomide and tiapride against the dyskinesias induced by long-term neuroleptic treatment in the primate. It would also be of considerable interest to investigate the actions of potential antidyskinetic drugs against the abnormal involuntary movements induced in primates by brain lesions and/or drug administration (review by Owen, 1979, for references to the work of Metler and Metler, 1942 ; Poirier, 1960 ; Wiles and Davis, 1969 ; Battista et al., 1973 ; Ng et al., 1973).

There is an obvious and continuing clinical need for drugs to more selectively antagonise the abnormal movements seen in pathological and drug-induced states. However, the improvement of animal models to detect drug action useful in the clinic will not be a simple task. Some difficulties are immediately obvious, the rodent and guinea-pig do not respond with the dystonic reactions to neuroleptic agents observed in man, indicating a fundamental difference in neuronal circuitry or sensitivity. Secondly, there are some differences in drug response between the guinea-pig and man : sulpiride, for example, is reported in one study to reduce tardive dyskinesias (Casey et al., 1979) and metolopramide may have a similar action (for references see Karp et al., 1981). Yet the antagonism is not shown in all patients. Does this variability in action reflect dopamine antagonist action on dopamine mechanisms of modified sensitivity, the sensitivity varying with the degree of pathophysiological change to dictate the drug response ? Is a potential sedative action contributory to "antidyskinetic action" ? In any event, sulpiride and metoclopramide do not antagonise dyskinesias in the guinea-pig model. With respect to the primate models, it has become of paramount importance that the dyskinesias which are induced by drug treatments should be reported with descriptive precision, and that the indexing of such behaviors should not obscure the development and antagonism of specific dyskinetic components which may be more or less sensitive to "antidyskinetic challenge". This becomes of increasing importance when some of the dyskinesias to acute neuroleptic challenge are very similar in appearance to those observed to chronic neuroleptic treatment - yet one dyskinesia (acute) is sensitive to atropine challenge whilst the other (tardive) is resistant.

Whatever the immediate difficulties in antidyskinetic drug design, a role for dopamine in the development of these disorders seems undisputed. The most important consequence of the last seven years' animal experimentation has been to encourage the belief that dyskinesias may be antagonised and, notwithstanding that human neurological disease states may involve extremely complex alterations in receptor-cellular activities, the most significant clue to an understanding and treatment of such disorders is that dopamine antagonists constitute their most effective treatment.

REFERENCES

Baldessarini, R.J., Tarsy D., *1978* — Tardive dyskinesia, In : *Psychopharmacology : A generation of progress* M.A. Lipton, A. Di Mascio, K.F. Killiam, (eds) pp. 993-1004, New York, Raven Press.

Bárány, S., Gunne L.M., *1979* — Pharmacological modification of experimental tardive dyskinesia. *Acta Pharmacol. Toxicol., 45* : 107-111.

Bédard, P., Parkes J.D., Marsden C.D., *1978* — Effect of new dopamine-blocking agent (oxiperomide) on drug-induced dyskinesias in Parkinson's disease and spontaneous dyskinesias. *Br. Med. J., 1* : 954-956.

Casey, D.E., Gerlach J., Simmelsgaard H., *1979* — Sulpiride in tardive dyskinesia. *Psychopharmacology, 66* : 73-77.

Casey D., Gerlach J., *1980* — Oxiperomide in tardive dyskinesia. *J. Neurol. Neurosurg. Psychiat., 43* : 264-267.

Costall, B., Naylor R.J., *1975* — Neuroleptic antagonism of dyskinetic phenomena. *Eur. J. Pharmacol, 33* : 301-312.

Costall, B., Naylor R.J., *1977* — Neuropharmacological indications for an antidyskinetic potential for tiapride. *Sem. Hôp. Paris, 53* : 72-76.

Costall, B., De Souza C.X., Naylor R.J., *1980* — Topographical analysis of the actions of 2-(N,N-dipropyl)amino-5,6-dihydroxytetralin to cause biting behaviour and locomotor hyperactivity from the striatum of the guinea-pig. *Neuropharmacology, 19* : 623-631.

Costall, B., Fortune D.H., Naylor R.J., *1978* — Differential activities of some benzamide derivatives on peripheral and intracerebral administration. *J. Pharm. Pharmacol, 30* : 796-798.

Costall, B., Fortune D.H., Naylor R.J., *1980* — Tiapride binds to mouse striatal tissue pre-exposed to dopamine stimulation. *J. Pharm. Pharmacol, 32* : 514-517.

Freedman, S.B., Poat J.A., Woodruff G.N., *1981* — (^{3}H)Sulpiride, a ligand for neuroleptic receptors. *Neuropharmacology, 20 : 1323-1326.*

Gunne, L.-M., Bárány S. *1976* — Haloperidol-induced tardive dyskinesia in monkeys. *Psychopharmacology, 50* : 237-240.

Jenner, P., Clow A., Theodorou A., Marsden C.D., *1978* — A behavioural and biochemical comparison of dopamine receptor blockade produced by haloperidol with that produced by substituted benzamide drugs. *Life Sci. 23* : 545-550.

Jenner, P., Marsden C.D., *1979* — The substituted benzamides — A novel class of dopamine antagonists. *Life Sci., 25* : 479-486.

Jenner, P., Marsden C.D., *1981* — Substituted benzamide drugs as selective neuroleptic agents. *Neuropharmacology, 20* : 1285-1293.

Justin-Besançon, L., Laville C., *1964* — Action anti-émétique du métoclopramide vis-à-vis de l'apomorphine et de l'hydergine. *C.R. Soc. Biol. (Paris), 158* : 723-727.

Karp, M.J., Perkel M.S., Hersh T., McKinney A.S., *1981* — Metoclopramide treatment of tardive dyskinesia. *JAMA, 246* : 1934-1935.

Lees, A.J., Lander C.M., Stern G.M., *1979* — Tiapride in levodopa-induced involuntary movements. *J. Neurol. Neurosurg. Psychiat., 42* : 380-383.

Lhermitte, F., Agid Y., Signoret J.-L., Studler J.M., *1977* — Les dyskinésies de « début et fin de dose » provoquées par la L-dopa. *Rev. Neurol. (Paris), 133* : 297-308.

Liebman, J., Neale R., Moen N.J., *1978* — Differential behavioural effects of sulpiride in the rat and squirrel monkey. *Eur. J. Pharmacol., 50* : 377-383.

Marsden, C.D., Tarsy D., Baldessarini R.J., *1975* — Spontaneous and drug induced movement disorders in psychotic patients. *In : Psychiatric aspects of neurologic disease.* D.F. Benson, D. Blumer (eds), pp. 219-266, New York, Grune and Stratton.

Meldrum, B.S., Anlezar G.M., Marsden C.D., *1977* — Acute dystonia as an idiosyncratic response to neuroleptics in baboons. *Brain, 100* : 313-326.

Neale, R., Fallon S., Gerhardt S., Liebman J.M., *1981* — Acute dyskinesias in monkeys elicited by halopemide, mezilamine and the "antidyskinetic" drugs oxiperomide and tiapride. *Psychopharmacology, 75* : 254-257.

Owen, R.T. *1979* — Dyskinesias, *Med. Act/Drugs of Today, 15* : 65-80.

Puech, A.J., Simon, P., Boissier, J.R., *1978* — Benzamides and classical neuroleptics : comparison of their actions using 6 apomorphine-induced effects. *Eur. J. Pharmacol, 50* : 291-300.

Porsolt, R.D., Jalfre, M., *1981* — Neuroleptic-induced acute dyskinesias in Rhesus monkeys. *Psychopharmacology, 75* : 16-21.

Price, P., Parkes J.D., Marsden C.D., *1978* — Tiapride in Parkinson's disease. *The Lancet, ii* : 1106.

Sahyoun, H.A., Costall B., Naylor R.J., *1982* — Benzamide action at α_2-adrenoceptors modifies catecholamine-induced contraction and relaxation of circular smooth muscle from guinea-pig stomach. *Naunyn-Schmiedeberg's Arch. Pharmacol.,* in press.

Stanley, Lautin M., A., Rotrosen J., *1979* — Antipsychotic efficacy of metoclopramide. *IRCS Med. Sci. Clin. Med, 7* : 322.

Weiss, B., Santelli S., Lusink G., *1977* — Movement disorders induced in monkeys by chronic haloperidol treatment. *Psychopharmacology, 53* : 289-293.

DISCUSSION

N. Matussek
What is your explanation regarding the mechanism of the anti-biting action of tiapride ? Is it cholinergic or something else ?

B. Costall
We do not think it is an anticholinergic effect, because this is not an effect we would expect on the acute dystonic reaction. So, I suppose we would have to say that it is a dopamine antagonist action.

N. Matussek
Is this a special dopamine antagonistic action ?

R. Naylor
Just a quick reply on this problem, because like many of the distinguished colleagues present at this meeting we have seen a number of dopamine receptors appearing, many many different types of dopamine receptors revealed at every conceivable level of investigation and I think that the most important task at the present moment is to determine those dopamine receptors. However, I fear this will be seen to be more an enthusiastic endeavour rather than a serious advancement of our subject, so I do not think we want at this particular time to say that we are dealing with yet another group of dopamine receptors. If we look back to a very early work, and now we are obviously going back 6 years or so, we talked about dopamine 1 and dopamine 2 receptors, this is a behavioral distinction ; the dopamine 1 receptors mediating the hyperactivity response and the dopamine 2 receptors mediating the dyskinetic response and in that terminology we clearly think of tiapride as acting on that second dyskinetic mechanism. Perhaps in retrospect, it may be now more useful just simply to think of it as an anti-dyskinetic agent and to think about future studies which may help us to more accurately define the nature of that particular dopamine mechanism without calling it dopamine 1, 2, 3, 4, 5, 6, 7 or whatever.

Ch. Eggers

My opinion is that your findings are in accordance with the ones of Ljungberg and Ungerstedt with regard to the atypical neuroleptics. I would like to know why very high doses of tiapride are used in your research, when our children with a tic syndrome are only given 5 mg/kg body weight. I believe the different kinds of pharmacokinetics play a large role, because the half-life periods are shorter in children than in adults.

B. Costall

I am sure that the answer indeed lies in the different pharmacokinetics. We certainly do require those larger doses in a guinea pig.

K. Fuxe

As you noted perhaps from one of my slides, in addition to dl-sulpiride we used tiapride in the lower dose range of 25 mg/kg, where obviously you did not get this anti-dyskinetic action. So, it would seem that in a low dosage we do not see any change of striatal dopamine turnover and possibly this means that in the higher dose range, tiapride affects some sites which are unknown. As pointed out previously, it is difficult to relate this to a special type of dopamine receptor. We also have data that tiapride mimics sulpiride in preferentially blocking the hyperactivity. Thus, it is similar to l-sulpiride and dl-sulpiride in this respect. Now we should use higher doses and see what happens to the various striatal dopamine systems.

"Atypical" neuroleptics : Behavioral arguments for a non necessarily univocal mode of action

Ph. Protais and J. Costentin

Laboratory of Pharmacodynamics and Physiology, Medicine and Pharmacy University of Rouen, France.

Summary : In order to develop tests for the selection of antipsychotic drugs which do not cause extrapyramidal symptoms, we have investigated various behavioral effects of apomorphine to see which are antagonized by "atypical" neuroleptics, and we have retained the following ones :
— The apomorphine-induced climbing behavior in mice (Protais et al. Psychopharmacology, 1976, 50, 1-6) as well as in rats.
— The apomorphine-induced hypothermia in mice, and in rats, where antagonists were injected directly in the brain.
— The yawning induced by low doses of apomorphine as well as its inhibition by higher doses of apomorphine.
— The apomorphine-induced penile erection in rats.
— The apormorphine-induced hypokinesia in mice.
In addition, we have observed some interactions of these "atypical" neuroleptics with morphine effects such as the running fit in mice, hypokinesia, or the potentiation of the catatonic cataleptic effects in rats. From these data, we suggest that the concept of "atypical" neuroleptics does not rest on a univocal mechanism, but on the contrary accounts for various types of interactions.

Introduction

The so-called "atypical" neuroleptics are dopamine antagonists which, in contrast to the "classical" neuroleptics, do not induce extrapyramidal side effects. This property, interesting from a therapeutical point of view, throws some discredit on screening methods for neuroleptics based on their cataleptogenic properties, since catalepsy in rats appears equivalent to extrapyramidal symptoms in man.

In order to develop new behavioral tests for easy screening of "atypical" neuroleptics, we have investigated in rats or mice various behavioral effects induced by apomorphine, to determine whether they were or not affected by the better known "atypical" neuroleptics : sulpiride, clozapine, thioridazine and mezilamine. In addition, we have examined their respective activities and compared them to those of the "classical" neuroleptic haloperidol. Our aim was also to better understand the mechanism(s) underlying their particular spectrum of activity.

Methods and animals

The tests used were :
— The apomorphine-induced climbing behavior in rats (Protais et al. submitted) : It concerns the use in male Wistar rats, of the test previously described in mice (Protais et al., 1976, Marçais et al., 1978). The climbing behavior elicited by

0.6 mg/kg of apomorphine was assessed by its duration in animals previously selected as responsive.

— The apomorphine-induced sniffing in male Wistar rats : It was assessed by its duration after the s.c. administration of the same 0.6 mg/kg apomorphine test dose.

— The apomorphine-induced licking in male Wistar rats : It was also assessed by its duration following the s.c. administration of the same 0.6 mg/kg apomorphine test dose.

— The apomorphine-induced yawning or inhibition of yawning. In male Wistar rats increasing doses of apomorphine, up to 0.1 mg/kg, induces a dose dependent increase in the yawning frequency ; higher apomorphine test doses decrease the yawning frequency also in a dose dependent manner, so that at 0.6 mg/kg, yawning is no longer observed during the hour following the s.c. injection.

— The physostigmine-induced yawning : In order to assess the anticholinergic component possibly connected with the tested neuroleptics which might account for the observed antagonism of the apomorphine-induced yawning (Holmgren et al., 1980, Yamada and Furukawa, 1980, have suggested that there might be a dopaminergic-cholinergic link in the yawning behavior), we have investigated the possible antagonism of yawning induced by 75 μg/kg of s.c. physostigmine ; for this purpose, each neuroleptic was tested at a dose corresponding to twice its ID_{50} opposed to 0.1 mg/kg apomorphine in the yawning test.

— The apomorphine-induced penile erections : The number of penile erections occurring in Wistar rats, during the hour following the s.c. administration of increasing doses of apomorphine shows a similar biphasic dose response curve, almost exactly superimposable on the preceding one. According to this observation, an 0.1 mg/kg apomorphine test dose was selected.

— The apomorphine-induced hypokinesia in mice : In this test, male Swiss mice (CD1 Charles River) were put into an actometer equipped with photoelectric cells, immediately after a s.c. injection of either saline or 0.15 mg/kg of apomorphine. The beams crossed between the 5th and the 20th min were counted. The spontaneous locomotor activity was decreased by about 60 % by apomorphine.

— The apomorphine-induced hypothermia in mice : At the end of preceding test, when the mice were taken away from the apparatus, their colonic temperature was measured. There was a decrease of approximately 3 °C in the body temperature.

The neuroleptics to be tested were administered i.p., 30 min. before the apomorphine injections, except sulpiride which was administered 90 min. before.

Results

We shall only consider here the main features of the data reported in the Table 1.

Among the tests performed in rats treated with a 0.6 mg/kg dose of apomorphine it appeared that sulpiride had a special antagonistic effectiveness in the climbing test, in contrast to the approximately 3.5 time higher doses required to inhibit the licking and the sniffing by 50 %.

Table 1 : *The antagonist efficacy of atypical neuroleptics
and haloperidol in comparison to various apomorphine-induced behaviors.*

Test (dose of Apomorphine mg/kg ; Animals)	Haloperidol	Sulpiride	Thioridazine	Clozapine	Mezilamine
Climbing (0.6 ; rats)	0.08 ± 0.01	26 ± 7	6.2 ± 0,5	26 ± 5	1 ± 0.2
Licking (0.6 ; rats)	0.08 ± 0.01	90 ± 9	7.3 ± 0.8	21 ± 3	1 ± 0.1
Sniffing (0.6 ; rats)	0.1 ± 0.01	90 ± 8	5.7 ± 0.7	24 ± 2	1.1 ± 0.1
Yawning inhibition (0.6 ; rats)	0.08 ± 0.01	∞	5.5 ± 0.5	∞	1 ± 0.1
Yawning induction 0.1 ; rats)	0.11 ± 0.01	26.5 ± 3,7	10.1 ± 1.3	5.4 ± 0.3	1 ± 0.1
Penile erection (0.1 ; rats)	0.08 ± 0.02	24 ± 9	7.4 ± 2.0	2.1 ± 0.4	1.1 ± 0.2
Hypokinesia (0.15 ; mice)	+(0.05)	+(0.5)	+(0.5)	∞	N.T.
Hypothermia (0.15 ; mice)	+(0.05)	+(5)	∞	∞	N.T.

The corresponding ID_{50} ± S.E.M. were calculated according to the Miller and Tainter's graphic method.
+ indicates a significant antagonism for the dose, in mg/kg, in brackets.
∞ indicates a lack of antagonism in the large range of the tested doses.
N.T. not tested.

In addition we observed that in contrast with other tested neuroleptics, it was not possible, in rats treated with 0.6 mg/kg apomorphine, to make the yawning reappear with sulpiride.

It was also impossible to make the yawning reappear with clozapine. This may be due to the anticholinergic activity of the drug, since, at a dose of 10 mg/kg, clozapine completely inhibited the physostigmine-induced yawning. An anticholinergic activity of thioridazine has been demonstrated (Miller and Hiley, 1974) but since 20 mg/kg of the drug did not antagonize the physostigmine-induced yawning, it does not seem to interfere in the yawning test and the antidopaminergic effect seems therefore to prevail.

From the test performed in mice it appears that, in contrast with most other apomorphine induced behaviors, the hypokinesia elicited in mice by 0.15 mg/kg of apomorphine is extremely sensitive to the antagonist effect of sulpiride since, with as little as 0.5 mg/kg, a significant antagonism of the hypokinesia was observed, which became virtually complete at 2 mg/kg. This marked efficacy does not depend on a peripheral localization of dopamine receptors. As a matter of fact a similar antagonism may be observed following the intracerebroventricular administration of 200 ng of sulpiride. This is also suggested by the different antagonistic effectiveness of haloperidol which easily crosses the blood brain barrier and of domperidone which does not (to be published). Clozapine does not antagonize the hypokinesia elicited by 0.15 mg/kg of apomorphine and even potentiates it slightly. This may be related to the fact that clozapine does not antagonize the apomorphine-induced hypothermia, but strongly potentiates it (paper submitted).

51

Thus 1.25 mg/kg of clozapine, which alone does not significantly affect the body temperature, caused a marked potentiation of the hypothermia elicited by 0.15 mg/kg of apomorphine ($-6.8\,^{\circ}$C $\pm\,0.4\,^{\circ}$C as compared with $-2.9\,^{\circ}$C $\pm\,0.2\,^{\circ}$C).

Thioridazine antagonizes the apomorphine-induced hypokinesia but does not affect the apomorphine-induced hypothermia. This indicates that these two effects, although occurring simultaneously, are not closely connected, although they may interact when hypothermia is increased (see above).

Discussion and conclusion

Taken together these data suggest that the concept of "atypical" neuroleptics cannot be explained only in terms of a specific blockade of a special dopamine receptor subtype. Such an explanation appears likely only for sulpiride. This agent seems to discriminate to some extent between the dopamine receptor subtype involved in several apomorphine-induced effects (such as the climbing behavior and the induction of yawning in rats, or the hypokinesia and the hypothermia in mice) and another dopamine receptor subtype involved in other effects of apomorphine (the sniffing, licking, or inhibition of yawning in rats), as well as in the cataleptogenic effect of neuroleptics. Sulpiride may have a higher affinity for the former than for the latter subtype. Binding studies, carried out by P. Sokoloff, M.P. Martres and J.C. Schwartz (in preparation) support this distinction between two such subtypes, designated D4 and D2 respectively. The other "atypical" neuroleptics tested, as well as haloperidol, apparently do not discriminate between the two dopamine receptor subtypes. The anticholinergic component of the clozapine and perhaps also of the thioridazine activity may be critical for their "atypical" character. None of these particularities can be retained for mezilamine. One should search in other directions for the explanation of its lack of cataleptogenic activity possibly in the noradrenergic agonist activity of the drug (Le Fur et al., 1979).

If the antipsychotic activity of neuroleptics depends on the blockade of the D4 dopamine receptor subtype and the extrapyramidal side effects of these agents depend on the blockade of the D2 dopamine receptor subtype, it is clearly of great importance to find agents with an even greater selectivity than sulpiride, and therefore to develop tests for such agents.

Acknowledgement
This investigation was supported by Grant, ATP 4176, from the Centre National de la Recherche Scientifique.

REFERENCES

Holmgren, B., Urba-Holmgren, R. *1980* — Interactions of cholinergic and dopaminergic influences on yawning behavior. *Acta Neurobiol. Exp, 40 :* 633-642.
Le Fur, G., Burgevin, M.C., Malgouris, C, Uzan, A. *1979* — Differential effects of typical and atypical neuroleptics on alphanoradrenergic and dopaminergic postsynaptic receptors. *Neuropharmacology, 18 :* 591-594.
Marçais, H, Protais, P., Costentin, J., Schwartz, J.C. *1978* — A gradual score to evaluate the climbing behaviour elicited by apomorphine in mice. *Psychopharmacology, 56 :* 233-234.
Miller, R.J., Hiley, C.R. *1974* — Antimuscarinic properties of neuroleptics and drug-induced parkinsonism *Nature, 248 :* 596-598.

Protais, P, Costentin, J., Schwartz, J.C. *1976* — Climbing behaviour induced by apomorphine in mice : a simple test for the study of dopamine receptors in striatum. *Psychopharmacology, 50* : 1-6.

Yamada, K., Furukawa T. *1980* — Direct evidence for involvement of dopaminergic inhibition and cholinergic activation in yawning. *Psychopharmacology, 67 :* 39-43.

DISCUSSION

G. Groß
Did you perform any experiments in animals pre-treated with 6-hydroxydopamine ? I think that would make it easier to decide which effect is pre-synaptic and which is post-synaptic in your behavioral experiments.

Ph. Protais
In which test ? Climbing, yawning, hypokinesia or hypothermia ?

G. Groß
For example yawning, for which you showed a bell-shaped dose/response curve. Have you any explanation for this ?

Ph. Protais
At the moment we have no explanation. It has been suggested in the literature that pre-synaptic dopamine receptors could be involved, but it has never been demonstrated.

G. Sedvall
Have you performed any studies with the d and l forms of sulpiride ?

Ph. Protais
We do not have the two forms of sulpiride. We hope that the Delagrange company will send it to us.

"Learned helplessness" as a model for human depression : A biochemical and pharmacological evaluation

W.H. Vogel, N.T. Gentile and R.M. Swenson

Department of Pharmacology and Department of Psychiatry and Human Behavior, Thomas Jefferson University, and Department of Psychiatry, University of Pennsylvania, Philadelphia, USA

Summary : Rats that could or could not cope with footshock were studied. Noncoping rats had higher plasma cate-cholamine and corticosterone concentration during stress and showed a slower return to baseline values after ter-mination of the stressor compared with coping animals. NE levels were decreased in the hypothalamus at the end of the session in the noncoping but not the coping animals. About 50 % of the noncoping animals showed a lear-ning deficit when tested later on an escape task. The learning impairment caused by the inability to control foots-hock is designated "learned helplessness". This escape deficit could be reduced by chronic imipramine treatment in half of the helpless animals. "Learned helplessness" in rats, because of its behavioral, biochemical and pharma-cological characteristics, may be a useful animal model for human depression.

Introduction

A number of investigators have tried to establish an animal model for depression. Reserpine treatment and social isolation have been used with varying success (Katz, 1981). A more promising model at present, however, seems to be the model of "learned helplessness" as originally formulated by Seligman (Maier and Seligman, 1971) and expanded more recently by others (Sherman et al., 1979 ; Weiss, 1980). In this model an animal is exposed first to an uncontrollable stressor and then tested later for possible consequences. Many of these animals experiencing inescapable stressors show a variety of symptoms that are similar to those seen in depressed patients. For instance, they show decreased locomotor activity, weight loss, and impaired acquisition or performance of a learned response, and this is unlike the effect seen in animals that can control the stressor (Maier and Seligman, 1971 ; Weiss, 1970 ; Weiss et al., 1979). Decreases in brain norepinephrine in noncoping versus coping rats have been reported (Weiss et al., 1979), and these neuroche-mical changes are in agreement with the biogenic amine hypothesis of depression. Chronic, but not acute, imipramine treatment has been claimed to reverse this syndrome (Sherman et al., 1979).

A crucial component in the development of "learned helplessness" is the inabi-lity of the animal to cope with the stressor. Because few data exist on the bioche-mistry of coping, we studied plasma catecholamines and corticosterone as well as brain catecholamine concentration in pairs of rats exposed to the same number of identical footshocks. One rat (the coping rat) could terminate the shock for both animals, whereas the other rat (the noncoping rat) had to endure the shock without control.

Methods

Footshock was given in a BRS/LVE (#RSC-044) rat shuttlebox modified by a metal partition bisecting the long axis of the cage. The floor was fixed in place, and two manipulanda (ceiling pole and wall paddle) were added to the left hand side. Two pole or paddle presses were required to terminate shock. Shock could not be avoided. The left hand compartment was used for all control shock subjects ; the right hand side was used for rats without control over shock. Grids in both compartments were wired in series to a shock scrambler and regulated shock source (LVE 113-04). Rats received 250 unpredictable footshocks (1 mA, 20 sec duration if not terminated, 10 sec inter-trial intervals, probability of onset 0.60). The duration of shock received by both rats depended on the speed with which the control rat terminated shock for both rats. Control rat responses were shaped for pole or paddle pressing during the first 15 minutes of the 1 hour trial, and typically, rats learned to terminate the shock within this time.

For blood measures, catheters were placed in the external jugular vein and passed into the vena cava (Upton, 1975 ; Pashko and Vogel, 1980). Blood samples were drawn while the rats were in the home cage (—15 min or 15 min prior to stressor onset), just before shock onset in the shock apparatus (0 min), during shock at 1, 5, 15, 30 and 60 min and 30 min (or 90 min into the experiment) after termination of the shock. Blood was also drawn from implanted rats that received no shock. A volume of 0.25 ml blood was removed via the catheter for catecholamine and corticosterone determinations, and the volume withdrawn was replaced with saline containing heparin.

For brain catecholamine determinations sets of rats were exposed to controllable or uncontrollable footshock and were decapitated at specified times. Control rats were placed in the box without shock. Brains were dissected on ice into hypothalamus and hippocampus. Samples were wrapped in foil and placed on dry ice immediately after dissection. Samples were stored at —70 °C until assay.

For behavioral and pharmacological studies, all rats were first tested for susceptibility to learned helplessness. These rats were given a similar set of 250 inescapable, unpredictable footshocks (1 mA, 2 sec duration, inter-trial interval = 10 sec, onset p = .60). Three hours later they were tested for escape latency in an unsignalled 2 way escape task. Rats received 20 trials with a reduced shock intensity (0.7 mA) lasting 20 seconds unless the rat made a hurdle jump to the temporary "safe" side of the apparatus. Rats with escape latencies of more than 8 seconds were arbitrarily designated as showing "learned helplessness". Only these rats were randomly assigned to one of two groups : saline or imipramine. Imipramine (10 mg/kg in saline vehicle) or saline was given 1 hour prior to inescapable shock as described above on day 0 of the study. Three hours following the termination of shock, they were tested for escape latencies as on day 0. On each of the subsequent 5 days of the study, injections of either saline or imipramine were made at approximately the same time of day. On the sixth day of the study, the procedure of day 0 was repeated ; rats were injected, subjected to inescapable shock, and later tested for escape latency in the shuttlebox.

Catecholamines were determined by the radioenzymatic technique using commercial kits (Upjohn Co., Cat-a-Kit[R], Kalamazoo, MI). Corticosterone was determined fluorometrically (Glick et al., 1964).

Results

To insure "learned helplessness" under our conditions, we tested rats after escapable and inescapable shock. In contrast to the coping condition, the inability to cope produced in some, but not all, rats an inability to learn to escape footshock in an unsignalled 2-way escape task. Approximately 50 % of our animals show this deficit, whereas the remaining animals, like coping animals, escape within a few seconds. Rats with delayed escape latencies respond rather consistently when tested repeatedly. This is shown in Table 1.

Table 1 — *Escape time after inescapable footshock at different days*

N	Mean Escape Time (sec)*	
Day 0 (6)	14.7 ± 1.6*	(11.0 ; 19.6)**
Day 1 (6)	14.4 ± 2.0	(8.9 ; 16.9)
Day 6 (6)	13.5 ± 2.0	(11.7 ; 20.0)

* Mean ± SEM
** Two individual animals displaying minimal or optimal « learned helplessness ».

Plasma norepinephrine (NE) and epinephrine (E) concentrations are shown in Tables 2 and 3. NE and E concentration do not change in nonshocked rats.

Table 2 — *Plasma norepinephrine levels (pg/ml) in rats receiving footshock*

Time (min)	NS $\overline{X}$ (SEM)N	C $\overline{X}$ (SEM)N	NC $\overline{X}$ (SEM)N
−15	177 (42) 5	170 (52) 4	154 (16) 11
5	230 (38) 5	402*(79) 6	818***(189) 11
15	172 (25) 5	460*(66) 6	868***(156) 11
60	266 (41) 6	414 (135) 6	546* (95) 11
90	214 (35) 5	401 (144) 6	363* (62) 11

Table 3 — *Plasma epinephrine levels (pg/ml) in rats receiving footshock*

Time (min)	NS $\overline{X}$ (SEM)N	C $\overline{X}$ (SEM)N	NC $\overline{X}$ (SEM)N
−15	62 (71) 5	105 (34) 5	128 (25) 10
5	170 (65) 5	323*(87) 5	876***(203) 11
15	129 (67) 5	502*(103) 5	920***(142) 11
60	184 (68) 5	141 (32) 5	538***(114) 11
90	141 (51) 5	87 (11) 5	318***(72) 10

* Comparison with - 15 min value ; $p < 0.05$;
** Comparison between coping (C) and noncoping (NC) animals ; $p < 0.05$ non-shocked (NS) animals were exposed only to the chamber without shock ;
| = Stress period ;
N = number of animals.

However, both coping and noncoping rats show marked rises in NE that persist throughout the stress period. Noncoping rats have higher NE concentration than coping rats during exposure to the stressor. After the stress period, noncoping rats remain high for the next 30 min, whereas coping rats show marked individual variations that make a statistical evaluation difficult ; some animals return quickly to baseline whereas others remain elevated. Differences become more marked with plasma E. Again, both animals show elevated levels during footshock, but coping rats return to normal by the end of the shock period. In noncoping rats, E concentration is significantly higher during and after the shock period.

Table 4 shows the plasma corticosterone concentration. Nonshocked rats have unchanged corticosterone concentration in plasma. Coping and noncoping rats have steroid levels higher than baseline during the stress period without a difference between both groups. Plasma corticosterone concentration in coping rats returns to baseline by 30 minutes after termination of the footshock. However, noncoping rats still are elevated markedly at this time.

Table 4 — *Plasma corticosterone (ug/100 ml) in rats receiving footshock*

Time (min)	NS $\bar{X}$ (SEM)N	C $\bar{X}$ (SEM)N	NC $\bar{X}$ (SEM)N
−15	22.3 (3.4) 5	14.4 (3.7) 5	18.0 (3.7) 9
5	19.0 (2.9) 4	30.7 (2.2)* 8	37.8* (4.2) 9
15	* 18.9 (3.6) 4	32.1 (2.5)* 5	33.3 (3.2) 11
60	20.4 (5.6) 4	28.6 (2.1)* 3	38.5* (3.0) 8
90	24.1 (2.7) 5	20.7 (4.8) 4	41.3*** (6.9) 6

* Comparison with −15 min value ; $p < 0.05$;
** Comparison between coping (C) and noncoping (NC) animals ; $p < 0.05$;
Non-shocked (NS) animals were exposed only to the chamber without shock ;
| = Stress period ;
N = number of animals.

Table 5 shows norepinephrine values in hypothalamus and hippocampus. Nonshocked rats (n = 6) have an average concentration of approximately 1600 ng/g in the hypothalamus. During and after stress, only noncoping rats show progressively lower norepinephrine concentrations in hypothalamus as compared with nonshocked or coping rats. In the hippocampus no changes are seen except low NE in the coping rats at the end of the stress period.

Table 5 — *Norepinephrine (ng/g) in hypothalamus and hippocampus in rats receiving footshock*

Time (min)	Hypothalamus C	NC	Hippocampus C	NC
0	1623 ± 72 (6)		133.4 ± 6.0 (6)	
10	1376 ± 151 (5)	1289 ± 129 (4)	117.8 ± 5.0 (5)	108.8 ± 12.0 (5)
60	1777 ± 82 (5)	1166 ± 126*(4)	96.9 ± 13.0* (4)	150.4 ± 26.0 (4)
90	1346 ± 155 (4)	962 ± 145*(4)	158.1 ± 28.0 (4)	130.6 ± 25.0 (5)

Values are means ± SEM.
* Comparison of values from coping (C) or noncoping (NC) rats with non-shocked controls ; $p < 0.05$;
| = Stress period ;
Numbers in parentheses denote number of animals

DA and E also were determined in these areas at the same times. No significant changes were noticed with the exception of DA in the hypothalamus which was low in noncoping (280 ± 23 ng/g; N = 4) rats at 10 min and low in coping (294 ± 39 ng/g; N = 7) rats at 90 min.

Table 6 shows the effects of imipramine on escape latencies. Chronic, but not acute, treatment produces significant improvement. However, this effect obviously does not occur in all rats.

Table 6 — *Effect of imipramine on « learned helplessness » in rats*

Saline	I	II	III	IV	V	VI	VII	Mean
Day 0**	19.6	18.3	15.0	13.6	11.0	11.0	—	14.8
Day 1	16.9	17.4	20.0	9.5	13.4	8.9	—	14.4
Day 6	20.0	10.7	17.6	13.2	10.7	11.7	—	14.0
Imipramine (10 mg/kg/day)								
Day 0**	17.7	9.0	10.6	8.3	11.4	20.0	14.6	13.0
Day 1	16.0	20.0	19.2	9.5	7.2	15.5	18.3	15.1
Day 6	20.0	9.7	10.2	7.0	6.0	9.1	2.7	9.2*

* Values are compared with saline data ; $p < 0.05$ (Mann Whitney U-Test) ;
** Day 0 is prior to saline or imipramine treatment.

Discussion

In this study, pairs of rats were exposed to electric footshock. Only one rat could terminate the shock for both rats. Thus, both animals received the same number of footshocks with the same intensities, but one animal could terminate or cope with the shock whereas the other animal had no control over or could not cope with the stressor.

Increases in plasma NE and E as well as corticosterone concentrations occurred in both coping and noncoping animals. Although some of the levels are higher in noncoping rats, the main difference seems to be in the return of the stress-induced changes to baseline levels. Plasma catecholamine and corticosterone concentrations return to baseline much more quickly in coping rats, whereas in noncoping rats these elevated levels continue considerably longer after termination of the stressor. This might indicate that the inability to cope is a more damaging experience-because its effects persist after the exposure to the stressor. The fact that noncoping rats, compared with coping rats, have higher concentrations of NE, E and, in particular, corticosterone is of interest to researchers studying human depression. Higher basal plasma cortisol concentration together with a disruption in cortisol rhythm have been reported in human depression (Carroll et al., 1976). Also, depressed patients have been shown to have higher NE and, in particular, E levels compared with healthy controls (Ackenheil et al., 1979).

Our brain values confirm and expand existing data. No significant changes are detected in the coping animals after terminating the stressor. In the noncoping animals, we confirm the finding of others who show that lower levels of NE in the hypothalamus follow termination of an inescapable stressor. In addition, we find

Table 7 - *Model of « learned helplessness »*

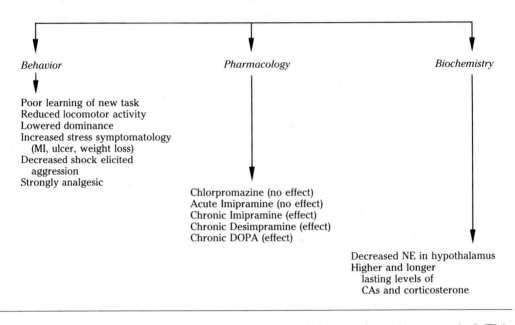

Inescapable Shock ("Life Event")

(Selective Effect)

Behavior

Poor learning of new task
Reduced locomotor activity
Lowered dominance
Increased stress symptomatology
   (MI, ulcer, weight loss)
Decreased shock elicited
   aggression
Strongly analgesic

Pharmacology

Chlorpromazine (no effect)
Acute Imipramine (no effect)
Chronic Imipramine (effect)
Chronic Desimpramine (effect)
Chronic DOPA (effect)

Biochemistry

Decreased NE in hypothalamus
Higher and longer
   lasting levels of
   CAs and corticosterone

that this reduction is present already at the end of the one hour stress period. This would be in agreement with a catecholamine deficiency theory of depression (Mendels et al., 1976). The decrease in NE in the hippocampus at the end of the stress period in coping animals could be interpreted as a learning and memory phenomenon involving the active development of an association between a response and shock termination. The hippocampus has been implicated in these processes (Thompson et al., 1981). This neurochemical change does not occur in the noncoping rats which do not have to remember a specific task.

The DA changes are more difficult to interpret. The decrease in DA at 10 min in the noncoping rats might be an early indication of increased NE turnover and demand on its precursor. Why noncoping rats have a higher DA content in hypothalamus 30 min after termination of the stressor is unclear at present, but this effect of inescapable shock on hypothalamic DA has been reported before (Weiss et al., 1979). Unlike changes in NE in hypothalamus, these changes in hypothalamic dopamine are not correlated to behavioral changes induced by inescapable shock.

Our pharmacological findings confirm previous data but add another component because of our more stringent criteria. We chose only animals that showed a certain degree of helplessness, that is, only animals taking longer than 8 sec to escape from shock during a 20 sec shock period. Animals that escaped in less than 8 sec were not labelled helpless and were not studied. Saline treatment produced only 1 out of 6 major responses (defined as an improvement of 15 % or better in escape behavior). Acute imipramine treatment caused 3 responses (average 35 %)

after one day of drug therapy and 4 responses (average 50 %) after 6 days of treatment with a relatively large dose (10 mg/kg) of the drug. Although these data are vague in scientific terms, they perhaps more closely resemble the human situation. Footshock will not cause an escape deficit in all but only in some animals ; similarly, "life events" will not precipitate a depressive episode in all but only in some individuals (Murphy and Brown, 1980). This depressive phase is self-limiting in some patients, and one out of 6 rats receiving only saline improved in escape behavior. Not all patients who receive imipramine will respond to the same degree. In a parallel fashion, not all rats receiving imipramine show improvement, and the improvement rate as with depressed patients increases with time. After 1 day, 3 rats responded moderately, and after 6 days, 4 animals improved markedly.

Thus, noncoping, in contrast to coping, can produce in rats a variety of behavioral and biochemical changes that are indicative of depression in humans. A summary of these effects, from the literature and from our studies, is shown in Table 7.

Although an animal model cannot demonstrate all of the behavioral characteristics seen in human depression, it can demonstrate some of them. More importantly, such a model may exhibit many of the neurochemical changes associated with depression. If so, this model may be useful in screening new antidepressant drugs and may lead to a better understanding of the biological abnormalities underlying a behavioral pathology.

Aknowledgements
This research was supported in part by NIMH Grant MH 14654.

REFERENCES

Ackenheil, M., Albus, M., Müller, F., Müller, Th., Welter, D., Zander, K., Engel, R. *1979* - Catecholamine response to short-term stress in schizophrenics and depressive patients. In E. Usdin, I. Kopin and J. Barchas (eds). *Catecholamines : Basic and Clinical Frontiers, Vol. 2.* New York, Pergamon Press, pp. 1937-1939.

Carroll, B.J., Curtis, G.C., Mendels, J. *1976* - Neurœndocrine regulation in depression ; I. Limbic system - adrenocortical dysfunction. *Arch. General Psychiat., 33 :* 1039-1044.

Glick, D., von Redlick, D., Levine, S. *1964* - Fluorometric determination of corticosterone and cortisol in 0.02-0.05 milliliters of plasma or submilligram samples of adrenal tissue. *Endocrinology, 74 :* 653-655L.

Katz, R.J. *1981* - Animal models and human depressive disorders. *Neurosci. Biobehavioral Rev., 5 :* 231-246.

Maier, S.F., Seligman, M.E.P. *1976* - Learned helplessness : Theory and evidence. *Jl. Exp. Psychol. General, 105 :* 3-46.

Mendels, J., Stern, S., Frazer, A. *1976* - Biochemistry of depression. *Dis. Nerv. System, 37 :* 3-9.

Murphy, E., Brown, G.W. *1980* - Life events, psychiatric disturbance and physical illness. *Br. J. Psychiat., 136 :* 326-338.

Pashko, S.M., Vogel, W.H. *1980* - Factors influencing the plasma levels of amphetamine and its metabolites in catheterized rats. *Biochem. Pharmacol., 29 :* 221-225.

Sherman, A.D., Allers, G.L., Petty, F., Henn, F. *1979* - A neuropharmacologically-relevant animal model of depression. *Neuropharmacol., 18 :* 981-893.

Thompson, R.F., Berger, J.W., Berry, S.D., Hœhler, F.K., Kettner, R.E.,Weiss, D.J. *1980* - Hippocampal substrate of classical conditioning. *Physiol. Psychol., 8 :* 262-279.

Upton, R.A. *1975* - Simple and reliable method for serial sampling of blood from rats. *J. Pharmac. Sci., 64 :* 112-114.

Weiss, J.M., *1970* - Somatic effects of predictable and unpredictable shock. *Psychosomatic Med., 32 :* 397-408.

Weiss, J.M., Glazer, H.I., Pohorecky, L.A., Barley, W.H., Schrœder, L.H. *1979* - Coping behavior and stress-induced behavioral depression : studies of the role of brain. *In :* E. Depue (ed.). *The psychology of the depressive disorder : implication for the effects of stress.* New York, Academic Press.

61

DISCUSSION

S. Z. Langer
I noticed on your slide, that 10 μg/kg was the dose of imipramine. Is that correct ?

W. H. Vogel
No, I am sorry, I should have pointed out that it means 10 mg/kg. I apologize for the omission.

S. Z. Langer
Did you try lower doses of imipramine ?

W.H. Vogel
No, we did not try lower doses, a group in Iowa has tried lower doses and they started to see an effect at approximately 5 mg/kg, at lower doses they did not see any effect.

S. Z. Langer
And was the dose of desimipramine also 10 mg/kg ?

W. H. Vogel
Yes, that is correct.

Ch. Eggers
In a publication I read recently, monkey infants who were separated from their mother at an early age showed a reduction in their noradrenaline levels of the hypothalamus. This corresponds with your results and to me as a child-psychiatrist these findings are very interesting. I believe that we have here a link between biochemical models and the development of psychological models of depression, this is because life experiences or earlier traumas according to Freud and Melanie Klein are relevant for the development of a depression in childhood, adolescence and adulthood.

W. H. Vogel
Yes, the monkey studies perhaps come closest to the human situation. On the other hand, it is quite expensive to use monkeys, it takes a long period of time. If our rat would simulate the monkey and the monkey would simulate the human, then within one hour we could produce the rat model which is much quicker.

D. Soulairac
Are you sure that your model is a model of true depression or only a model of anxiety ? And what are the actions of benzodiazepines ?

W. H. Vogel
Benzodiazepines have been shown by the Iowa group not to be effective. Unfortunately, they did not give a dose range, but only tested one particular dose. Is it a model of human depression ? I do not know. I thought and would wish that maybe a clinician would say, « that is what we see in humans ». If they say : « No, that is not what we see in humans », then of course it is not a model. I am particularly impressed by two facts : The first is, if every single animal would show these signs and symptoms, I would say it is not a good model, because not every single human being exposed to a life event will become depressed, only a certain number will. In addition, a second fact speaks for this : We repeated the experiments with old animals. Whereas in the young rats 3 to 4 months old, 50 % of these rats show « learned helplessness ». In older rats, one year to one and half years old, approximately 80 % to 85 % will show the learned helplessness. This goes hand in glove with the human situation. So, I think it is the selectivity which is important. You get similar effects with reserpine, but every single animal will show it. I think it is the selectivity which makes me hopeful that this model comes closer to the human situation.

S. Z. Langer
Did you look at the serotonin biochemistry in the brain ?

W. H. Vogel

We are now looking into it and I hope that it will be decreased.

S. Z. Langer

Have you tried any selective inhibitor of serotonin-uptake which does not affect the noradrenergic system in terms of its pharmacology ?

W. H. Vogel

This model is very new. Of course, a lot of studies have been done on stress, cold stress, immobilization and so forth, and of course serotonin is affected, GABA is affected, receptors are affected, but I think very little has been done in terms of actually exposing two animals to the same events, where one animal can cope with the stressor, whereas the other animal cannot cope with it. So, we are at the very beginning here as it comes to the CNS chemistry. However, in answer to your question, no, we have not done so.

M. Ackenheil

You asked me to comment on your results, especially to the adrenaline levels. Although, of course, we do not give foot-shocks to patients or to man, we select stress situations and the increase of the ratio noradrenaline : adrenaline depends on the kind of stress situation according to the Funkenstein hypothesis. In situations where one acts actively, there is an increase in noradrenaline, in other situations, which are more passively experienced, an increase in adrenaline is found. In depressive patients the ratio noradrenaline : adrenaline generally is lower and this ratio fits well with your hypothesis. Furthermore, as far as the symptoms of stress are concerned, we have some investigations in patients with sepsis shock : In comparing the two groups, the group of patients who were dying had much higher adrenaline levels than other group of survivors. The noradrenaline levels of both groups did not show such a big difference, however, I would assume that the adrenaline levels are a more secondary phenomenon of stress, because psychotropic drugs influence the adrenaline release less than the noradrenaline release.

W. H. Vogel

I think the adrenaline responds to both and you see this in that the « coping » animal will also show an increase, whilst it is in the non-coping animal where the increases are a little higher and where, in particular, increases seem to be longer lasting. I do not know how long it will carry over, at least it will carry over for three hours. It might actually carry over more and it might perhaps be irreversible if we expose the rat not only once to one hour, but if we repeatedly expose the animal.

K. Fuxe

I was also interested in the 5-HT biochemistry, however, it would also be nice to know if you have done something about regional studies on noradrenaline, because it would be useful to see if there is a differential regional action on noradrenaline, if you have a general stress or other types of stress. This is a very special type of model which you have shown so beautifully here ; it would be good to find out if they might have a very certain profile in a special part of the noradrenaline system.

W. H. Vogel

This model is very new — at least in our laboratory — and at the moment we are still at a sort of turning point, because if I get the feeling that I have a very interesting, but only scientific model here, then I am not sure if I am going to continue it. On the other hand, if I get the feeling, this is not only of scientific interest, but it really seems to simulate a human condition, then I would really carry on in full swing, because the catheterization of the animal and looking at the plasma level would allow us, for instance, to make selective breeding studies. If it is possible that we can selectively breed for high and low responders, then we can take these animals, sacrify them, look at the brain chemistry and see how they differ in their brain chemistry.

N. Matussek

In my opinion this is a good model for exogenous depression, but not for the endogenous one, because life events are important for reactive and neurotic depression. Until now we have no clear data saying that life events are also important for endogenous depression. Therefore, I think, it could help us to understand better the neurotic-reactive type of depression, but I doubt that this is a good model for endogenously depressive patients.

W. H. Vogel

I think the only way we might perhaps come close to this would be by selectively breeding animals, which over-respond to an exogenous event, thus bringing out special qualities which disposes the animal to « learned helplessness » and we may come closer to the animal model where the depression is exogenous.

J. S. Kim

You told me that the serotonin system is decreased, where did you measure it ?

W. H. Vogel

In this model we did not look at serotonin. I was talking in general terms ; if you expose an animal to cold, to immobilization, then the serotonin decreases.

J. S. Kim

This is certainly possible, because your data and that of other researchers show that after the shock-model plasma cortisol levels increased, then liver pyrrolase increases and plasma tryptophane decreases. So, it would be interesting to measure the serotonergic system in your model.

J. Mendlewicz

From the clinical point of view, I would tend to agree with Prof. Matussek and I would even go further. Some of the symptoms, the behavioral symptoms you describe may be seen in some forms of schizophrenia and even in some very severe phobic neuroses, so I think we have to be quite careful about the clinical extrapolation. The other thing, which may be interesting to look at, is if you could find some other biological disturbances which have been described in human depression, such as cortical steroid binding globuline and REM latency. Is it reduced in some of your non-coping rats ? And if you have hypercortisol secretion, then it may be interesting to look at the dexamethasone suppression test.

W. H. Vogel

That is hopefully what my student is doing at the moment. Yes, we do want to test this. Now what you said about the schizophrenic reaction, you are absolutely correct. On the other hand, I feel a little bit confident that chlorpromazine really does not do anything. As a matter of fact, it makes the animals worse. I do not know what happens if you have a depressed patient who is not schizophrenic and you give this patient chlorpromazine, i.e. whether he would show no response or would get worse. This makes me a bit confident that we might not necessarily look at psychotic reactions.

C. Gennari

I was very impressed by your model, it is very interesting. You said that you have observed many effects, one of which is analgesia. In this respect, I would like to ask you if you have measured the plasma levels of β-endorphin and endogenous opioids and would you think that it could be interesting to pre-treat animals with naloxone, an opioid antagonist ?

W. H. Vogel

We only measured the tail-flick in the animal, in which the tail is put into hot water and the time is measured until the animal flicks its tail out. Our coping rats do not show any effects, they have normal tail-flick. Therefore, it is not surprising that our non-coping rats show the expected latency, that the endorphin levels in the brain increase and that can partially block the analgesia with naloxone. Apparently, the analgesia and particularly the stress-induced analgesia is due to the endorphin, as well as a serotonin-mediated mechanism. If you block the endorphin, you get a partial antagonism, but you do not achieve a complete antagonism, because of the serotonin involvement.

P. Grof

It seems that you have an animal model of some human condition and that the question is whether it is a model of depression or of anxiety ? I was thinking that one of the first things you should do now, would simply be to return to the same model and just try very different dosages of the same drug. If you look at the literature from the early sixties', you will find that chlorpromazine was described as an antidepressant when given in a very low dosage.

W. H. Vogel
We only used the high dose as is used for antipsychotic studies.

P. Grof
Similarly, it would be interesting to go into high doses of imipramine to see what would happen in your model.

Ch. Eggers
It is too bad that the adult-psychiatrist has often little knowledge about child-psychiatry. From the point of view of developmental psychology, there are relations between early life events, early life experiences in children and later neurotic, reactive and endogenous depression. I would just like to mention that Melanie Klein's and Winnicotts's research in child psychology is at this point in accordance with the work of Hubertus Tellenbach and Wolfang Loch, two adult-psychiatrists.

W. H. Vogel
Thank you very much for your suggestions, I now hope that the NIMH is going to support me.

Changes in behavior and neurotransmitter metabolism in the rat following acute and chronic sulpiride administration. *

F. Hasan and B.E. Leonard,

Pharmacology Department, University College, Galway, Republic of Ireland.

Summary : Following the acute and chronic administration of ($\pm$) sulpiride, the hypermotility induced by low acute doses of apormorphine (0,10 mg/kg i.p.) in the "open field" apparatus was attenuated. The effect of chronic sulpiride was less than that seen after an acute dose of the neuroleptic which suggests that a desensitization of pre-synaptic dopamine receptors may have occurred. There is evidence that the behavioral effects of ($\pm$) sulpiride are primarily due to the ($-$) isomer. Sulpiride did not antagonize the enhanced locomotor behavior induced by high doses of apomorphine (1.0 mg/kg).

The turnover of dopamine, serotonin and noradrenaline in four regions of the brains of the rats was also examined. Both acute and chronic sulpiride attenuated the increase in dopamine turnover caused by acute apomorphine in the striatum but did not affect the increased turnover of noradrenaline in the limbic regions of the brain caused by the dopamine agonist. The concentration of serotonin in the midbrain and limbic regions was reduced by both acute and chronic sulpiride administration.

These results suggest that sulpiride has a complex effect on central neurotransmission which cannot be explained only in terms of a specific blockade of pre-synaptic dopamine receptors.

Introduction

It is widely assumed that the antipsychotic action of neuroleptic drugs is attributable to their ability to decrease the activity of the dopaminergic system. Such an assumption is supported by the finding that all well-established antipsychotic drugs block post-synaptic dopamine receptors whereas drugs such as amphetamine, which stimulate the release of dopamine, can produce a toxic psychosis which closely resembles acute paranoid schizophrenia (Beamish and Kiloh, 1960). Post-mortem data implicating an abnormality in dopamine synthesis release, or in post-synaptic receptor activity, is equivocal however with some groups of investigators demonstrating an increase in the concentration of the neurotransmitter in some brain regions (Bird et al., 1977), whereas others found no change in dopamine turnover (Kleinman et al., 1979). Owen et al. (1978) and Lee et al. (1978) have independently reported that the dopamine receptor sensitivity is increased in the basal ganglia of non-drug treated schizophrenic patients. Other studies of post mortem material have shown that the concentration of noradrenaline is raised in some regions of the schizophrenic brain (Bird et al., 1979 ; Crow et al., 1979, Kleinman et al., 1980) but the regions in which these changes were found differed. It is not the purpose of this article to discuss the possible aetiology of schizophrenia but

* Some of the studies mentioned in this review were communicated to the Summer Meeting of the British Association of Psychopharmacology (Hasan and Leonard, 1981).

merely to stress that an abnormality in brain dopamine metabolism in this condition is by no means proven.

Evidence that neuroleptic drugs act as antagonists of post-synaptic dopamine receptors in the brain has been provided by the detailed *in vitro* receptor binding studies of Snyder et al. (1974) and Seeman and Lee (1975) among others. Such findings have been confirmed *in vivo* by, for example, the ability of these drugs to antagonize amphetamine-induced stereotyped behavior in rats (Randrup and Munkvad, 1972) and apomorphine-induced gnawing behavior (Janssen et al., 1978). However, the question arises as to whether these effects are causally or coincidentally related to the anti-psychotic action of the drugs. For example, the anti-psychotic agent clozapine shows minimal activity in both the *in vitro* and acute *in vivo* tests for neuroleptic activity whereas thiethylperazine is a potent dopamine receptor antagonist in all animal tests yet shows little antipsychotic activity in man (Barchas et al., 1978). More recently, Greenblatt et al. (1980) reported that the indoline derivative CL 77, 328, a putative neuroleptic was devoid of effect on the dopaminergic system in the brain as assessed by both biochemical (e.g. reduction in dopamine sensitive adenylate cyclase activity) and behavioral studies.

A critical consideration of such studies thus leads one to the view that changes in central dopaminergic activity may be of relevance in evaluating the potency, and extrapyramidal side effects potential, of an antipsychotic agent that is structurally related to the "classical" neuroleptics but may be of only limited value in the discovery of a new class of compounds with antipsychotic activity. It is against this background that we have attempted to evaluate the pharmacological properties of the benzamide neuroleptic sulpiride. This drug is structurally unrelated to the "classical" neuroleptics of the phenothiazine and butyrophenone class and has been shown to be an effective antipsychotic agent which apparently produces only minimal extrapyramidal side effects (Mouren et al., 1970 ; Bouvier et al., 1971). The structure is shown in Figure 1.

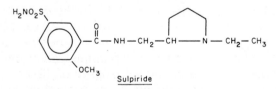

Sulpiride

The purpose of our study was to investigate the acute and chronic sulpiride on central neurotransmitter systems *in vivo* by studying changes in behavior thought to be mediated by one or more of these transmitter systems. Whereas emphasis has been placed on the antipsychotic profile of the drug, some attention will also be given to its antidepressant potential, as evidence has indicated that sulpiride may have such properties (Niskanen et al., 1975).

Studies on the action of sulpiride on dopamine receptors in the rat brain in vivo : Behavioral effects.

There is experimental evidence to suggest that there are at least two distinct populations of dopamine receptors in the striatum. One population appears to be located post-synaptically and is responsible for eliciting the locomotor and other behavioral responses that occur following the release of the neurotransmitter or following the administration of high doses (> 1.0 mg/kg) of the dopamine agonist apomorphine (Schwartz et al., 1978). The other population of dopamine receptors appears to be located pre-synaptically whose function involves the inhibition of dopamine release (Kehr et al., 1972). By using low (< 0.1 mg/kg) or high (> 0.5 mg/kg) doses of apomorphine, and observing the behavior of the rat it is possible to differentiate the effects of pre- and post-synaptic stimulation of these receptors. Thus low doses of apomorphine attenuate while high doses facilitate locomotor activity (Harrison-Reed, 1980).

In the initial investigation, we studied the effects of sulpiride on the behavior of rats treated with either low or high doses of apomorphine. In the *first experiment*, groups of 10 rats (male, Sprague-Dawley, 200 - 220 g) were injected with different doses of apomorphine (0.05 — 10.0 mg/kg i.p.) and placed in the "open field" apparatus 10 min after drug treatment. The animals were observed for 3 min and the ambulation, rearing, grooming and defaecation scores recorded. The results of this experiment are shown in Table 1.

Table 1 - *The effect of single, acute, doses of apomorphine (APO) on the ambulation and rearing scores in the "open field" apparatus.*

Treatment	Ambulations	Rearings
Controls (saline treated)	92 ± 6	11.5 ± 1.2
APO - 0.05	$33 \pm 4**$	$7.9 \pm 0.8*$
0.10	$53 \pm 5*$	$7.7 \pm 0.9*$
0.25	65 ± 6	9.0 ± 0.7
0.50	67 ± 8	8.2 ± 0.5
1.00	78 ± 4	10.0 ± 1.2
5.00	113 ± 7	12.2 ± 0.7
10.00	120 ± 6	14.0 ± 1.1

*p <0.05
**p <0.02 versus controls.

From this experiment it is clear that low doses of apomorphine (0.05 and 0.1 mg/kg) attenuate locomotor activity in the "open field" apparatus whereas higher doses (> 1.0 mg/kg) had little effect. In the *second experiment* the interaction between sulpiride and apomorphine was assessed. Groups of rats were injected either acutely or chronically (14 days) with sulpiride (20 mg/kg i.p.). 30 min after the last dose of sulpiride, groups of rats were injected with either the "low" or "high" dose of apomorphine and their behavior in the "open field" apparatus determined 10 min later. The results are summarized in Table 2.

From this experiment, it can be seen that a single dose of sulpiride antagonizes the effect of the low dose of apomorphine on the ambulation and rearing scores in the "open field" without affecting the higher dose. However, when sulpiride was given chronically, the antagonistic effect was considerably diminished. This suggests that the sensitivity of the pre-synaptic dopamine receptors may increase following the prolonged administration of the neuroleptic. Other investigators have also shown that chronic sulpiride treatment increases the number of dopamine binding sites in the striatum and enhances apomorphine induced stereotypy (Jenner et

Table 2 - *The effects of sulpiride, given acutely and chronically, on the ambulation and rearing scores in the "open field" apparatus following the acute administration of apomorphine.*

| | Saline | | Apomorphine | | | |
| | | | 0.10 mg/kg | | 1.00 mg/kg | |
	Ambulations	Rearings	Ambulations	Rearings	Ambulations	Rearings
Saline	96 ± 8	13.7 ± 1.9	43 ± 3*	5.5. ± 0.6*	88 ± 6	14.8 ± 1.1
Sulpiride (acute)	89 ± 7	12.0 ± 1.0	87 ± 9**	12.8 ± 0.9**	92 ± 5	13.2 ± 1.2
Sulpiride (chronic)	78 ± 6	10.0 ± 1.2	59 ± 6***	8.8. ± 0.3***	85 ± 0	11.0 ± 0.8

*p <0.02 versus controls
**p <0.02 versus APO (0.1)
***p <0.05 versus APO (0.1)

al., 1982) which shows that sulpiride, like the classical neuroleptic haloperidol, induces behavioral and biochemical supersensitivity of dopamine receptors in the rat brain.

In the *third experiment*, an attempt was made to determine the duration of treatment necessary for the onset of pre-synaptic dopamine receptor sensitivity to occur. Groups of rats were treated with sulpiride (10 mg/kg i.p.) daily for 1, 7 and 14 days and their behavior in the "open field" apparatus assessed at the end of the treatment period in the presence or absence of a low acute dose of apomorphine. The results of this study are given in Table 3.

Table 3 - *Effect of the duration of sulpiride treatment on the reduction in ambulation and rearing behavior in the "open field" apparatus following the acute administration of apomorphine.*

| Days of sulpiride treatment : | 1 | | 7 | | 14 | |
treatment :	Ambulations	Rearings	Ambulations	Rearings	Ambulations	Rearings
Saline	88 ± 9	11.2 ± 0.7	92 ± 7	10.7 ± 1.1	81 ± 8	9.1 ± 0.8
Apomorphine, acute (0.1)	39 ± 3**	6.0 ± 0.5**	41 ± 5**	5.8 ± 0.7	36 ± 3**	2.4 ± 0.4**
Sulpiride (10) + Apomorphine	75 ± 5***	8.3 ± 0.9***	62 ± 4***	8.3 ± 0.8	65 ± 3***	6.7 ± 0.9***

*p <0.05 ;
**p <0.01 versus controls
***p <0.05 versus APO.

From this experiment, it can be seen that the reversal of the effect of apomorphine by sulpiride is less after 7 days of treatment than it is after acute treatment. This suggests that the hypersensitivity of the pre-synaptic dopamine receptors is already manifest after only 7 days of treatment with the neuroleptic. This experiment was extended to determine the effects of different doses of sulpiride, given acutely and chronically (14 days), on the performance of rats in the "open field" apparatus after an acute low dose of apomorphine. Groups of rats were given 10, 20 or 50 mg/kg sulpiride, either acutely or chronically and the reversal of the hypomotility induced by apomorphine determined. The results are summarized in Table 4.

From these results it can be seen that there is little quantitative difference between the lowest and highest acute dose of sulpiride in reversing the hypomotility caused by apomorphine. However, following chronic administration, the reversal of the acute effect of apomorphine is greater with the lowest dose of sulpiride and

Table 4 - *Effect of different doses of sulpiride, given acutely and chronically, on the reduction in ambulation following the acute administration of apomorphine*

	Acute	Chronic
Control (Saline).. 100 %		
Apomorphine (0.1)... 36 %*		
APO+Sulpiride (10)	81 %**	75 %**
APO+Sulpiride (20)	90 %**	61 %**
APO+Sulpiride (50)	83 %**	58 %***

All results expressed as a percentage control value.
  *p < 0.01 versus control ;
 **p < 0.01 ;
***p < 0.05 versus APO.

least with the highest dose suggesting that the higher doses of sulpiride cause a more pronounced supersensitivity of the pre-synaptic dopamine receptors.

In the *fourth experiment* the effects of different low doses of chlorpromazine on the ambulation and rearing scores of rats in the "open field" apparatus were assessed. This experiment was undertaken to compare the effects of sulpiride with a "classical" neuroleptic whose pharmacological activity has been attributed to a blockade of post-synaptic dopamine receptors. In this experiment, groups of 10 rats were injected with chlorpromazine (0.5 — 5.0 mg/kg i.p.) either in the presence or absence of apomorphine (0.05 mg/kg). One hour after the injection of chlorpromazine, and 10 min after apomorphine, their behaviors in the "open field" apparatus was determined. The results are given in Table 5.

Table 5 - *Effect of acute doses of chlorpromazine, alone and in combination with apomorphine (0.05 mg/kg i.p.) on the ambulation and rearing scores of rats placed in the "open field" apparatus.*

		Saline		Apomorphine (0.05 mg/kg)	
		Ambulations	Rearings	Ambulations	Rearings
Controls (Saline)		68 ± 6	10.5 ± 1.1	22 ± 4**	1.8 ± 0.6**
Chlorpromazine	0.5	52 ± 3	9.4 ± 0.7	27 ± 5**	2.2 ± 04**
	1.0	45 ± 7	10.2 ± 1.2	26 ± 4**	3.1 ± 0.6*
	2.0	22 ± 4**	3.5 ± 0.7**	12 ± 2**	1.5 ± 0.4**
	5.0	12 ± 3	1.4 ± 0.5**	15 ± 2**	0.9 ± 0.4**

 *p < 0.05 ;
**p < 0.01 versus controls.

From this study, it can be concluded that even low doses of chlorpromazine do not antagonize the hypomotility that results from the administration of a low dose of apomorphine. This suggests that these drugs may not interact at the same dopamine receptor sites *in vivo*.

Studies on the action of sulpiride on neurotransmitter metabolism in the rat brain in vivo

From the behavioral studies summarized above, it may be concluded that sulpiride reverses the hypomotility caused by low doses of apomorphine by antagonizing the effect of the dopamine agonist on pre-synaptic receptors. In an attempt to obtain more direct verification of the action of these drugs on the dopaminergic system in the various regions of the rat brain, we have studied changes in dopamine, noradrenaline and serotonin metabolism in the striatum, mid-brain and amygdaloid cortex and olfactory tubercles. These regions were selected so that changes in neurotransmitter metabolism in both limbic and non-limbic regions could be assessed.

In the *first experiment,* the effects of acute (20 mg/kg i.p.) and chronic (20 mg/kg i.p. for 14 days) dose of sulpiride, administered either alone or together with a low dose of apomorphine (0.1 mg/kg i.p.) were determined. In these and subsequent experiments reported in this section, the concentrations of the neurotransmitters and metabolites were assayed fluorimetrically, following separation on columns of Sephadex G-10, by the method of Earley and Leonard (1978). The results of this study are summarized in Table 6.

The results of this experiment clearly demonstrate that a low, acute dose of apomorphine significantly affects all three neurotransmitter systems. The raised concentration of dopamine in the striatum, together with those of the dopamine metabolites, suggests that the release of the neurotransmitters may be reduced by apomorphine, and the intraneuronal metabolism facilitated. Whereas the concentration of noradrenaline was unchanged, that of serotonin was increased in the cortex ; as the concentration of its metabolite was unchanged it would appear that apomorphine may reduce the release of serotonin in that brain region.

Acute sulpiride diminished the effects of apomorphine on both the dopaminergic and serotonergic systems ; in general, the neuroleptic tended to overcompensate for the effects of apomorphine on these neurotransmitter systems.

Not surprisingly, chronic sulpiride caused changes in dopamine and serotonin qualitatively similar to that caused by acute administration of the drug. In addition, it lowered the noradrenaline concentration in both the mid-brain and cortex. The combination of chronic sulpiride with acute apomorphine produced changes which would not have been predicted from the effects of either drug alone. Thus the effect of apomorphine on the dopamine concentration in the striatum was unaffected by chronic sulpiride, whereas the increase in DOPAC and HVA was significantly reduced. Similarly, the rise in serotonin in the cortex caused by apomorphine is antagonized by chronic sulpiride treatment. However, the concentration of noradrenaline in both the cortex and limbic regions is increased by the combined drug treatment.

From this study, it is difficult to conclude whether the primary actions of apomorphine and sulpiride are on dopaminergic, serotonergic or noradrenergic function. Whatever the final explanation, it cannot be assumed that the behavioral effects of these drugs are explicable only in terms of their well-established action on the dopaminergic system.

In the *second experiment,* the effect of a low acute dose of chlorpromazine (0.5 mg/kg i.p.) on neurotransmitter metabolism in three regions of the rat brain was studied. In this experiment, groups of 10 rats were killed 1 hour after chlorpromazine administration or, in the case of the groups treated with apomorphine alone or in combination with chlorpromazine, 15 min after the injection of the dopamine agonist. The results of this experiment are summarized in Table 7.

Table 6 - *Changes in the concentrations of some neurotransmitters and their metabolites following the acute and chronic administration of sulpiride interaction with a low acute dose of apomorphine.*

	DA	DOPAC	HVA	NA	5-HT	5-H1AA
			Controls			
Striatum	100 ± 8	100 ± 7	100 ± 14	100 ± 8	100 ± 6	100 ± 8
	(3.67 ± 8)	(0.31 ± 0.02)	(0.21 ± 0.03)	(0.49 ± 0.04)	(0.68 ± 0.04)	(0.36 ± 0.03)
Mid-brain	100 ± 7	100 ± 13	100 ± 12	100 ± 8	100 ± 9	100 ± 7
	(0.56 ± 0.04)	(0.28 ± 0.03)	(0.24 ± 0.02)	(0.48 ± 0.03)	(0.35 ± 0.02)	(0.33 ± 0.02)
Amygdala + olf. tub.	100 ± 5	100 ± 4	100 ± 8	100 ± 7	100 ± 8	100 ± 8
	(0.58 ± 0.05)	(0.24 ± 0.01)	(0.19 ± 0.02)	(0.37 ± 0.02)	(0.21 ± 0.02)	(0.45 ± 0.03)
Cortex	100 ± 9	100 ± 12	100 ± 10	100 ± 5	100 ± 9	100 ± 10
	(0.46 ± 0.04)	(0.33 ± 0.04)	(0.31 ± 0.04)	(0.38 ± 0.03)	(0.30 ± 0.02)	(0.30 ± 0.03)
			Apomorphine (0.1)			
Striatum	$145 \pm 5^*$	$145 \pm 6^*$	$138 \pm 4^*$	100 ± 8	94 ± 8	92 ± 9
Mid-brain	100 ± 7	108 ± 8	87 ± 6	107 ± 8	113 ± 9	121 ± 8
Amygdala + olf. tub.	93 ± 8	100 ± 12	$147 \pm 4^*$	116 ± 9	105 ± 5	95 ± 5
Cortex	84 ± 11	94 ± 10	116 ± 6	95 ± 9	$139 \pm 10^*$	114 ± 8
			Acute sulpiride (20)			
Striatum	86 ± 10	77 ± 12	100 ± 12	$73 \pm 6^*$	82 ± 5	94 ± 9
Mid-brain	71 ± 8	$64 \pm 16^*$	$46 \pm 18^*$	$58 \pm 10^*$	$137 \pm 6^*$	$121 \pm 5^*$
Amygdala + olf. tub.	116 ± 9	$147 \pm 9^*$	$132 \pm 12^*$	89 ± 10	$262 \pm 10^{**}$	89 ± 5
Cortex	109 ± 11	65 ± 20	$71 \pm 14^*$	$79 \pm 7^*$	87 ± 9	$70 \pm 10^*$
			Acute sulpiride + Apomorphine.			
Striatum	$123 \pm 9^{* \bullet}$	$56 \pm 5^{* \bullet}$	$64 \pm 10^{* \bullet}$	108 ± 10	100 ± 6	92 ± 7
Mid-brain	95 ± 8	107 ± 10	93 ± 8	94 ± 9	$66 \pm 4^{* \bullet}$	106 ± 6
Amygdala + olf. tub.	100 ± 6	71 ± 12	86 ± 21	116 ± 10	$71 \pm 13^{* \bullet}$	104 ± 6
Cortex	107 ± 7	100 ± 8	103 ± 11	111 ± 10	$93 \pm 8^{\bullet}$	90 ± 8
			Chronic sulpiride			
Striatum	114 ± 7	90 ± 14	100 ± 12	96 ± 6	99 ± 6	83 ± 7
Mid-brain	$64 \pm 6^*$	$54 \pm 13^*$	75 ± 22	$69 \pm 10^*$	$191 \pm 6^{**}$	$133 \pm 10^*$
Amygdala + olf. tub.	121 ± 7	83 ± 15	105 ± 15	114 ± 5	$219 \pm 7^{**}$	84 ± 9
Cortex	80 ± 10	$48 \pm 19^*$	$35 \pm 18^*$	$68 \pm 15^*$	$127 \pm 9^{**}$	103 ± 10
			Chronic sulpiride + Apomorphine			
Striatum	$145 \pm 8^*$	$73 \pm 10^{* \bullet}$	$64 \pm 13^*$	94 ± 6	103 ± 5	100 ± 9
Mid-brain	94 ± 8	100 ± 6	100 ± 13	105 ± 8	$57 \pm 5^*$	105 ± 9
Amygdala + olf. tub.	$132 \pm 12^{* \bullet}$	111 ± 6	$68 \pm 20^{* \bullet}$	$146 \pm 5^{* \bullet}$	100 ± 7	96 ± 6
Cortex	117 ± 7	108 ± 10	96 ± 12	$148 \pm 9^{* \bullet}$	$100 \pm 10^{\bullet}$	108 ± 10

All values expressed as % control $\pm$ SEM
*p < 0.05
**p < 0.01 versus control
•p < 0.05 versus APO.
Absolute values for the concentrations of amines and their metabolites in control group given in parenthesis.
DA = dopamine, DOPAC = dihydroxyphenylacetic acid, HVA = homovanillic acid, NA = noradrenaline, 5-HT = serotonin, 5-H1AA = 5-hydroxyindoleacetic acid.

Table 7 - *Effect of an acute low dose of chlorpromazine on the changes in neurotransmitter metabolism induced by a low dose of apomorphine.*

	DA	DOPAC	HVA	NA	5-HT	5-H1AA
Controls						
Striatum	100 ± 7	100 ± 7	100 ± 11	100 ± 9	100 ± 8	100 ± 5
Olf. tub. + amyg.	100 ± 7	100 ± 7	100 ± 5	100 ± 8	100 ± 5	100 ± 6
Mid-brain	100 ± 10	100 ± 10	100 ± 15	100 ± 7	100 ± 5	100 ± 5
Apomorphine (0.05 mg/kg)						
Striatum	120 ± 6	$119 \pm 8^*$	75 ± 11	$142 \pm 6^*$	100 ± 8	86 ± 6
Olf. tub. + amyg.	$129 \pm 7^*$	$126 \pm 8^*$	$58 \pm 18^*$	118 ± 6	$67 \pm 8^*$	100 ± 6
Mid-brain	107 ± 11	100 ± 10	167 ± 10	100 ± 7	$80 \pm 5^*$	$74 \pm 10^*$
Chlorpromazine (0.5 mg/kg)						
Striatum	98 ± 8	107 ± 9	100 ± 12	100 ± 9	105 ± 6	105 ± 7
Olf. tub. + amyg.	100 ± 7	95 ± 10	116 ± 7	107 ± 7	$74 \pm 5^*$	80 ± 6
Mid-brain	$73 \pm 15^*$	114 ± 8	96 ± 16	91 ± 10	96 ± 5	91 ± 10
Apomorphine (APO) + Chlorpromazine (CPZ)						
Striatum	94 ± 6	105 ± 14	92 ± 10	107 ± 6	98 ± 5	100 ± 5
Olf. tub. + amyg.	$106 \pm 9^\bullet$	118 ± 12	$100 \pm 10^\bullet$	114 ± 5	$68 \pm 8^*$	88 ± 6
Mid-brain	92 ± 10	118 ± 8	$77 \pm 15^\bullet$	83 ± 13	96 ± 5	83 ± 6

*p <0.05 versus controls
$^\bullet$p <0.05 versus APO.
The absolute concentrations of the neurotransmitter and their metabolites in the control group were quantitatively similar to those shown for the controls in Table 6.

It is apparent from this study that the dose of apomorphine used (0.05 mg/kg) is associated with quantitatively different changes in neurotransmitter metabolism to that observed with the slightly higher dose (0.1 mg/kg).

These results show that chlorpromazine has only a slight effect on the changes induced by apomorphine. Thus, pre-treatment with a low dose of chlorpromazine prevents decrease in dopamine turnover in the limbic regions (olfactory tubercles and amygdala) which occurs following the administration of the dopamine agonists ; chlorpromazine also attenuated the elevation of noradrenaline in the striatum. It is not without significance that a low dose of chlorpromazine that does not reverse the hypomotility caused by a low acute dose of apomorphine has little effect on the reduction in the turnover of dopamine caused by apomorphine in the striatum. By contrast, all doses of sulpiride studied (10-100 mg/kg) were found to reverse both the behavioral effects of apomorphine and the reduction in dopamine turnover in the striatum. These results suggest that the antagonism of the effects of apomorphine by sulpiride must be partially attributable to the action of the neuroleptic on the pre-synaptic dopamine receptors in the striatum but clearly other neurotransmitter systems are also associated with the behavioral and neurochemical changes caused by both apomorphine and sulpiride.

The dopaminergic system and affective disorders : The effects of sulpiride on some animal models of depression

Studies supporting the role of dopamine in affective disorders arose out of the observation that the "classical" neuroleptics were effective in reducing the symptoms of mania. In the case of depression, however, the role of dopamine in the aetiology of the disease is less certain with some investigators showing a decrease in the concentration of the dopamine metabolite, homovanillic acid (HVA), in the CSF of depressed patients (Van Praag and Korf, 1973), while others could find no change (Bowers, 1974). It could be argued that the changes in the CSF-HVA concentration, when they occurred, were more a reflection of the degree of psychomotor retardation, presumably involving a reduction in activity in the basal ganglia, than a direct biochemical correlate of the depressed affect seen in the patient. Furthermore, the concentration of HVA may vary with the gender of the patient and the assay method used (Post and Murphy, 1979).

More recently there has been a renewed interest in the possible involvement of the dopaminergic system in the aetiology of depression following the observation by Randrup and Braestrup (1977), that many tricyclic and non-tricyclic antidepressants inhibit the re-uptake of tritiated dopamine into synaptosomal fractions from the rat brain. Furthermore, Serra et al. (1979) have shown that chronic treatment of rats with either amitriptyline or mianserin prevents the hypomotility of rats subsequently injected with a low dose of apomorphine (0.05 mg/kg). These authors explain their results by suggesting that chronic antidepressant treatment causes a subsensitivity of pre-synaptic dopamine receptors. The findings of Serra et al. (1979) have been extended by Chiodo and Antelman (1980) who showed that the ability of apomorphine to selectively depress the spontaneous electrical activity of dopaminergic neurons located in the zona compacta of the substantia nigra was attenuated following the chronic administration of imipramine, amitriptyline or iprindol. The possible significance of these observations was provided by the finding that rats showing dopamine autoreceptor subsensitivity following prolonged antidepressant therapy also showed enhanced responsiveness to an environmental stimulus (tail-pressure). This may simulate the enhanced responsiveness of patients to environmental stimuli following prolonged antidepressant medication.

In the previous section of this article, it was shown that both the acute and chronic treatment of rats with sulpiride results in a reversal of the hypomotility caused by a low acute dose of apomorphine. By contrast, chlorpromazine did not reverse the effect of apomorphine, a finding which contrasts with that of Serra et al. (1979) who showed that chlorpromazine also reversed the hypomotility caused by apomorphine. The effect of chronic sulpiride treatment on apomorphine-induced hypomotility might be a reflection of its novel neuroleptic action and/or its potential antidepressant activity. To test the latter possibility, we compared the effect of the chronic administration of sulpiride with a number of different types of antidepressants on the apomorphine response.

In this experiment, groups of 10 rats were injected once daily for 14 days with sulpiride, β-flupenthixol, salbutamol, reserpine or one of the antidepressants shown in Table 8. On the day following treatment, half of the animals in each group were injected with a low dose of apomorphine (0.05 mg/kg) and 15 minutes after injec-

Table 8 - *Effect of chronic neuroleptic or antidepressant drug treatment on the hypomotility caused by a low acute dose of apomorphine.*

Drug	Dose (mg/kg)	Class	Effect on motility in open field : alone + APO (0.05 mg/kg)	
Apomorphine	0.05 (acute)	DA-agonist	35 %*	—
Amitriptyline	5.0 × 14d.	Tricyclic A.D.	80 %	74 %**
Citalopram	10.0 b.d. × 14d	Nontricyclic A.D.	88 %	61 %**
Trazodone	75 × 14d	Nontricyclic A.D.	67 %	59 %**
Nomifensin	5 × 14d	Nontricyclic A.D.	135 %*	85 %**
Mianserin	5 × 14d	Nontricyclic A.D.	82 %	59 %**
Salbutamol	5 b.d. × 14d	β-agonist	85 %	80 %**
Reserpine	0.1 × 14d	Antihypertensive	83 %*	38 %
Sulpiride	20 × 14d	Neuroleptic	81 %	61 %**
β-flupenthixol	0.1 × 14d	Neuroleptic	104 %	38 %**

All results expressed as % saline injected control (= 100 %)
*p < 0.05 versus control
**p < 0.05 versus acute APO.

tion their behavior in the "open field" apparatus assessed. The remaining animals were not treated with apomorphine and their activity in the « open field » was also assessed 24 hours after the last dose of the neuroleptic or antidepressant. The results are summarized in Table 8.

The results of this experiment, clearly demonstrate that, irrespective of the structure of the antidepressant used, all drugs which have been shown to be clinically effective antidepressants (Leonard, 1981, for review) reverse the hypomotility of apomorphine treated rats in the "open field" apparatus. These results thus confirm and extend those of Serra et al. (1979). Of the two neuroleptics investigated, β-flupenthixol has been shown also to have antidepressant properties while a preliminary report shows that sulpiride may have some antidepressant effects (Niskanen et al., 1975).

Only sulpiride was shown to be effective in reversing the apomorphine induced hypomotility however. To investigate the potential antidepressant properties of sulpiride in more detail we therefore decided to see what effect the chronic administration of the drug had on the behavior of the olfactory bulbectomized rat model of depression.

A detailed review of the behavioral and biochemical changes which occur following the bilateral ablation of the olfactory lobes of the rat has been published elsewhere (Leonard and Tuite, 1981). In summary, it has been shown that this surgical lesion causes permanent behavioral deficits that may be specifically ameliorated following the chronic treatment of the animals with antidepressants ; the acute administration of antidepressants, or the chronic administration of any psychotropic drug which lacks antidepressant activity in man, does not reverse the behavioral deficit. In the "open field" apparatus, bulbectomized rats show a characteristic hypermotility which can be reversed by chronic antidepressant treatment.

In this experiment, groups of 10 Sprague-Dawley rats (male 280-300 g) were either bilaterally bulbectomized or sham operated and allowed to recover from the surgery for 14 days. Following recovery, the animals were either injected with saline (controls), sulpiride (20 mg/kg i.p.) or with the novel antidepressant mianserin (5 mg/kg i.p.) for 14 days. Twenty-four hours after the last drug treatment, the rats were placed in the "open field" apparatus and observed for 3 min. The results of this study are summarized in Table 9.

Table 9 - *Effect of the chronic administration of sulpiride and mianserin on the behavior of olfactory bulbectomized rats in the "open field" apparatus. Score per 3 min.*

	Ambulation	Rearing	Grooming
Sham + Saline	100 ± 6	100 ± 10	100 ± 11
	(91.5 ± 5.5)	(14.3 ± 1.5)	(5.1 ± 0.6)
Sham + Mianserin	81 ± 12	102 ± 11	90 ± 7
Sham + Sulpiride	82 ± 8	91 ± 18	121 ± 20
OB + Saline	143 ± 7*	185 ± 7*	25 ± 3*
OB + Mianserin	116 ± 9**	142 ± 5**	80 ± 5**
OB + Sulpiride	83 ± 7**	129 ± 17**	159 ± 19**

All results expressed as % controls (= 100). Absolute values for controls (sham + saline) given in parenthesis. OB = Olfactory bulbectomized. *p <0.05 versus controls. **p <0.05 versus OB.
It can be seen that sulpiride like mianserine, attenuates the hypermotility and enhanced rearing behavior of the bulbectomized rats.

Discussion

Effect of sulpiride on dopamine receptors

One of the major differences between sulpiride and neuroleptics of the phenothiazine, thioxanthine and butyrophenone classes lies in the fact that sulpiride does not block the effects of dopamine on dopamine sensitive adenylate cyclase in either the striatum or the limbic system (Trabucchi et al., 1975). Such a finding has led Kebabian and Calne (1979) to the suggestion that there are at least two types of dopamine receptors in the brain, one of which is linked to adenylate cyclase and is unaffected by sulpiride (D_1) while the other is blocked by sulpiride but not linked to the cyclase system (D_2). The behavioral effects of such dopamine receptor agonists as apomorphine may be explained in terms of their selective action on D_1 receptors (which leads to increased locomotor activity and stereotypy), or D_2 receptors (which causes a decrease in locomotor activity which follows the diminished release of dopamine). The findings reported here, which confirm those of other investigators, suggest that sulpiride by blocking the pre-synaptic dopamine receptors, may actually enhance dopaminergic neurotransmission in the rat brain. Detailed studies by Costall et al. (1980) of the acute effects of the isomers of sulpiride on the locomotor activity induced by the bilateral injection of (+)-amphetamine into the nucleus accumbens, clearly showed that sulpiride was 4 — 8 times more effective on pre- as compared with post-synaptic dopamine receptors, the (-) isomer of sulpiride being the active form of the drug. More recent studies by Memo et al. (1981), in which rats were chronically treated with sulpiride or haloperidol for 21 days, also showed that sulpiride produced a selective supersensitivity of the pre-synaptic (D_2) receptors whereas haloperidol selectively affected the post-synaptic (D_1) receptors only. Our results for the effect of sulpiride on the change in locomotor activity induced by a low dose of apomorphine confirm the findings of Memo et al. (1981).

So far, the assumption has been made that changes in locomotor activity that occur following the administration of apomorphine, either alone or together with a neuroleptic, are causally related to changes in dopaminergic activity in the striatum. However, there is good evidence to show that mesolimbic areas of the rat brain are directly involved in the regulation of general motor activity (Galey and Le Maal, 1976). Detailed studies by Jones et al. (1981) have shown that motor activity is under the control of the dopaminergic, serotonergic and GABA-ergic systems. Furthermore, projections from cell bodies containing these neurotransmitters terminate in the nucleus accumbens, an area of the mesolimbic system which may be intimately involved in regulating motor activity. While caution must be exercised in extrapolating from the crude neurochemical findings reported here, it is not without interest to note that both apomorphine and sulpiride cause changes in dopamine and serotonin metabolism in the mesolimbic areas that we studied. There is also evidence that sulpiride increases the concentration of the inhibitory transmitter GABA in these brain regions (unpublished) which might also help to explain the action of the drug in reversing the hypomotility that occurs following the acute administration of a low dose of apomorphine. It is, of course, still a matter of speculation whether these changes in locomotor activity in the rat have any bearing on the neuroleptic action of sulpiride but it is assumed that the neurochemical changes occurring in the rat and man after sulpiride are qualitatively similar, it is not unreasonable to speculate that the novel profile of sulpiride lies more in the mechanism whereby it normalizes defective neurotransmission in the limbic region of the brain rather than in specifically blocking D_2 receptors.

If it is assumed that all neuroleptics owe their clinical efficacy to an ability to modify dopaminergic activity, then we are faced with a paradox. Thus the "classical" neuroleptics by blocking the D_1 receptors impede dopaminergic activity whereas sulpiride facilitates dopaminergic activity due to its selective blockade of D_2 receptors. If, as has been implied by several groups of investigators (see Introduction), there is an overactivity of the dopaminergic system in the brain of the schizophrenic, one would anticipate that sulpiride would enhance the symptoms of the disease rather than attenuate them ! As there is good evidence to show that sulpiride is an effective antipsychotic agent and like all "classical" neuroleptics raises the concentration of HVA in the CSF of patients following drug treatment (Sedvall et al., 1978), one must look for explanations of its neuroleptic activity elsewhere.

Pinnock, et al. (1979) have shown that, in spite of its lack of dopamine receptor blocking activity when tested on dopamine-sensitive adenylate cyclase, sulpiride is a potent antagonist of the physiological response to dopamine when applied microiontophoretically to the substantia nigra. In vivo studies of the effect of sulpiride on the metabolism of dopamine in the striatum of rats by Hoffmann et al. (1979) and by ourselves clearly show that the effects of sulpiride on dopamine synthesis are slight, possibly due to the poor penetration of the blood brain barrier. These findings confirm the autoradiographic study of Benakis and Rey (1976) who showed that ^{14}C sulpiride only accumulated appreciably in those brain regions in which the blood-brain barrier is incomplete (for example, the pituitary gland and chemoreceptor trigger zone). Thus one explanation for the apparent lack of effect of sulpiride on dopamine sensitive adenylate cyclase activity may be due to its inability to penetrate the receptor sites in the brain, at least under the experimental conditions that have been used to study its action. Support for this view comes from the studies of Woodruff et al. (1980) who showed that drugs will block the D_1 receptor sites only if they have a sufficiently high oil/water partition coefficient and have dopamine receptor antagonist activity. Of course, these findings do not, as yet, explain why sulpiride acts as a neuroleptic. Nevertheless, apart from its apparent inability to block dopamine sensitive adenylate cyclase activity, it shares with conventional neuroleptics an ability to stimulate prolactin secretion and to act as an antiemetic (Mielke et al., 1977). Perhaps the explanation lies in its action on other neurotransmitter systems which may indirectly modulate central dopaminergic activity. In support of this view, Nicoletti et al. (1981) have shown that the chronic administration of the drug results in a substantial increase in the concentration of GABA in both the substantia nigra and corpus striatum ; haloperidol, administered under the same conditions, only raised the concentration of the inhibitory neurotransmitter in the corpus striatum. Whether this effect on striatal GABA can provide an explanation for the ability of sulpiride to suppress tardive dyskinesia (Casey et al. 1979) is a matter of speculation. Regarding the action of sulpiride on dopamine receptors, all current evidence suggests that while the functional effects of sulpiride and the related benzamides closely resemble those of "classical" neuroleptics, the mechanisms whereby their effects are brought about differ. As Jenner and Marsden (1979) have concluded in their review of the benzamide neuroleptics, perhaps this mechanism involves important distinctions between different population of dopamine receptors in the brain.

Sulpiride as a potential antidepressant

Clinical evidence for the antidepressant effect of sulpiride and related benzamide neuroleptics is so far limited. Thus a single-blind study of twelve randomly selected depressed patients by Niskanen et al. (1975) showed that sulpiride was slightly better than amitriptyline in ameliorating the depressive symptoms. Apart from this study there appears to be little objective evidence to suggest that sulpiride has antidepressant properties although there are clinical impressions which support this view (e.g. Collard and Dufrasne, 1972). Nevertheless, cognisance must be taken of the fact that the neuroleptic flupenthixol has well established antidepressant properties (Young et al., 1976).

It is generally agreed that the aetiological basis of depression resides in a disorder of noradrenergic and/or serotonergic activity (Leonard, 1981, for review). One would therefore anticipate that treatment with sulpiride would result in changes in the metabolism of these amines should the drug have any action on these monoamines in the human brain. However, Bjerkenstedt et al. (1979) could show no change in the concentration of the main serotonin and noradrenaline metabolites, MOPEG and 5-H1AA, following the administration of sulpiride to psychotic women. It is of course, possible that sulpiride would produce changes in the concentration of these metabolites in depressed patients whose neurotransmitter status would presumably differ from that of psychotic patients but so far evidence is not forthcoming and one must rely on extrapolation from animal models of depression.

Of the animal models available, the apomorphine antagonism and bulbectomy models described in this article have an advantage over all others in that they show a high degree of selectivity in detecting only clinically effective antidepressants and, more importantly, antidepressant drugs can be detected only following chronic administration. Furthermore, the period of chronic drug treatment necessary before a positive response is obtained approximates to that required for a therapeutic response (i.e. about 14 days). In both animal models, sulpiride was shown to have a qualitatively similar effect to both the conventional tricyclic antidepressants, as exemplified by amitriptyline, and the non-tricyclic type exemplified by mianserin.

Conclusion

Evidence has been presented from behavioral studies to suggest that sulpiride differs from the « classical » neuroleptics in that it selectively antagonizes the effects of low doses of apomorphine on the motility of the rat. Preliminary studies of the changes in biogenic amine metabolism in both limbic and striatal regions suggest that these behavioral effects are associatied with changes in dopamine, noradrenaline and serotonin metabolism. It therefore seems unlikely that the neuroleptic activity of sulpiride is only attributable to its ability to modify central dopaminergic transmission.

Behavioral studies in two animal models of depression have also shown that sulpiride produces changes which are qualitatively similar to those seen following chronic antidepressant treatment. There is some evidence to suggest that the « antidepressant » activity of sulpiride may be associated with a change in noradrenaline and serotonin metabolism in the limbic system (unpublished). In trying to ascribe the pharmacological activity of sulpiride to any one neurotransmitter system, perhaps it is as well to take cognisance of the view expressed by Richardson (1974) who stressed that, instead of a particular neurotransmitter having a particular behavioral effect, it is rather the balance between several neurotransmitter systems that determines behavior. Thus although specific behavioral patterns might be associated with the predominance of a single neurotransmitter, other transmitter systems are necessary for the successful completion of the behavioral pattern.

Acknowteagements
The authors wish to thank Chemitechna Ltd. (U.K.) for supplying the sulpiride used in these studies and for financial support towards part of the project.

REFERENCES

Barchas, J.D., Berger, P.A., Matthysse, S., Wyatt, R.J. *1978* — The biochemistry of affective disorders and schizophrenia. *In : Principles of Psychopharmacology* W.G. Clarke, and J. del Guidice, (eds.) pp. 105-131. New York, Academic Press.

Beamish, P., Kiloh, L. *1960* — Psychosis due to amphetamine consumption. *J. Ment. Sci., 106* : 337-343.

Benakis, A., Rey, C. *1976* — Etude autoradiographique du sulpiride 14C chez la souris et le rat. *J. Pharmac., 7* : 367-378.

Bird, E.D., Spokes, E.G., Barnes, J., Mackay, A.V.P., Iversen, L.L., Shepherd, M. *1977* — Increased brain dopamine and reduced glutamate and decarboxylase activity in schizophrenia and related psychoses. *Lancet, ii* : 1157-1159.

Bird, E.D., Spokes, E.G., Iversen, L.L. *1979* — Brain norepinephrine and dopamine in schizophrenia. *Science, 204* : 93-94.

Bjerkenstedt, L., Harnryd, C., Sedvall, G. *1979* — The effect of sulpiride on monoaminergic mechanisms in psychotic women. *Psychopharmac., 64* : 135-139.

Bouvier, C., Masquin, A., Amieux, M.C. *1971* — Indications psychiatriques du sulpiride a propos de 60 observations. *J. Méd. Lyon., 52* : 519-533.

Bowers, M.G. *1974* — Central dopamine turnover in schizophrenic syndromes. *Arch. Gen. Psychiat. 31* : 50-54.

Casey, D.E., Gerlach, J., Simmelsgaard, H. *1979* — Sulpiride in tardive dyskinesia. *Psychopharmac., 66* : 73-77.

Chiodo, L.A., Antelman, S.M. *1980* — Repeated tricyclics induce a progressive dopamine auto-receptor subsensitivity independent of daily dose. *Nature, 287* : 451-454.

Collard, J., Dufrasne, M. *1972* — Sulpiride et monoamides cérébrales. *In : Compte Rendu de Psychiatrie et de Neurologie de Langue Française. LXX Session* : pp. 1639-1642.

Costall, B., Huis, C, Naylor, R.J. *1980* — Differential actions of substituted benzamides on pre-and post-synaptic dopamine receptor mechanisms in the nucleus accumbens. *J. Pharm. Pharmacol. 32* : 594-596.

Crow, T.J., Baker, H.F., Cross, A.J., Joseph, M.H. *1979* — Monoamine mechanisms in chronic schizophrenia : post mortem neurochemical findings. *Br. J. Psychiat., 134* : 249-256.

Earley, C.J., Leonard, B.E. *1978* — Isolation and assay of noradrenaline, dopamine, 5-hydroxytryptamine and several metabolites from brain tissues using disposable Bio-Rad columns packed with Sephadex G-10. *J. Pharmac. Meth., 1* : 67-79.

Galey, D., Le Moal, M. *1976* — Locomotor activity after various radio-frequency lesions of the limbic midbrain area in the rat. Evidence for a particular role of the ventral mesencephalic tegmentum. *Life Sci., 19* : 677-684.

Greenblatt, E.N., Coupet, J., Rauh, E., Szucs-Myers, A.A. *1980* — Is dopamine antagonism a requisite of neuroleptic activity ? *Arch. Int. Pharmacology, 248* : 105-119.

Harrison-Reed, P.E. *1980* — Behavioural evidence for increased dopaminergic activity after long-term lithium pretreatment in rats. *I.R.C.S. Med. Sci, 8* : 313.

Hasan, F., Leornard, B.E. *1981* — Studies on the action of (±) sulpiride on dopamine receptors in the rat brain *in vivo. Neuropharmacol., 20* : 1327-1330.

Hoffman, M., Jommi, G.C., Montefusco, O., Tonon, G.C., Spano, P.F., Trabucchi, M. *1979* — Stereospecific effects of (-) sulpiride on brain dopamine metabolism and prolactin release. *J. Neurochem., 32* : 1547-1550.

Janssen, P.A., Van Bever, W.F.M. *1978* — Pre-clinical pharmacology of neuroleptics. *In : Principles of psychopharmacology*. W.G. Clark and J. del Guidice (ed) pp. 279-295. New York, Academic Press.

Jenner, P., Marsden, C.D. *1979a* — Mini review : The substituted benzamides — a novel class of dopamine antagonists. *Life Sci., 25* : 479-486.

Jenner, P., Marsden, C.D. *1979b* — The mechanism of action of substituted benzamide drugs. *In : Sulpiride and other benzamides*, Spano, P.F., Trabucchi, M., Corsini, G.U. and Gessa, G.L. (eds) pp. 119-147. Milan, Italian Brain Res. Found. Press.

Jones, D.L., Mogenson, G.L., Wu, M. *1981* — Injections of dopaminergic, serotonergic and GABAergic drugs into the nucleus accumbens : effects on locomotor activity in the rat. *Neuropharmacol, 20* : 29-37.

Kebabian, J.W. and Calne, D.B. *1979* — Multiple receptors for dopamine. *Nature, 277* : 93-96.

Kehr, W., Carlsson, A., Lindqvist, M., Magnusson, T., Attack, C. *1972* — Evidence for a receptor mediated feedback control of striatal tyrosine hydroxylase activity. *J. Pharm. Pharmacol, 24* : 744-747.

Kleinman, J.E., Potkin, S., Rogol, A., Buchsbaum, M.S. Murphy, D.L., Gillin, J.C., Nasrallah, H.A. and Wyatt, R.J. *1979* — A correlation between platelet monoamine oxidase activity and plasma prolactin concentrations in man. *Science, 206,* 489-481.

Lee, T., Seeman, P., Tourtellotte, W.W., Farley, I.J., Hornykiewicz, O. *1978* — Binding of ^{3}H-neuroleptics and ^{3}H-apomorphine in schizophrenic brain. *Nature, 274* : 897-900.

Leonard, B.E. *1980* — Pharmacological properties of some "second generation" antidepressant drugs. *Neuropharmacol, 19* : 1175-1183.

Leonard, B.E., Tuite, M. *1981* — Anatomical, physiological and behavioural aspects of olfactory bulbectomy in the rat. *Int. Rev. Neurobiol., 22* : 251-286.

Memo, M., Battaini, F., Spano, P.F., Trabacchi, M. *1981* — Sulpiride and the role of dopaminergic receptor blockade in the antipsychotic activity of neuroleptics. *Acta Psychiat. Scand., 63* : 314-324.

Mielke, D.H., Gallant, D.M., Kessler, C. *1977* — An evaluation of unique new antipsychotic agent, sulpiride : Effects on serum prolactin and growth hormone levels. *Am. J. Psychiat., 134* : 1371-1375.

Mouren, P., Majet, J., Larrieu, A. *1970* — Essai clinique d'une molécule nouvelle : le sulpiride en pratique psychiatrique. *Sem. Hôp. Paris 46* : 87-103.

Nicoletti, F., Patti, F., Condorelli, D.F., Rampello, L. Giammona, G., Scapagnini, U. *1981* — Comparative effects of chronic haloperidol and sulpiride treatment on nigral and striatal GABA content. *J. Neurochem., 37* : 1048-1051.

Niskanen, P., Tamminen, T., Viukari, M. *1975* — Sulpiride vs. amitriptyline in the treatment of depression. *Curr. Therap. Res., 17* : 281-284.

Owen, F., Cross, A.J., Longden, A., Poulter, M., Riley, G.J. *1978* — Increased dopamine receptor sensitivity in schizophrenia. *Lancet, ii* : 223-226.

Pinnoch, R.D., Woodruff, G.H., and Turnbull, M.J. *1979* — Sulpiride blocks the action of dopamine in the rat substantia nigra. *Eur. J. Pharmac., 56,* 413-414.

Post, R.M., Gerner, R.H., Carman, J.S., Gillin, J.C., Jimerson, D.C., Goodwin, F.K. and Bunney, W.E. *1979* — Effects of a DA agonist piribedil in depressed patients : Relationship of pre-treatment HVA to antidepressant response. *Arch. Gen. Psychiat., 35,* 609-615.

Randrup, A., Munkvad, I. *1972* — Influence of amphetamine on animal behaviour : stereotypy, functional impairment and possible animal human correlations. *Psychiat. Neurol. Neurochem., 75* : 193-292.

Randrup, A., Braestrup, C. *1977* — Uptake inhibitors of biogenic amines by newer antidepressant drugs : relevance to the dopamine hypothesis of depression. *Psychopharmac., 53* : 309-314.

Richardson, J.S. *1974* — Basic concepts of psychopharmacological research as applied to the psychopharmacological analysis of the amygdala. *Acta Neurobiol. Exp., 34* : 543-562.

Schwartz, J.C., Costentin, J., Maltres, M.P., Protais, P., Baudry, M. *1978* — Modulation of receptor mechanisms in the CNS : hyper- and hyposensitivity to catecholamines. *Neuropharmacol., 17* : 665-685.

Sedvall, G., Bjerkenstedt, L., Lindstrom, L., Wode-Helgodt, B. *1978* — Clinical assessment of dopamine receptor blockade. *Life Sci., 23* : 425-430.

Seeman, P., Lee, T. *1975* — Antipsychotic drugs : direct correlation between clinical potency and pre-synaptation in dopamine neurons. *Science, 188* : 369-373.

Serra, G., Argiolas, A., Klimek, V., Fadda, F., Gessa, G.L. *1979* — Chronic treatment with antidepressants prevents the inhibitory effect of small doses of apomorphine on dopamine synthesis and motor activity. *Life Sci., 25* : 415-424.

Snyder, S., Banerjee, S., Yamamusa, H., Greenberg, D. *1974* — Drugs, neurotransmitters and schizophrenia. *Science, 184* : 1243-1253.

Trabucchi, M., Longoni, R., Fresia, P., Spano, P.F. *1975* — Sulpiride : a study of the effects on dopamine receptors in rat neostriatum and limbic forebrain. *Life Sci., 17 : 1551-1556.*

Van Praag, H.M. Korf, J. *1973* — Monoamine metabolism in depression : clinical application of the probenecid test. In : *Serotonin and behaviour*, J. Barchas and E. Usdin (eds.). pp. 457-462. New York, Academic Press.

Woodruff, G.N., Freedman, S.B., Poat, J.A. *1980* — Why does sulpiride not block the effect of dopamine on the dopamine-sensitive adenylate cyclase ? *J. Pharm. Pharmacol., 32* : 802-803.

Young, J.P.R., Hughes, W.C., Lader, M.H. *1976* — A controlled comparison of flupenthixol and amitriptyline in depressed out patients. *Br. Med. J., 1* : 1116-1118.

DISCUSSION

S.Z. Langer
How long after the last injection of sulpiride following the chronic treatment did you test the effects of apomorphine and its blockade by sulpiride ?

B.E. Leonard
In most cases 12 hours after the last dose of sulpiride. We have also done the experiment after 6 hours and get essentially the same effects, so it seems unlikely that we are observing a rebound effect that may follow the elimination of sulpiride from the brain.

S.M. Langer
The other possibility is that after chronic treatment you may have a residual sulpiride in the brain which may be responsible for the subsensitivity of the blockade. This could mask a supersensitivity to apomorphine that you might see if you test your animals much later. This might be an interesting experiment to try.

B.E. Leonard
Yes, we are in the process of doing this now.

Substituted benzamides and other neuroleptics : Do they block a common dopamine receptor ?

G. Bartholini, B. Zivkovic, B. Scatton J. Dedek, P. Worms and K.G. Lloyd.

Research Department, LERS, Synthélabo Paris, France.

Summary : A heterogeneity of cerebral dopamine (DA) receptors (D_1 and D_2) has been proposed on the basis of *in vitro* experiments. However, the functional implications of these DA receptor subtypes for the action of neuroleptics is not yet clear. The present pharmacological analysis of the effects of a variety of neuroleptics on behavioral and biochemical parameters related to DA receptor function in rodents indicates that neuroleptics which block D_2 receptors (benzamides) do not differ qualitatively from those which act on both receptor subtypes. Thus, the relative potencies of neuroleptics (1) to increase striatal DA neuron activity, (2) to block DA post-synaptic receptors on cholinergic neurons, and (3) to antagonize the behavioral effects of apomorphine, are very strongly correlated. Moreover, irrespective of their selectivity for DA receptor subtypes, neuroleptics given repeatedly induce similar adaptive changes in DAergic transmission. These results suggest that the impairment of DAergic transmission by different classes of neuroleptics involves a single DA receptor (probably the D_2 type). The difference in the pharmacological spectrum between classes of neuroleptics is probably related to properties other than DA receptor blockade.

Introduction

In recent years, a new class of neuroleptic drugs, with atypical pharmacological and clinical spectra has emerged. Among these drugs special attention·has been given to substituted benzamides, particularly to sulpiride, because this drug exerts an antipsychotic action with less frequent side effects than classical neuroleptics like the phenothiazines and butyrophenones (Borenstein et al., 1969).

Pharmacological and biochemical experiments show that substituted benzamides block dopaminergic transmission, but in contrast to other neuroleptics, these drugs fail to antagonize dopamine-induced stimulation of adenylate cyclase (Trabucchi et al., 1975 ; Scatton et al., 1977). These findings, along with the discovery that some dopamine receptor agonists (e.g. bromocriptine, lisuride, lergotrile) do not stimulate the cAMP generating system in the dopamine neuron innervated regions (Kebabian et al., 1977 ; Schmidt and Hill, 1977 ; Goldstein et al., 1978), are taken as evidence for the existence of multiple forms of dopamine receptors and is used as a basis for their classification : D_1 receptor which is coupled to adenylate cyclase and D_2 receptor which is not (Spano et al., 1979 ; Kebabian and Calne, 1979).

Similarities between substituted benzamides and other neuroleptics

As the essential difference between substituted benzamides and other neuroleptics lies in their ability to antagonize dopamine-sensitive adenylate cyclase, the question arises as to whether adenylate cyclase blockade by neuroleptics plays a role in the impairment of dopaminergic transmission caused by these drugs.

To answer this question, one has to compare the potencies of neuroleptics with a wide range of antagonistic activity on adenylate cyclase, using a variety of parameters indicative of dopaminergic transmission (namely the activity of dopaminergic neurons).

In recent studies (Zivkovic et al., 1980 ; Zivkovic et al., 1982), we analysed the effects of 13 neuroleptics of various chemical classes (Table 1) on dopaminergic neurons (striatal tyrosine hydroxylase activity and homovanillic acid levels) and post-synaptic events, some of biochemical (change in striatal acetylcholine concentration) and of functional (apomorphine induced climbing) nature. All the neuroleptics tested in this study, irrespective of their ability to antagonize dopamine-sensitive adenylate cyclase, produced dose-dependent effects on all the measured parameters. Thus, phenothiazines and thioxanthenes, which are potent antagonists of dopamine-sensitive adenylate cyclase, produced effects qualitatively similar to those induced by butyrophenones which are weak inhibitors of this enzyme (Clement-Cormier et al., 1974) or substituted benzamides which lack completely this activity. Moreover, the correlation coefficients obtained by plotting the potencies (ED_{50}) of neuroleptics for one parameter against the others are highly significant while the slopes are close to unity (Table 1).

Table 1 - *Correlation coefficients and slopes obtained by plotting the potencies (ED_{50}) of neuroleptics to induce various biochemical and behavioral effects.*

Correl. Coeff. Slope	TH	HVA	Ach	AA
TH		0.989	0.863	0.929
HVA	1.01		0.869	0.932
Ach	0.96	0.99		0.939
AAC	0.93	0.92	1.04	

ED_{50} values were obtained graphically from dose-effect relationships for the following neuroleptics : haloperidol, spiperone, pimozide, (+) butaclamol, mezilamine, (α)-flupenthixol, clozapine, chlorpromazine, thioridazine, sulpiride, metoclopramide, flubepride and sultopride.
Abbreviations : TH = kinetic activation of striatal tyrosine hydroxylase ; HVA = increase in the striatal level of homovanillic acid ; Ach = decrease in the striatal level of acetylcholine ; AAC = antagonism of the apomorphine-induced climbing in mice. All the correlation coefficients are significant at 0.01 %.

These results indicate that the neuroleptic-induced alterations in the measured indices of impaired dopaminergic transmission are related to the blockade of dopamine receptors possessing very similar — if not identical — pharmacological properties. The qualitative similarities between the effects induced by those neuroleptics which antagonize dopamine sensitive adenylate cyclase, and those which do not, suggest that the blockade of this enzyme does not play an important role in the changes of dopaminergic transmission induced by these drugs.

Therefore, according to the above classification of dopamine receptor subtypes, changes in dopaminergic transmission induced by neuroleptics appear to be related to the D_2 receptor blockade. These pharmacological and biochemical results are supported by dopamine receptor binding studies. When using neuroleptic ligands which we preferentially label the D_2 receptor (^{3}H-spiperone, ^{3}H-haloperidol), the relative displacing potencies of neuroleptics, including benzamides, correlate with their potencies to induce pharmacological effects in experimental animals (Creese et al., 1976), and with the average daily doses used clinically to treat schizophrenics (Seeman, 1977). On the contrary, the potencies of neuroleptics to displace ligands which bind predominantly to the recognition site of the D_1 receptor (e.g. ^{3}H-flupenthixol) fail to show any correlation with pharmacological effects but correlate highly with their potencies to inhibit dopamine-induced stimulation of adenylate cyclase (Hyttel, 1978 ; Cross and Owen, 1980). For example, sulpiride, which does not antagonize dopamine-sensitive adenylate cyclase, is 200 times more potent in inhibiting ^{3}H-haloperidol binding than in displacing ^{3}H-flupenthixol, whereas piflutixol, which is a potent antagonist of adenylate cyclase, is 3 times more potent in displacing ^{3}H-flupenthixol than ^{3}H-haloperidol (Hyttel, 1978).

Interaction of benzamides and other neuroleptics with dopamine receptors in vivo

Although all these results support the idea that substituted benzamides are selective antagonists of the D_2 receptor, a property common to all neuroleptics, recent studies comparing binding characteristics of ^{3}H-spiperone and ^{3}H-sulpiride have revealed some essential differences between these two neuroleptics. Thus, in contrast to spiperone, sulpiride binding shows an absolute dependency on sodium ions (Jenner and Marsden, 1981). This *in vitro* finding is interpreted as an indication that sulpiride acts on a subpopulation of D_2 receptors.

Table 2 - *Effect of LY — 141865 and SKF-38393 on the tritium content in rat brain regions after intracarotid injection of ^{3}H-NPA.*

Treatment	Dose mg/kg, i.v.	^{3}H-NPA (dpm/mg tissue)		
		Striatum	Olfactory tubercle	Nucleus accumbens
Saline		213 ± 10	107 ± 7	72 ± 6
LY-141865	0.05	219 ± 5	94 ± 10	73 ± 8
	0.3	123 ± 12***	67 ± 8**	49 ± 6*
	1	67 ± 3***	37 ± 5***	34 ± 4***
	3	36 ± 1***	32 ± 2***	29 ± 2***
SKF-38393	10	255 ± 21	132 ± 9	85 ± 3

Rats received various doses of LY-141865 or SKF-38393 15 min before intracarotid pulse injection of ^{3}H-NPA (5 ng in 10 μl ; 1 μCi). Animals were sacrificed 20 min after the injection of the ligand. Each value is the mean with SEM obtained from 5 rats.
* $p < 0.05$; **$p < 0.01$; *** $p < 0.001$ as compared to saline treated rats.

In order to study the interaction of dopamine receptor agonists and antagonists *in vivo*, we recently developed a method which involves labelling brain receptors by a pulse injection of tritiated ligand into the internal carotid artery of the rat (D'Ambrosio et al., 1982). Using this method, it was possible to demonstrate

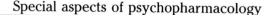

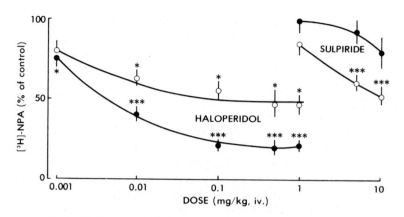

Fig. 1 - Displacement by haloperidol and sulpiride of ³H-NPA binding to striatum (●) and nucleus accumbens (o). Rats received intravenous injection of various doses of the neuroleptics 15 min before intracarotid pulse injection of ³H-NPA (5 ng in 10 µl ; 1 µCi). Rats were sacrificed 20 min after the ligand application. Each point with vertical bars represents the mean with SEM of five experimental values.
* p<0.05 ; *** p<0.001 versus saline injected controls (100 %).

binding of ³H-N-propylnorapomorphine (NPA) to dopamine receptor *in vivo*. In order to characterize the type of dopamine receptor to which NPA binds, we studied the effect of specific D_1 and D_2 agonists SKF-38393 and LY-141865, respectively (Table 2). Ten mg/kg of SKF-38393 given intravenously failed to affect tritium retention in striatum, olfactory tubercle and nucleus accumbens at 20 min after the intracarotid injection of ³H-NPA (5 ng ; 1 µCi). By contrast, LY-141-865 antagonized the binding of ³H-NPA to dopamine neuron innervated regions in a dose-dependent manner. Three mg/kg of this compound given intravenously decreased by more than 80 % the ³H-NPA binding in the striatum. These results indicate that under these experimental conditions ³H-NPA selectively labels D_2 receptors.

Binding of ³H-NPA *in vivo* is also antagonized by haloperidol and sulpiride (Fig. 1). Both neuroleptics produced a dose dependent decrease in the tritium content in the striatum and in the nucleus accumbens. Haloperidol was several hundred times more potent than sulpiride. However, these neuroleptics were not equally effective in displacing ³H-NPA binding in the two brain regions : Although haloperidol was more effective in striatum than in nucleus accumbens (maximal inhibition ~ 80 vs ~ 50 % respectively) its potency was the same in the two regions (ED_{50} = dose producing 50 % of the maximal effect = 0.005 mg/kg). In contrast, both efficacy and potency of sulpiride to displace ³H-NPA were greater in the nucleus accumbens than in the striatum : Thus, 10 mg/kg of the compound decreased the ³H-NPA binding by 50 and 20 % respectively. The ED_{50} was 1,7 mg/kg for nucleus accumbens and 6,4 mg/kg for striatum.

These results indicate that both haloperidol and sulpiride block D_2 dopamine receptors. Haloperidol, however, appears to be more effective in antagonizing ³H-NPA retention in the striatum as compared to nucleus accumbens, while the reverse is true for sulpiride. It is interesting to note that similar results were obtained when ^{3}H-spiperone was used to label dopamine receptors *in vivo* (Köhler et al., 1979). These findings are consistent with biochemical results which show that sulpiride preferentially increases tyrosine hydroxylase activity (Zivkovic et al., 1975) and dopamine metabolism (Bartholini, 1976 ; Scatton et al., 1979) in the limbic system whereas haloperidol acts predominantly in the striatum.

It is not yet understood why sulpiride preferentially affects the limbic system while haloperidol is more effective in striatum. Differential brain distribution of haloperidol does not seem to be involved, as this neuroleptic is equally distributed in the brain after its intravenous injection (Laduron et al., 1978). Although *in vitro* experiments failed to demonstrate that neuroleptics have different affinities for dopamine receptors in different brain regions, they did not exclude the possibility that this may be the case *in vivo*. In view of recent findings that some peptides, such as cholecystokinins, may influence neuroleptic binding to dopamine receptor (Fuxe et al., 1981) and the fact that these peptides are unequally distributed in dopamine neuron innervated regions (Hökfelt et al., 1980), it is possible that *in vivo* dopamine receptors in discrete regions do display different affinities for neuroleptics.

Nevertheless, these *in vivo* binding studies indicate that the regional biochemical effects of neuroleptics are related to a differential degree of dopamine receptor blockade in various dopamine neuron innervated regions. Moreover, these results may explain the differences between neuroleptics in their potency to induce catalepsy and to alleviate psychosis. Thus, based on the hypothesis that limbic dopamine receptor blockade is responsible for the antipsychotic action of neuroleptics whereas blockade of striatal dopamine receptors is responsible for extrapyramidal side effects, it could be presumed that neuroleptics which preferentially block limbic dopaminergic transmission exhibit antipsychotic action at doses which only moderately affect extrapyramidal function.

Concluding remarks

Our extensive studies comparing the biochemical effects of substituted benzamides and other neuroleptics to a variety of behavioral parameters indicative of the functional state of dopaminergic transmission failed to reveal any substantial difference between these classes of neuroleptics. The ability of classical neuroleptics to antagonize dopamine-sensitive adenylate cyclase does not appear essential for the pharmacological and clinical profile of these drugs.

The impairment of dopaminergic transmission induced by substituted benzamides as well as by other neuroleptics is related to the blockade of the dopamine receptor which is not coupled to adenylate cyclase. The functional consequences of inhibition of this enzyme by some neuroleptics are still unknown.

RÉFÉRENCES

Bartholini, G. *1976* - Differential effect of neuroleptic drugs on dopamine turnover in extrapyramidal and limbic system. *J. Pharm. Pharmacol., 28 :* 429-433.

Borenstein, P., Champion, C., Cujo, A., Gekiere, F., Oliverstein, C., Kranarz, P. *1969.* — Un psychotrope original : le sulpiride. *Sem. Hôp. Paris, 45 :* 1301-1314.

Clement-Cormier, Y.C., Kebabian, J.W., Petzold, G.L. Greengard, P. *1974* - Dopamine sensitive adenylate cyclase in mammalian brain : a possible site of action of antipsychotic drugs. *Proc. Nat. Acad. Sci. 71 :* 1113-1117.

Creese, I., Burt, D.R., Snyder, S.H. *1976* - Dopamine receptor binding predicts clinical and pharmacological potencies of antischizophrenic drugs. *Science, 192 :* 481-483.

Cross, A.J., Owen, F. *1980* - Characteristics of ^{3}H-cis-flupenthixol binding to calf brain membranes. *Eur. J. Pharmacol., 65 :* 341-347.

D'Ambrosio, A., Zivkovic, B. Bartholini, G. *1982 —* ^{3}H-haloperidol labels brain receptors after its injection into the internal carotid artery. *Brain Res., 238 :* 470-474.

Fuxe, K., Agnati, L.F., Benefenati, F., Cimmino, M., Algeri, S., Hökfelt, T., Mutt, V. *1981* - Modulation by cholecystokinins of ^{3}H-spiroperidol binding in rat striatum : evidence for increased affinity and reduction in the number of binding sites. *Acta Physiol. Scand., 113 :* 567-569.

Goldstein, M., Lew., J.Y., Nakamura, S., Battista, A.F., Liberman, A., Fuxe, K. *1978* - Dopamine-philic properties of ergot alkaloids. *Fed. Proc., 37 :* 2202-2206.

Hökfelt, T., Rehfeld, J.F., Skriboll, L., Ivemark, B., Goldstein, M., Markey, K. *1980.* Evidence for coexistence of dopamine and CCK in mesolimbic neurons. *Nature, 285 :* 476-477.

Hyttel, J. *1978 -* Effects of neuroleptics on ^{3}H-haloperidol and ^{3}H-cis(Z)-flupenthixol binding and on adenylate cyclase activity in vitro. *Life Sci., 23 :* 551-556.

Jenner, P., Marsden, C.D. *1981* - Substituted benzamide drugs as selective neuroleptic agents. *Neuropharmacology, 20 :* 1285-1293.

Kebabian, J.W., Calne, D.B. *1979* - Multiple receptors for dopamine. *Nature, 277 :* 93-96.

Kebabian, J.W., Calne, D.B., Kebabian, P.R. *1977* - Lergotrile mesylate : An in vivo dopamine agonist which blocks dopamine receptors in vitro. *Com. Psychopharmacol., 1 :* 311-318.

Köhler, C., Ögren, S.-O., Haglund, L., Ängeby, T. *1979 -* Regional displacement by sulpiride of ^{3}H-spiperone binding in vivo. Biochemical and behavioural evidence for a preferential action on limbic and nigral dopamine receptors. *Neurosci. Lett., 13 :* 51-56.

Laduron, P.M., Janssen, P.F.M., Leysen, J.E. *1978* - Spiperone : a ligand of choice for neuroleptic receptors. 2 : Regional distribution and in vivo displacement of neuroleptic drugs. *Biochem. Pharmacol., 27,* 317-321.

Scatton, B., Bischoff, S., Dedek, J., Korf, J. *1977* - Regional effects of neuroleptics on dopamine metabolism and dopamine-sensitive adenylate cyclase activity. *Eur. J. Pharmacol., 44 :* 287-292.

Scatton, B., Worms, P., Zivkovic, B., Depoortere, H., Dedek, J., Bartholini, G. *1979* - On the neuropharmacological spectra of « classical » (haloperidol) and « atypical » (benzamide derivatives) neuroleptics. *In : Sulpiride and other Benzamides,* P.F. Spano, M. Trabucchi, G.U. Corsini and G.L. Gessa (eds) pp. 53-66. New York, Raven Press.

Schmidt, M.J., Hill, L.E. *1977* - Effects of ergots on adenylate cyclase activity in the corpus striatum. *Life Sci., 20 :* 789-798.

Seeman, P. *1977* - Anti-schizophrenic drugs - Membrane receptor sites of action. *Biochem. Pharmacol., 26 :* 1741-1748.

Spano, P.F., Stefanini, E., Trabucchi, M., Fresia, P. *1979* - Stereospecific interaction of sulpiride with striatal and neostriatal dopamine receptors. *In : Sulpiride and other Benzamides.* P.F. Spano, M. Trabucchi, G.U. Corsini and G.L. Gessa (eds), pp. 11-31. New York, Raven Press.

Trabucchi, M., Longoni, R., Fresia, P., Spano, P.F. *1975* - Sulpiride : A study of the effects on dopamine receptors in rat neostriatum and limbic forebrain. *Life Sci., 17 :* 1551-1556.

Zivkovic, B., Guidotti, A., Revuelta, A., Costa, E. *1975* - Effect of thioridazine, clozapine and other antipsychotics on the kinetic state of tyrosine hydroxylase and on the turnover rate of dopamine in striatum and nucleus accumbens. *J. Pharmacol. Exp. Ther., 194 :* 37-47.

Zivkovic, B., Scatton, B., Dedek, J., Worms, P., Lloyd, K.G., Bartholini, G. *1980* - Involvement of different types of dopamine receptors in the neuroleptic action. *12th CINP Congress,* Abstr. 729, Göteborg.

Zivkovic, B., Worms, P., Scatton, B., Dedek, J., Oblin, A., Lloyd, K.G., Bartholini, G. *1983* - Functional similarities between benzamides and other neuroleptics. *In : Advances in Biochemical Psychopharmacology.* E. Costa and G. Biggio (eds), New York, Raven Press (in press).

DISCUSSION

R. Naylor
That was an immensely interesting talk and you should be congratulated on a very nice technique. I wonder about the SKF results ; SKF does induce some behavioral changes, albeit not in the model that you described. For example, in the turning model, I wonder what receptor system we should describe as the action of SKF, too. Or in other words, what dopamine receptor does SKF stimulate to cause the behavioral changes that it causes, for example circling ?

G. Bartholini
In our experience, SKF 38393 in doses up to 10 to 30 mg/kg does not cause either behavioral effects, nor biochemical changes in terms of NPA displacement or Ach release, nor does it modify the levels of HVA. Therefore, we think that the D_1 site does not correspond to a functional DA receptor subtype. If behavioral effects (i.e. rotation after nigral 6-OHDA) are observed with high doses of the SKF compound, they could be attributed to stimulation of D_2 sites, but there is no evidence of that as yet.

N. Matussek
Dr. Bartholini, do you think that for the prolactin release of neuroleptics D_2 receptors are more important than D_1 receptors ?

G. Bartholini
Yes, but I am not able to answer the question.

K. Fuxe
Certainly SKF 38393 does not reduce prolactin secretion for instance. There is little doubt that the DA receptor controlling prolactin secretion is very much of the D_2 type.

G. Sedvall
In the chronic experiments with sulpiride that you described where the HVA elevation was actually reversed, what kind of effects do you find on the acetylcholine release during these conditions ? I was wondering, as the dose you used there was very high at 100 mg/kg of sulpiride, do you have the same problems with lower doses of sulpiride ? I ask this question, because we do not find in this time-course this type of tolerance to the HVA in patients.

G. Bartholini
As far as the first part of the question is concerned, we observe tolerance to sulpiride of the acetyl-choline release as it occurs after "classical" neuroleptics. As for the tolerance to sulpiride of the HVA increase, one has indeed to administer very high doses (e.g. 100 mg/kg i.p.) ; lower, systemic doses virtually do not affect the striatum.

M. Goldstein
I would like to ask about the potency of LY on the post-synaptic receptors as measured by the inhibition of the release of acetylcholine. How does it compare with other dopamine agonists ?

G. Bartholini
I think LY-141865 is a powerful agent, as it induces a strong inhibition of the « in-vitro » Ach release with IC_{50} of the maximal effect of 0,14 μM. This is comparable to the potency of apomorphine.

K. Fuxe
The data which we reported in Stockholm with SKF-38393 showed a rather poor penetration of

SKF-38393 into the brain. However, when we injected SKF-38393 intraventricularly ranging from 100 μg up to 500 μg and analysed the various dopamine nerve terminals, we got indications of a rather widespread reduction in dopamine turnover. So, our interpretation was that there must be a D_1—like dopamine receptor, which can regulate the dopamine turnover in most forebrain dopamine nerve terminal systems, in addition to the D_2 type of dopamine receptor. Maybe there are both D_1 and D_2 types of dopamine receptor regulating turnover of dopamine.

G. Bartholini

This relates to the question of Dr. Naylor. In principle, I agree with you that one cannot exclude that high doses of the SKF compound have some effect on the D_2 subtype. However, in the in-vitro experiments where one can operate with high concentrations, no effect whatsoever is observed on post-synaptic cholinergic cells which are known to possess D_2 type sites ; and this up to 100 μM SKF.

K. Fuxe

What do you suggest ; that it may well be that these D_1 or D_2 receptors are regulating different types of post-synaptic responses in view of the results obtained in our model on acetylcholine release and that both of them regulate dopamine turnovers in a similar way ?

G. Bartholini

I agree, obviously we cannot exclude that there are other effects induced by SKF 38393, which we do not measure ; however, for the « classical » and known in-vivo parameters, such as the decrease in HVA and the displacement of NPA, as well as the inhibition of Ach release *in-vitro,* there is no effect of SKF.

K. Fuxe

We also observed this lack of action *in-vivo* in our studies on ^{3}H-NPA binding *in-vivo* following systemic treatment. Maybe this is related to the poor penetration of SKF-38393 into the brain ? At least, that is our feeling.

G. Bartholini

This possibility might apply to the blockade of tyrosine hydroxylase activity or the changes in HVA, although we gave doses of SKF as high as 30 mg/kg i.p. ; however, this possibility does not hold true for the *in-vitro* experiments when we used concentrations up to 100 μM without effect.

K. Fuxe

Yes, I think that is a very good observation and I tend to feel that we have here an important differentiation between D_1 and D_2 agonists.

R. Naylor

The problems of brain penetration do not arise when we consider the very nice experiment, where Dr. Bartholini showed that sulpiride causes a selective displacement of tritiated NPA from limbic brain areas as distinct from the striatal areas. I think he showed about a ten-fold difference in the ability of sulpiride to displace tritiated NPA from accumbens as distinct from striatum. Have you attempted the same experiment by using a compound like metoclopramide ?

G. Bartholini

No, we did not try this with metoclopramide, but you surely know metoclopramide behaves like a classical neuroleptic as far as its behavioral and biochemical effects are concerned : It induces catalepsy, it antagonizes apomorphine or other dopamine agonists and it causes an increase in dopamine metabolism which is greater in extrapyramidal than in limbic regions similar to SL-74 205 the other orthomethoxy-benzamide I have shown ; this is exactly the pattern of, for instance, haloperidol, apart from its blockade of adenylate cyclase.

K. Fuxe

I would like to answer your comment, Dr. Naylor. There is no disagreement whatsoever about the possibilities that dl-sulpiride preferentially displaces *in-vivo* binding in the limbic area. This is well in line with our data and Dr. Bartholini's data.

Effect of atypical neuroleptic drugs on central and peripheral noradrenergic mechanisms in rats

Gerhard Groß

Institute of Pharmacology of the University of Essen, Federal Republic of Germany

Summary: The effects of some neuroleptic drugs (sulpiride, clozapine, thioridazine, haloperidol, levomepromazine) on cerebral and cardiac noradrenergic mechanisms have been investigated. All compounds tested enhanced ^{3}H-noradrenaline efflux from electrically stimulated cortical brain slices and antagonized the clonidine induced inhibition of tachycardia during electrical stimulation of sympathetic heart nerves in pithed rats. These actions seem to be partly due to a blockade of pre-synaptic α-autoreceptors. Long-term treatment with clozapine and thioridazine decreased cortical as well as cardiac β-adrenoceptors. Sulpiride, had no influence on β-adrenoceptor density. The relevance of these results, with respect to changes in noradrenergic neurotransmission induced by neuroleptics is discussed.

Most antipsychotic drugs, especially atypical and low potency neuroleptics, display a broad spectrum of pharmacological actions. Their antipsychotic effect in man has been related to dopamine receptor antagonism or inhibition of dopamine stimulated adenylate cyclase in the striatum and in limbic areas of the brain (Carlsson and Lindqvist, 1963 ; Andén et al., 1970 ; Miller et al., 1974). Several neuroleptic drugs, however, interfere also with central nervous and peripheral noradrenergic mechanisms. An inhibition of the noradrenaline sensitive cAMP generating system in the limbic forebrain seems to contribute to behavioral effects of some neuroleptic drugs (Blumberg et al., 1976). A blockade of the α-adrenoceptors may cause sedation (Peroutka et al., 1977 ; Snyder et al., 1978) as well as unwanted side effects mediated by the peripheral autonomic nervous system (Göthert et al., 1977). Neuroleptics have been reported to enhance noradrenaline turnover in the brain (Andén et al., 1970 ; Bartholini et al., 1973 ; Bürki et al., 1975 ; Nybäck and Sedvall, 1970) and to increase noradrenaline plasma levels in man (Ackenheil, 1980). Although the mechanism of this turnover acceleration is not completely understood, a blockade of pre-synaptic α-adrenoceptors may be involved. Arbilla et al. (1978) found an increase in potassium stimulated ^{3}H-noradrenaline release from brain tissue in the presence of chlorpromazine or clozapine. This enhancement of transmitter release may in turn result in an increased noradrenaline synthesis. An increased concentration of noradrenaline can cause a down regulation of post-synaptic adrenergic receptors. In contrast to several high potency antipsychotics some low potency and atypical neuroleptic drugs possess antidepressant properties. According to Sulser et al. (1978) an antidepressant action may be linked to a reduction of cerebral β-adrenoceptors. The present study was performed to further analyse the mechanisms by which atypical

91

neuroleptic drugs alter the noradrenaline release from central and peripheral neurons and to find out whether β-adrenoceptor changes occur during long term treatment. The effects of clozapine, thioridazine, and sulpiride on noradrenergic neurotransmission were investigated using (1) electrically stimulated rat brain slices preloaded with ^{3}H-noradrenaline, (2) cardiovascular responses in pithed rats, and (3) a β-adrenoceptor binding assay. In some experiments classical neuroleptic or antidepressant drugs were included for comparison.

Effect of neuroleptic drugs on release and uptake of ^{3}H-noradrenaline in rat brain slices

Slices from the parietooccipital cortex were preincubated with 10^{-7}M (-) ^{3}H-noradrenaline, subsequently superfused with physiological buffer solution and stimulated twice for 2 min by electrical pulses of 2 msec at 3 Hz, 12 mA, beginning at the 45th and 85th min of superfusion. The stimulation induced transmitter overflow was calculated as percent of the ^{3}H content of the slices at the beginning of the stimulation period and called S_1 or S_2, respectively. In control experiments the ratio S_2/S_1 amounted to 0.94 ± 0.02 (n = 40). The drugs were added 20 min before S_2.

The noradrenaline uptake by brain slices was estimated by determining their ^{3}H content after preincubation with 10^{-7}M (-) ^{3}H-noradrenaline for 10 min. The drugs were added 30 min before ^{3}H-noradrenaline.

All the neuroleptic drugs tested enhanced the electrically stimulated ^{3}H-noradrenaline release (Fig. 1 A). Already at 1 μM, sulpiride significantly increased the ^{3}H-efflux by 18 %, thioridazine, levomepromazine, haloperidol by 23 — 30 % and clozapine by 66 %. At higher concentrations, sulpiride again showed the weakest action ; clozapine proved to be the most potent drug. The basal ^{3}H-efflux was enhanced by all neuroleptics at 100 μM indicating an unspecific toxic action. In ^{3}H-noradrenaline uptake experiments (Fig. 1B) clozapine was almost as active as the reference compound cocaine. In contrast, sulpiride was completely ineffective.

Figure 1 clearly shows the differences between the abilities of neuroleptics to increase ^{3}H-noradrenaline release on the one hand, and to inhibit neuronal transmitter uptake on the other hand. The increase in ^{3}H-efflux from electrically stimulated brain slices due to 1 μM clozapine (+ 66 %) was attenuated, but remained significant (+ 33 %), when noradrenaline uptake was blocked by a high concentration of cocaine (Fig. 2).

Clonidine reduced the ^{3}H-noradrenaline efflux from electrically stimulated brain slices by activation of pre-synaptic α_2-adrenoceptors. Clozapine and levomepromazine, present throughout the superfusion, clearly antagonized this effect of clonidine (Table 1). Although other possibilities cannot be completely ruled out, a blockade of pre-synaptic α_2-adrenoceptors by neuroleptic drugs seems to contribute to the enhancement of noradrenaline release during electrical stimulation.

Effect of neuroleptic drugs on noradrenergic mechanisms in pithed rats

The pithed rat is an appropriate model to test pre- and post-synaptic adrenoceptor mediated responses of the cardiovascular system *in vivo*. Spinal as well as supraspinal reflexes are eliminated. Both vagus nerves were cut, and the

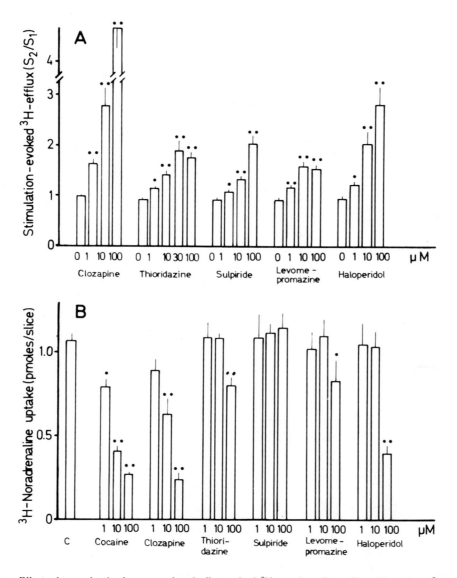

Fig. 1 — Effect of neuroleptic drugs on electrically evoked ^{3}H-noradrenaline efflux (A) and on ^{3}H-noradrenaline uptake (B) of cortical brain slices of the rat.

A. After preincubation with 10^{-7}M (-) ^{3}H-noradrenaline the slices were stimulated twice for 2 min (3Hz, 1 msec, 12 mA) after 45 (S_1) and 85 min (S_2) of superfusion. Drugs were added 20 min before S_2.

B. Uptake of (—) ^{3}H-noradrenaline was estimated as ^{3}H retained in cortical brain slices at 37 °C after 10 min of incubation with ^{3}H-noradrenaline. Drugs were added 30 min before ^{3}H-noradrenaline.

Given are means ± SEM

n ⩾ 6 (A) ; n ⩾ 5 (B)

∗p < 0.05, ∗∗p < 0.005 compared with controls (Student's t-test). For further details see Gross and Schümann (1980)

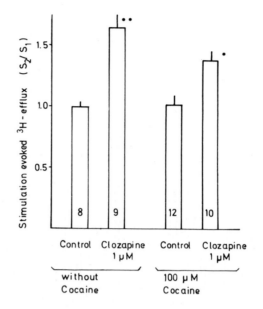

Fig. 2 — Effect of clozapine on electrically evoked
^{3}H efflux from rat brain slices preincubated with
^{3}H-noradrenaline.
Clozapine was added 20 min before S$_2$; cocaine was
present throughout the superfusion. For details see
legend to Fig. 1
*p < 0.05, **p < 0.0005

Table 1. - *Effect of clozapine and levomepromazine on the clonidine*
induced inhibition of ^{3}H efflux from brain slices during electrical stimulation

Drugs added	Stimulated ^{3}H-efflux (S$_2$/S$_1$)	n
Control	0.92 ± 0.05	9
Clonidine (10nM)	0.63 ± 0.04	22
Clonidine (10nM) + clozapine (1μM)	0.93 ± 0.03*	10
Clonidine (10nM) + levomepromazine (10μM)	0.87 ± 0.07*	10
Clonidine (100nM)	0.38 ± 0.03	15
Clonidine (100nM) + clozapine (1μM)	0.67 ± 0.08*	10
Clonidine (100nM) + levomepromazine (10μM)	0.70 ± 0.10*	8

The slices were preincubated with 10^{-7}M ^{3}H-noradrenaline and stimulated twice after 45 (S$_1$) and 85 min (S$_2$) of
superfusion. Clonidine (10 or 100 μM) was added 20 min before S$_2$. In the experiments with clozapine and
levomepromazine, these drugs were present throughout the superfusion.
p<0.005 compared with the respective clonidine experiments without neuroleptic drug.

muscarinic acetylcholine receptors were blocked by atropine. The electrical stimulation of the C7-T1 preganglionic sympathetic nerves increased the heart rate by 124 ± 8 beats/min (n = 7). Clonidine reduced this tachycardia due to its pre-synaptic α_2-adrenergic action. The pre-synaptic effects of atypical neuroleptics on sympathetic heart nerves were assessed as inhibition of the clonidine induced decrease in heart rate. Clozapine, thioridazine, and sulpiride clearly antagonized this bradycardia (Table 2). Typical neuroleptics (levomepromazine and haloperidol)

Table 2 - *Pithed rat : Effect of neuroleptic drugs on the clonidine induced inhibition of tachycardia during electrical stimulation of sympathetic heart nerves*

| Drug | | n | Decrease in heart rate (Δ beats/min) Clonidine (nM/kg) | | | |
			1	*3*	*10*	*30*
Control		8	11 ± 2	24 ± 3	44 ± 3	73 ± 7
Clozapine	1 μM/kg	6	0*	10 ± 3*	38 ± 3	67 ± 5
	10 μM/kg	6	0*	0*	23 ± 4*	54 ± 6*
Thioridazine	10 μM/kg	6	0*	16 ± 4	35 ± 4	69 ± 9
	30 μM/kg	6	0*	2 ± 1*	28 ± 4*	56 ± 8
Sulpiride	1 μM/kg	6	0*	13 ± 3*	37 ± 5	58 ± 5
	10 μM/kg	6	0*	2 ± 1*	21 ± 4*	51 ± 7*

The preganglionic heart nerves at C7-T^1 were stimulated (0.5 Hz, 1 msec, 28 V).
The drugs were injected 20 min before clonidine.
Means $\pm$ SEM of n animals. *$p < 0.05$ compared with controls.

were active in the same dose range (data not shown). Clozapine and sulpiride further enhanced the increase in heart rate due to single electrical pulses in the presence of cocaine (Fig. 3). The tachycardia induced by administration of ex-

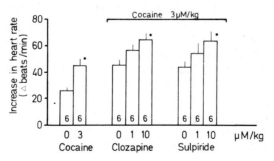

Fig. 3 — Pithed rat : effect of cocaine, clozapine, and sulpiride on the increase in heart rate due to electrical stimulation with single pulses.
Stimulation parameters : 1 msec, 28V
*p < 0.05, compared with the respective control.

ogenous noradrenaline could be increased by inhibition of the neuronal noradrenaline uptake with cocaine. Atypical neuroleptics, however, had no effect in these experiments (Table 3). Thus, an antagonism at the pre-synaptic α_2-adrenoceptor level seems likely. The post-synaptic vascular α-adrenoceptors, which mediate the increase in diastolic blood pressure due to noradrenaline (in the presence of bupranolol at 30 μM/kg) were blocked to a considerable extent by clozapine, thioridazine, and levomepromazine (1 — 10 μM/kg) but not by sulpiride and haloperidol (data not shown).

Table 3. - *Pithed rat : Effect of cocaine and neuroleptic drugs*
on the noradrenaline induced increase in heart rate in pithed rats

Drug			Increase in heart rate (Δ beats/min) Noradrenaline (nM/kg)			
		n	*0.3*	*1*	*3*	*10*
Control		4	16 ± 4	43 ± 5	60 ± 2	85 ± 4
Cocaine	1μM/kg	4	$26 \pm 3*$	51 ± 3	$70 \pm 2*$	85 ± 1
	10 μM/kg	4	$49 \pm 2*$	$64 \pm 1*$	$80 \pm 4*$	84 ± 5
Control		4	6 ± 1	43 ± 5	78 ± 5	114 ± 4
Clozapine	10μM/kg	4	10 ± 1	39 ± 5	78 ± 4	106 ± 5
Control		4	8 ± 3	41 ± 7	59 ± 5	83 ± 3
Thoridazine	10μM/kg	4	10 ± 3	38 ± 5	59 ± 7	84 ± 4
Control		4	31 ± 6	54 ± 11	70 ± 10	103 ± 6
Sulpiride	10μM/kg	4	25 ± 4	45 ± 8	70 ± 7	99 ± 3

The drugs were injected 20 min before noradrenaline.
Means $\pm$ SEM of n animals ; *p$<$0.05 compared with respective controls.

Effect of chronic treatment with atypical neuroleptic drugs on β-adrenoceptors in the cerebral cortex and myocardium of rats

Drugs, which increase the noradrenaline release or turnover by neuronal uptake inhibition or by pre-synaptic α-adrenoceptor antagonism, induce a down regulation of post-synaptic cerebral β-adrenoceptors (Wiech and Ursillo, 1980). If long term treatment with atypical neuroleptic drugs also caused a sustained increase in noradrenaline concentration at the post-synaptic site, a down regulation of β-adrenoceptors should be expected. Rats were injected i.p. twice daily with clozapine, thioridazine, and sulpiride for 18 days ; the antidepressant drugs desipramine and trazodone were tested as reference compounds. The doses of desipramine, trazodone, and thioridazine were equimolar (60 μM/kg/day). The dose chosen for clozapine was lower (30 μM/kg/day), since at higher doses the animals lost weight ; sulpiride, which was well tolerated, was given at a higher dose (120 μM/kg/day). The density and affinity of β-adrenoceptors was determined in a crude membrane fraction of the rat cerebral cortex and heart using the ^{3}H-dihydroalprenolol binding assay as described by Bylund and Snyder (1976) with minor modifications. The Scatchard analysis of specific ^{3}H-dihydroalprenolol binding revealed a single binding site and was used to estimate the maximal number of binding sites (B_{max}) and the equilibrium dissociation constant (K_D). As expected, chronic desipramine treatment resulted in a 52 % loss of ^{3}H-dihydroalprenolol binding sites in the cortex. The affinity was slightly increased. After chronic administration of clozapine and thioridazine, B_{max}-values were reduced by 24 and 21 %, respectively in the cortex, and by 28 and 24 % in the myocardium. Like trazodone, sulpiride failed to alter the β-adrenoceptor density in both tissues (Table 4).

Table 4. - *Density and affinity of ³H-dihydroalprenolol binding sites in the cortex and heart of rats after long term treatment with antidepressant and neuroleptic drugs*

Treatment (18 days)	Dose (mg/kg/day)	Cortex			Heart		
		n	B_{max} fmol/mg	K_D nM	n	B_{max} fmol/mg	K_D nM
Control	—	10	6.89 ± 0.35	1.6	7	2.26 ± 0.12	1.0
Desipramine	18	10	3.30 ± 0.26**	1.1*	8	2.03 ± 0.11	1.3
Trazodone	24	11	6.52 ± 0.51	1.6	8	2.07 ± 0.07	1.1
Clozapine	10	11	5.25 ± 0.27**	1.5	8	1.63 ± 0.10**	1.1
Thioridazine	24	10	5.46 ± 0.40*	1.5	8	1.71 ± 0.11*	1.0
Sulpiride	40	10	6.51 ± 0.50	1.6	8	1.96 ± 0.09	1.0

The membranes were incubated at 25°C for 30 min with 8 - 9 concentrations of ³H-dihydroalprenolol ranging from 0.1 - 5 nM. The maximal number of binding sites (B_{max}) and the equilibrium dissociation constants were determined by Scatchard analysis. Means ± SEM of n experiments. *$p < 0.025$, **$p < 0.005$ compared with controls.

Conclusions

All the neuroleptic drugs tested enhanced the electrically stimulated ³H-noradrenaline efflux from cortical brain slices. This effect could already be demonstrated at concentrations which failed to inhibit ³H-noradrenaline uptake by brain slices.

Clozapine increased the stimulated transmitter efflux when the noradrenaline uptake was already blocked by cocaine.

Clozapine and levomepromazine antagonized the pre-synaptic α-adrenergic effect of clonidine in brain slices.

In pithed rats all neuroleptics inhibited the clonidine induced decrease in heart rate during electrical stimulation. This effect also cannot be explained by an inhibition of neuronal noradrenaline uptake.

The α-adrenoceptor mediated pressor response was clearly blocked by clozapine, thioridazine, and levomepromazine, but not by sulpiride or haloperidol.

The data presented above demonstrate that clozapine exerted the most distinct influence on noradrenergic neurotransmission, whereas sulpiride displayed the weakest action. This is in agreement with the clinical experience that clozapine and thioridazine produce more pronounced autonomic side effects, such as tachycardia and orthostatic hypotension, than sulpiride.

In the case of clozapine, the increased noradrenaline release could be attributed to an antagonism at the pre-synaptic α-adrenergic autoreceptor level and to an inhibition of neuronal uptake. In the case of thioridazine and sulpiride the blockade of pre-synaptic α-adrenoceptors provides the most likely explanation.

There seem to be no fundamental differences between the effects of typical and atypical neuroleptic drugs with regard to their effect on noradrenergic neurotransmission. The doses and plasma levels of atypical neuroleptics, however, are usually higher than those of high potency phenothiazines or butyrophenones.

Chronic treatment with clozapine and thioridazine reduced the β-adrenoceptor density in the cerebral cortex as well as in the myocardium, probably as a consequence of an increased noradrenaline release. The down regulation of β-adrenoceptors, which has been related to an antidepressant action of drugs (Sulser et al., 1978), was reported to depend on intact pre-synaptic noradrenergic nerve terminals (Schweitzer et al., 1979). Sulpiride and trazodone, however, failed to decrease the cortical β-adrenoceptor density in our experiments. Their antidepressant properties must be explained by other mechanisms.

Acknowledgements
The skilful technical assistance of Miss U. Jansen, Miss M. Hagedorn and Mr. E. Hagelskamp is gratefully acknowledged.

REFERENCES

Ackenheil, M. *1980* — Biochemical effects (in men) *In : Psychotropic Agents, Part I Handbook of Exp. Pharmacol pp. 213-223*. Hoffmeister F., Stille G. (eds). Heidelberg, Springer Verlag.

Andén, N.E. Butcher, S.G., Corrodi H., Fuxe K., Ungerstedt U. *1970* — Receptor activity and turnover of dopamine and noradrenaline after neuroleptics. *Eur. J. Pharmacol., 11* : 303-314.

Arbilla, S., Briley, M.S., Dubocovich, M.L., Langer, S.Z. *1978* — Neuroleptic binding and their effects on the spontaneous and potassium-evoked release of ^{3}H-dopamine from the striatum and of ^{3}H-noradrenaline from the cerebral cortex. *Life Sci, 23* : 1775-1780.

Bartholini, G., Keller, H.H., Pletscher, A. *1973* — Effect of neuroleptics on endogenous norepinephrine in rat brain. *Neuropharmacol., 12* : 751-756.

Blumberg, J.B., Vetulani, J., Stawarz, R.J., Sulser, F. *1976* — The noradrenergic cyclic AMP generating system in the limbic forebrain : pharmacological characterization in vitro and possible role of limbic noradrenergic mechanism in the mode of action of antipsychotics. *Eur. J. Pharmacol., 37* : 357-366.

Bürki, H.R., Ruck, W., Asper, H. *1975* — Effect of clozapine, thioridazine, perlapine and haloperidol on the metabolism of biogenic amines in the brain of the rat. *Psychopharmacol., 41* : 27-33.

Bylund, D.B., Snyder, S.H. *1976* — Beta-adrenergic receptor binding in membrane preparations from mammalian brain. *Mol. Pharmacol., 12* : 568-580.

Carlsson, A., Lindqvist, M. *1963* — Effect of chlorpromazine or haloperidol on formation of 3-methoxytyramine and normetanephrine in mouse brain. *Acta pharmacol., 20* : 140-144.

Göthert, M., Lox, H.-J., Rieckesmann, J.-M. *1977* — Effects of butyrophenones on sympathetic nerves of the isolated rabbit heart and on the postsynaptic α-adrenoceptors of the isolated rabbit aorta. *Naunyn-Schmiedeberg's Arch. Pharmacol., 300* : 255-265.

Groß G., Schümann, H.J. *1980* — Enhancement of noradrenaline release from rat cerebral cortex by neuroleptic drugs. *Naunyn-Schmiedeberg's Arch. Pharmacol., 315* : 103-109.

Miller, R.J., Horn, A.S., Iversen, L.L. *1974* — The action of neuroleptic drugs on dopamine-stimulated adenosine cyclic 3', 5'-mono-phosphate production in rat neostriatum and limbic forebrain. *Mol. Pharmacol., 10* : 759-766.

Nybäck, H., Sedvall, G. *1970* — Further studies on the accumulation and disappearence of catecholamines formed from tyrosine-^{14}C in mouse brain. Effect of some phenothiazine analogues. *Eur. J. Pharmacol., 10* : 197-205.

Peroutka, S.J., U'Prichard, D.C., Greenberg, D.A., Snyder, S.H. *1977* — Neuroleptic drug interactions with norepinephrine alpha-receptor binding sites in rat brain. *Neuropharmacol., 16* : 549-556.

Schweitzer, J.W., Schwartz, R., Friedhoff, A.J. *1979* — Intact presynaptic terminals required for beta-adrenergic receptor regulation by desipramine. *J. Neurochem., 33* : 377-379.

Snyder, S.H., U'Prichard, D.C., Greenberg, D.A. *1978* — Neurotransmitter receptor binding in the brain. *In : Psychopharmacology : A generation of progress pp. 361-370*. Lipton M.A., DiMascio A., Killam K.F. (eds). New York, Raven Press.

Sulser, F., Vetulani, F., Mobley, P. *1978* — Mode of action of antidepressant drugs. *Neuropharmacol., 27* : 257-261.

Wiech, N.L., Ursillo, R.C. *1980* — Acceleration of desipramine-induced decrease of rat corticocerebral β-adrenergic receptors by yohimbine. *Comm. Psychopharmacol., 4* : 95-100.

DISCUSSION

M. Ackenheil
I would like to ask you if you measured the noradrenaline efflux after DMI ? How would you explain that most neuroleptics enhance the noradrenaline efflux ? After long-term treatment a difference can be seen between sulpiride, clozapine and thioridazine due to adaptation. Why is there no down-regulation of ß-receptors after sulpride, because enhancement of noradrenaline release can result in such an effect ?

G. Groß
To the last question, I think the effect of sulpiride is a very weak one. You have seen that in brain slices it only enhances the ^{3}H-noradrenaline overflow by 18 % at the lowest concentration. It may be that this is enough to enhance the neurotransmission, but it is certainly not enough to decrease the number of ß-adrenoreceptors. To the first question about DMI.

S.Z. Langer
In your experiment, did you use the racemic or the S-isomere of sulpride ?

G. Groß
Racemic only, as I do not have the isomeres.

S.Z. Langer
And would you conclude from your data that sulpiride is enhancing a noradrenergic neurotrans-mission through the blockade of pre-synaptic alpha-2-adrenorecepters like clozapine, or would you think that another mechanism might be involved ?

G. Groß
I am relatively sure in the case of clozapine and thioridazine, but not in the case of sulpiride, therefore, I have reported these results with caution. But the enhancement of ^{3}H-noradrenaline overflow is not explained by ^{3}H-uptake inhibition, on the other hand, in pithed rats it antagonizes the clonidine action. So, I cannot exclude an α-blocking effect and I think LeFur and co-workers have shown a relatively high affinity of sulpiride to clonidine binding sites.

S.Z. Langer
Did you try the combination of chronic sulpiride and chronic DMI on ß-adrenoreceptor binding ? It is known that when you combine an alpha-2-adrenoreceptor antagonist with an inhibitor of noradren-aline uptake you accelerate or potentiate down-regulation of ß-1-adrenoreceptors in the brain. If that is the case, if you were to combine sulpiride with DMI and perhaps look even at shorter time inter-vals than the one you have employed you may have a clear answer. Did you try that ?

G. Groß
I know these experiments with yohimbine and DMI, but I think if there is an effect of sulpiride it would be so small in comparison with DMI, that it would be difficult to interpret such experiments.

S.Z. Langer
I think in that case you should use a lower dose of DMI which may facilitate the interpretation of the data. Perhaps a dose that by itself does not down-regulate. Then the addition of sulpiride to that treatment in a dose that is inactive on its own could be helpful.

W.H. Fennell
In the cardiac accelerator nerve preparation in dogs, where they have also undergone spinal section, we have given S-sulpiride and found that there is no increase in coronary sinus noradrenaline sec-

retion above control with stimulation. However, for phentolamine there was a marked increase. I wonder if your effects may be due to ganglion stimulation due to R-sulpiride which is included in sulpiride.

G. Groß
Which receptor in the ganglions?

W.H. Fennell
I do not know exactly.

N. Matussek
I will come back to Dr. Langer's question regarding the combination of an alpha-2-receptor antagonist with an inhibitor of noradrenaline uptake in my presentation tomorrow. But I would like to ask you, Dr. Groß, since you think that clozapine in some aspect has a profile like an antidepressant and that in its structure it is also more similar to antidepressant than to neuroleptic drugs : Is it known that it has antidepressant properties in patients as well ? Actually, fluponex, the successor of clozapine, has a most striking effect on the affect in chronic schizophrenic patients. Has the antidepressant effect of clozapine and of its successor been clinically investigated ?

G. Groß
As far as I know, there are no clinical studies concerning the antidepressant effect of clozapine, but I think that the hypothesis of Sulser, that the down-regulation of ß-adrenoreceptors is linked with an antidepressant action, is not very valid.

N. Matussek
Have you investigated mianserine ? Mianserine should also be a pre-synaptic adrenoreceptor blocking agent.

G. Groß
This has been done by Baumann and Maître and in pithed rats by Doxey and others and it has a pre-synaptic alpha-adrenoreceptor blocking property.

M. Ackenheil
With reference to Prof. Matussek's question, it was described that clozapine has some antidepressant effects, but that these depend on the dosage. In this context, I would like to ask Dr. Groß, if there is a shift between the blockade of pre-synaptic receptors to the post-synaptic receptor site ? All results with these increased noradrenaline levels were found in acute experiments, however, increased noradrenaline levels in humans can be seen under rest conditions only after chronic treatment with neuroleptics of 5 to 10 years. There are differences between the different neuroleptics, for instance, already at the beginning of treatment clozapine increases noradrenaline levels, whereas at this point in time the other neuroleptics do not increase noradrenaline levels. I have the impression that first a pre-synaptic blockade of neuroleptics occurs and later on after chronic treatment probably more a blockade of the post-synaptic noradrenaline receptors. Also, from the clinical point of view there is a difference with regard to behavioral effects. The mentioned results are probably an explanation that in the beginning neuroleptics have other clinical effects than after longer treatment. In this context, one should bear in mind that schizoprenia as a whole cannot be considered as an unique illness. Dr. Lecrubier will perhaps discuss in his presentation that one should consider the minus and the plus symptomatics, and that neuroleptics act generally in the usual dosage more on the plus symptomatics.

G. Groß
We have not done acute experiments, but I think it is not so easy to compare clinical experiments with those done *in-vitro* or acutely *in-vivo*, since in patients pharmacokinetic aspects have to be considered which may explain such actions.

G. Bartholini
I just want to recall the well-known fact, which was established about 15 or 20 years ago, that

neuroleptics in low doses have some antidepressant activity ; this is not a property which is peculiar to clozapine or orthomethoxy-benzamides, but refers to all neuroleptics tested. This action may be related to what Prof. Ackenheil has recalled, namely, a pre-synaptic action of these agents.

N. Matussek
Dr. Bartholini, can you really show me one controlled study in endogenously depressive patients dealing with antidepressant properties of neuroleptic drugs ?

G. Bartholini
The reason there are no controlled studies, is that the changes are not dramatic ; however, every good clinician, and I think you agree with me, knows that at low doses patients are somewhat improved.

J. Mendlewicz
Why did you say that the hypothesis of the down-regulation of the ß-receptors may have nothing to do with the action of the antidepressant ?

G. Groß
I do not want to say that it has nothing to do with it, but I think not all antidepressants cause a down-regulation and an antidepressant effect is not always combined with this down-regulation and I think I have shown it.

K. Fuxe
You gave a very nice talk here with regard to the properties of ß-adenoreceptor binding sites after sulpiride treatment. In this experiment, did you ever have a chance to study the adenylate cyclase regulation by noradrenaline receptors? Perhaps the coupling was changed, although there is no change in the recognition sites. Did you study this ?

G. Groß
No, we did not.

P. Grof
I think these studies may have tremendous importance for understanding of the issue of antidepressant action of neuroleptics. There are controlled studies in the literature, such as Hollister's and Nahunek and his group, documenting clearly that with neuroleptics one can produce improvement in depressed patients. However, the difficulty is that you have to suppress the extrapyramidal symptoms and therefore, you also have to use anticholinergics. I think that raises one basic question : If you want to understand the effects of neuroleptics in depressed patients, you probably have to look not only at noradrenergic mechanisms, but also at the same time at the cholinergic and dopaminergic profiles. Only from an integrated study might you be able to get some understanding of what is going on.

S.Z. Langer
You showed a very interesting result in your down-regulation of ß-adrenoreceptor's study, namely, that when you down-regulate the ß-1-adrenoreceptors in the brain after chronic DMI you do not down-regulate the ß-adrenoreceptors in the heart. Could you tell us how do you interpret these results, because you have noradrenergic nerves, you inhibit re-uptake and in both cases you have a narrow synaptic gap, you have post-synaptic ß-adrenoreceptors and why do you not down-regulate in the heart ?

G. Groß
This was only the case with DMI, the other drugs had similar results in the cortex as in the heart, so, for DMI I think it may be a pharmacokinetic question. Plasma levels during long-term treatment are lower than those found in the brain near the receptor site.

S.Z. Langer
Yes, that is possible.

Y.Lecrubier

I would like to come back to that antidepressant effect of neuroleptics, because I think it is quite misleading. Of course, thioridazine is useful in some depressed patients, but this does not mean that it is an antidepressant ; benzodiazepines are also useful in some depressed patients and you can find a lot of drugs with a lot of different mechanisms of action, which could show some improvement in depressed patients ; but what is the specificity of the patients and of the drug ? With neuroleptics you do not find any controlled study really proving that other drugs would not be equally effective in the patients where it was proved that neuroleptics were effective and in saying so I am in agreement with Prof. Matussek.

Stereoselective blockade by sulpiride of the effects of dopamine agonists on the release of dopamine, noradrenaline and acetylcholine.

S.Z. Langer, S. Arbilla, A-M. Galzin and R. Cantrill.

Biology Department, LERS Synthélabo, Paris, France.

Summary : Dopamine inhibitory pre-synaptic receptors of the D_2 subtype modulate the release of dopamine, acetylcholine and noradrenaline. These receptors can be demonstrated through the inhibitory effects of dopamine receptor agonists on transmitter release and its selective blockade by specific D_2 dopamine receptor antagonists like S-sulpiride. In slices of several regions of the rabbit brain, low concentrations of sulpiride facilitate stereoselectively the release of dopamine but not acetylcholine or noradrenaline suggesting that endogenously released dopamine activates dopamine autoreceptors possibly located on dopaminergic nerve terminals. Inhibition by endogenous dopamine of acetylcholine release may occur through the activation by amphetamine of a reserpine-resistant pool of recently synthetized transmitter. The potential use of selective dopamine receptor antagonists at dopamine receptors modulating the release of dopamine and acetylcholine and the importance of these experimental models for the study of drugs used in the treatment of schizophrenia are discussed.

Introduction

Stimulation of dopamine receptors of the D_2 subtype reduces the release of various neurotransmitters in the peripheral and in the central nervous system (Langer et al., 1982).

In the peripheral nervous system, dopamine receptor agonists reduce the release of noradrenaline and the end-organ responses to postganglionic sympathetic stimulation both under *in vitro* and *in vivo* experimental conditions (Enero and Langer, 1975 ; Dubocovich and Langer, 1980 ; Massingham et al., 1980 ; Shepperson et al., 1982).

The inhibition of the electrically-evoked release of ^{3}H-noradrenaline in the central nervous system can be demonstrated with dopamine receptor agonists using superfused brain slices (Galzin et al., 1982). These inhibitory effects of dopamine receptor agonists on central noradrenergic neurotransmission are more clearly seen when the α_2-adrenoceptors are blocked (Galzin et al., 1982).

The release of dopamine in the striatum of various species is modulated by inhibitory dopamine autoreceptors, which are probably located pre-synaptically (for review, see Langer, 1980). In contrast to the dopamine receptors that inhibit the release of noradrenaline, the dopamine autoreceptors that regulate the release of dopamine appear to play a physiological role in dopaminergic neurotransmission (Kamal et al., 1981 ; Arbilla and Langer, 1981 ; Lehmann et al., 1981).

Dopamine receptor agonists inhibit the electrically-evoked release of ^{3}H-acetylcholine from the cholinergic interneuron in the striatum of various species (Hertting et al., 1980 ; Scatton, 1982 ; Lehmann et al., 1982). This inhibitory dopa-

103

mine receptor is of D_2 subtype and appears to be the target of endogenously released dopamine.

The present article reviews the release of modulating dopamine receptors and provides evidence for the physiological role of some of these dopamine receptors, as judged from the effect of dopamine receptor antagonists on the release of the neurotransmitter.

Influence of the stereoisomers of sulpiride on peripheral noradrenergic neurotransmission

In support of the view that the pre-synaptic dopamine receptors which inhibit the release of noradrenaline are of the D_2 subtype, it has been shown that S-sulpiride, but not the R-enantiomed, blocks the inhibitory effects of dopamine receptor agonists on the release of noradrenaline, both under in vitro as well as under in vivo conditions (Dubocovich and Langer, 1980 ; Massingham et al., 1980 ; Shepperson et al., 1982).

It is of interest to note that in the concentration range of S-sulpiride, in which there is complete antagonism of the inhibitory effects of dopamine receptor agonists on noradrenaline release, there is no increase by S-sulpiride on its own in transmitter release elicited by nerve stimulation (Dubocovich and Langer, 1980 ; Massingham et al., 1980 ; Shepperson et al., 1982). These results indicate that the peripheral pre-synaptic dopamine receptors that inhibit noradrenaline release do not play a physiological role in the regulation of noradrenergic neurotransmission. In contrast to the failure of blockade of dopamine receptors with sulpiride to enhance noradrenaline release, it is well established that blockade of pre-synaptic inhibitory α_2-adrenoceptors by yohimbine, RX 781094 or phentolamine enhances the release of the noradrenergic neurotransmitter during nerve stimulation (for review, see Langer, 1980). Consequently, in contrast to the pre-synaptic α_2-adrenoceptors, the pre-synaptic inhibitory dopamine receptors do not play a physiological role in the regulation of peripheral noradrenergic neurotransmission. Nevertheless, these pre-synaptic inhibitory dopamine receptors are attractive targets for agonists which produce hypotensive and bradycardic actions through the reduction of noradrenaline output in the peripheral sympathetic system.

Influence of the stereoisomers of sulpiride on central noradrenergic neurotransmission

The calcium-dependent, electrically-evoked release of ^{3}H-noradrenaline from slices of the hypothalamus or the cerebral cortex is inhibited by dopamine receptor agonists like apomorphine and pergolide (Galzin et al., 1982). These effects are more clearly seen when the α_2-adrenoceptors are blocked with yohimbine or phentolamine (Galzin et al., 1982). Sulpiride or butaclamol block stereoselectively the inhibitory effects of dopamine receptor agonists, but in the same range of concentrations they do not enhance by themselves the electrically-evoked release of ^{3}H-noradrenaline (Galzin et al., 1982).

When the S- and R-stereoisomers of sulpiride are tested for their own effects on the electrically-evoked release of ^{3}H-noradrenaline, an increase in transmitter overflow is obtained in the range of concentrations 3 to 30 μM for S-sulpiride and

Table 1.- *Effects of (S) and (R) sulpiride on the spontaneous and electrically-evoked release of ^{3}H-noradrenaline from slices of rabbit hypothalamus.*

	μM	n	S_1	S_2/S_1	Sp_2/Sp_1
Control		10	0.96 ± 0.10	0.99 ± 0.06	0.81 ± 0.02
S-sulpiride	1	4	0.75 ± 0.15	1.21 ± 0.07	0.81 ± 0.03
S-sulpiride	3	4	0.74 ± 0.16	1.74 ± 0.11 (a)	0.84 ± 0.02
S-sulpiride	10	6	0.91 ± 0.10	1.96 ± 0.28 (a)	0.86 ± 0.02
S-sulpiride	30	5	0.83 ± 0.10	2.86 ± 0.34 (a)	0.86 ± 0.02
R-sulpiride	1	8	0.71 ± 0.10	1.25 ± 0.11	0.77 ± 0.02
R-sulpiride	3	4	0.86 ± 0.16	1.33 ± 0.16	0.77 ± 0.02
R-sulpiride	10	6	0.90 ± 0.12	1.68 ± 0.12 (a)	0.78 ± 0.01
R-sulpiride	30	4	0.90 ± 0.20	2.07 ± 0.20 (a)	0.83 ± 0.02

Slices of rabbit hypothalamus were labelled with ^{3}H-noradrenaline and continuously superfused with Krebs' medium.
S_1 corresponds to the percent of total tissue radioactivity released by the first period of electrical stimulation (5 Hz, 2 min) and S_2 to the second one obtained 44 min later. (R) or (S) sulpiride in the concentrations indicated were added to the superfusion medium 20 min before S_2.
Sp_2/Sp_1 represents the ratio of the spontaneous outflow of total radioactivity. Sp_1 corresponds to the fraction of total tissue radioactivity released spontaneously in the 4 min sample before S_1 and Sp_2 is the fraction of total tissue radioactivity released spontaneously in the 4 min sample preceding S_2 and during exposure to the drug.
Values are mean $\pm$ S.E.M. of n experiments per group.
(a) $p < 0.005$, when compared with the control group.

with 10 to 30 μM for R-sulpiride (Table 1). This increase in ^{3}H-noradrenaline overflow is obtained under conditions in which neither S- nor R-sulpiride modify the basal outflow of radioactivity (Table 1). It is unlikely that the increase by sulpiride of ^{3}H-noradrenaline release from the hypothalamus is related to antagonism at the level of dopamine receptors because these effects of sulpiride are observed in concentrations higher than those required for blockade of dopamine receptors (Table 2). In addition, S-sulpiride in a concentration of 10 μM (producing a two-fold increase in ^{3}H-noradrenaline overflow) does not antagonize the α_2-adrenoceptor mediated inhibition of ^{3}H-noradrenaline overflow elicited by clonidine or adrenaline (Galzin et al., 1982). Consequently, the enhancement by sulpiride of the electrically-evoked release of ^{3}H-noradrenaline from rabbit hypothalamic slices does not seem to involve blockade of pre-synaptic α_2-adrenoceptors. It is of interest that the facilitation by sulpiride of central noradrenergic neurotransmission does not seem to be stereospecific, because the R-isomer of sulpiride was only slightly less active than the S-isomer (Table 1). On the other hand, there is a 10-fold difference in potency when the S and the R-stereoisomers of sulpiride are tested for their potency in blocking the dopamine autoreceptor in slices of the rabbit caudate nucleus (Table 2).

Influence of the stereoisomers of sulpiride on central dopaminergic neurotransmission

In perfused slices of the rabbit caudate, the electrically-evoked release of ^{3}H-dopamine is enhanced by low concentrations of S-sulpiride (Table 2). These effects of S-sulpiride are due to blockade of the pre-synaptic dopamine autoreceptors that regulate the calcium-dependent electrically-evoked release of dopamine

Table 2.- *Effects of the stereoisomers of sulpiride on the spontaneous and electrically-evoked release of* [3]*H-dopamine from slices of the rabbit caudate nucleus.*

	μM	n	S_1	S_2/S_1	Sp_2/Sp_1
Control		10	3.69 ± 0.18	0.89 ± 0.02	0.87 ± 0.02
S-sulpiride (S_2)	0.01	6	4.41 ± 0.26	0.96 ± 0.02	0.91 ± 0.06
	0.1	5	4.53 ± 0.50	1.20 ± 0.02 (a)	0.82 ± 0.03
	1	6	5.67 ± 0.25	1.38 ± 0.04 (a)	0.81 ± 0.02
R-sulpiride (S_2)	0.01	6	4.31 ± 0.38	0.87 ± 0.06	0.90 ± 0.02
	0.1	7	4.43 ± 0.39	0.92 ± 0.03	0.83 ± 0.02
	1	3	5.45 ± 0.57	1.19 ± 0.03 (a)	0.85 ± 0.02
Apomorphine	0.1	9	5.42 ± 0.23	0.42 ± 0.02 (a)	0.84 ± 0.03
S-sulpiride ($S_1 + S_2$) +Apomorphine (S_2)	0.01 0.1	7	5.20 ± 0.34	0.71 ± 0.04 (b)	0.91 ± 0.05
R-sulpiride ($S_1 + S_2$) +Apomorphine (S_2)	0.1 0.1	4	5.07 ± 0.23	0.40 ± 0.07 (a)	0.96 ± 0.03

Slices of rabbit caudate nucleus were labelled with ^{3}H-dopamine and continuously superfused with Krebs' medium.

S_1 corresponds to the percent of total tissue radioactivity released by the first period of electrical stimulation (3 Hz, 2 min) and S_2 to the second one obtained 44 min later. Drugs in the concentrations indicated were added to the superfusion medium 20 min before S_2. When the antagonism by sulpiride was examined, (S) or (R) sulpiride were added 20 min before S_1 and kept in the medium throughout the experiment.

Sp_2/Sp_1 represents the ratio of the spontaneous outflow of total radioactivity. Sp_1 represents the fraction of total tissue radioactivity released spontaneously in the 4-min sample before S_1 and Sp_2 is the fraction of total tissue radioactivity released spontaneously in the 4-min sample preceding S_2 and during exposure to the drug.

Values are mean $\pm$ S.E.M. of n experiments per group.

(a) $p < 0.001$, when compared with the control group.

(b) $p < 0.001$, when compared with apomorphine 0.1 μM alone.

(for review, see Langer, 1980). As shown in Table 2, blockade of dopamine auto-receptors by sulpiride is clearly stereo-selective, and similar results have been obtained with the stereoisomers of butaclamol (Arbilla and Langer, 1981).

Concentrations of S-sulpiride as low as 10 nM (Table 2) can antagonize the inhibitory actions of apomorphine on ^{3}H-dopamine release elicited by electrical stimulation. Yet, the R-isomer of sulpiride at a 10-fold higher concentration (100 nM) failed to antagonize the inhibitory action of apomorphine on ^{3}H-dopamine release (Table 2).

As shown in Table 2, with 1 μM S-sulpiride, there is already a maximal enhancing effect on dopaminergic neurotransmission while this concentration of S-sulpiride does not modify the release of ^{3}H-noradrenaline elicited by electrical stimulation (Table 1). The concentrations of S-sulpiride, which enhance noradrenergic neurotransmission (3, 10, and 30 μM, Table 1) do not produce additional increases in the release of ^{3}H-dopamine elicited by electrical stimulation in the rabbit caudate (data not shown). Therefore, the facilitation of central noradrenergic neurotransmission by high concentrations of sulpiride appears to be selective for noradrenaline, because in the range of 1 to 30 μM sulpiride there are no additional increases in the overflow of ^{3}H-dopamine elicited by electrical stimulation.

Effects of sulpiride on the electrically-evoked release of ^{3}H-acetylcholine from the rabbit caudate nucleus

In contrast to the results obtained with S-sulpiride for ^{3}H-dopamine release from the caudate nucleus (Table 2), the electrically-evoked release of

Table 3.- *Effects of S-sulpiride, apomorphine and (d)-amphetamine on the spontaneous and electrically-evoked release of ^{3}H-acetylcholine from slices of the rabbit caudate nucleus.*

	μM	n	S_1	S_2/S_1	Sp_2/Sp_1
Control		13	3.94 ± 0.13	0.80 ± 0.02	0.56 ± 0.02
S-sulpiride (S_2)	0.01	4	3.70 ± 0.58	0.85 ± 0.05	0.50 ± 0.03
	0.1	4	3.93 ± 0.67	0.86 ± 0.02	0.50 ± 0.02
	1	4	4.31 ± 0.27	0.88 ± 0.01 (a)	0.54 ± 0.01
S-sulpiride ($S_1 + S_2$)	0.1	6	4.23 ± 0.12	0.86 ± 0.02	0.53 ± 0.02
Apomorphine (S_2)	0.1	4	3.61 ± 0.37	0.21 ± 0.03 (b)	0.41 ± 0.02(b)
S-sulpiride ($S_1 + S_2$) Apomorphine (S_2)	0.1 0.1	4	4.00 ± 0.15	0.72 ± 0.03 (c)	0.53 ± 0.04
(d)-Amphetamine (S_2)	0.1	4	3.46 ± 0.29	0.77 ± 0.02	0.47 ± 0.02
	0.3	3	3.83 ± 0.25	0.66 ± 0.01 (b)	0.47 ± 0.02
	1	4	3.24 ± 0.26	0.39 ± 0.05 (b)	0.52 ± 0.02
S-sulpiride ($S_1 + S_2$) +(d)-Amphetamine (S_2)	0.1 1	4	3.24 ± 0.37	0.72 ± 0.03 (d)	0.52 ± 0.03

Slices of rabbit caudate nucleus were labelled with ^{3}H-choline and continuously superfused with Krebs' medium. S_1 corresponds to the percent of total tissue radioactivity released by the first period of electrical stimulation (1 Hz, 2 min) and S_2 to the second one obtained 44 min later. Drugs in the concentrations indicated were added to the superfusion medium 20 min before S_2. When the antagonism by sulpiride was examined, S-sulpiride was added 20 min before S_1 and kept in the medium throughout the experiment.
Sp_2/Sp_1 represents the ratio of the spontaneous outflow of total radioactivity. Sp_1 represents the fraction of total tissue radioactivity released spontaneously in the 4-min sample before S_1 and Sp_2 is the fraction of total tissue radioactivity released spontaneously in the 4-min sample preceding S_2 and during exposure to the drug.
Values are mean $\pm$ S.E.M. of n experiments per group.
(a) $p < 0.005$, (b) $p < 0.001$, when compared with the control group.
(c) $p < 0.001$, when compared with apomorphine 0.1 μM alone.
(d) $p < 0.001$, when compared with (d)-amphetamine 1 μM alone.

^{3}H-acetylcholine was not enhanced in the presence of 0.01 to 1 μM S-sulpiride (Table 3). Nevertheless, 0.1 μM S-sulpiride significantly antagonized the inhibition by apomorphine of the electrically-evoked release of ^{3}H-acetylcholine (Table 3). The failure of S-sulpiride on its own to enhance the electrically-evoked release of ^{3}H-acetylcholine suggests that under our experimental conditions there is no physiological interaction of dopaminergic neurotransmission on acetylcholine release. Yet, when neuronal uptake of dopamine is inhibited by nomifensine, the electrically-evoked release of ^{3}H-acetylcholine is inhibited (data not shown) indicating that released dopamine can reach the pre-synaptic dopamine receptors that modulate acetylcholine release when inactivation of the released dopamine through neuronal uptake is inhibited by nomifensine.

Exposure to (d)-amphetamine (0.1 to 1 μM) inhibited in a concentration-dependent manner the release of ^{3}H-acetylcholine elicited by electrical stimulation (Table 3). The inhibition by amphetamine of ^{3}H-acetylcholine release elicited by depolarization was antagonized by S-sulpiride (Table 3), indicating that it involves the activation of dopamine receptors. In contrast to these results, the inhibition by amphetamine of the electrically-evoked release of ^{3}H-dopamine in the caudate nucleus is not blocked by dopamine receptor antagonists (Kamal et al., 1983).

107

When the antagonist, S-sulpiride, has on its own a facilitating effect on transmitter release, then the corresponding dopamine receptors are likely to play a physiological role in the regulation of the release of the neurotransmitter. This is the case for the dopamine autoreceptor which regulates dopaminergic neurotransmission in the caudate of several species. On the other hand, the dopamine receptors that modulate the release of noradrenaline in the peripheral and in the central nervous system do not seem to play a physiological role, but can be acted upon by dopamine receptor agonists to inhibit noradrenaline release.

Effects of d-amphetamine on the electrically-evoked release of ^{3}H-acetylcholine from the rat caudate nucleus

The inhibition by amphetamine of ^{3}H-acetylcholine release elicited by electrical stimulation has also been obtained in the rat striatum (Table 4). In contrast to the results obtained with amphetamine, at concentrations as high as 10 μM tyramine only slightly inhibited the release of ^{3}H-acetycholine (Table 4). In the rat striatum, the effects of amphetamine on ^{3}H-acetylcholine release are not reduced by depletion of the endogenous stores of dopamine by a pretreatment with reserpine (Table 4), while the inhibitory effect of tyramine was abolished after reserpine treatment (Table 4). It appears that in contrast to tyramine, amphetamine inhibits the electrically-evoked release of ^{3}H-acetylcholine through the release of dopamine from a special pool which is resistant to pretreatment with reserpine. In support of this view, it was found that : a) after pretreament with reserpine, the inhibition by amphetamine of ^{3}H-acetylcholine release is antagonized in the presence of the inhibitor of tyrosine hydroxylase activity, α-methylparatyrosine (Cantrill R., Arbilla S. and Langer S.Z., unpublished observations) and b) chemical denervation with 6-hydroxydopamine reduces the inhibitory effects of amphetamine on the release of ^{3}H-acetylcholine in the rat striatum (Cantrill R., Arbilla S., Zivkovic B. and Langer S.Z., unpublished observations).

Table 4.- *Differences between the inhibitory actions of (d)-amphetamine and tyramine on the electrically-evoked release of ^{3}H-acetylcholine from slices of the rat striatum.*

Drug before S_2	μM	n	Untreated S_1	Untreated S_2/S_1	n	Reserpine 5 mg/kg S_1	Reserpine 5 mg/kg S_2/S_1
None	—	20	3.25 ± 1.24	0.92 ± 0.13	20	3.70 ± 1.27	0.90 ± 0.05
d-Amph	0.1	4	5.00 ± 1.24	0.80 ± 0.05	4	4.09 ± 0.88	0.86 ± 0.06
d-Amph	1.0	5	4.53 ± 1.12	0.59 ± 0.03 (b)	14	4.06 ± 0.87	0.50 ± 0.09 (c)
d-Amph	10.0	4	5.08 ± 1.50	0.23 ± 0.12 (c)	5	4.20 ± 0.47	0.14 ± 0.05 (c)
Tyramine	1.0	5	3.67 ± 0.69	0.85 ± 0.04	5	4.25 ± 0.57	0.88 ± 0.02
Tyramine	10.0	8	3.38 ± 0.80	0.62 ± 0.02 (a)	5	4.75 ± 1.24	0.91 ± 0.04

When indicated, rats received 5 mg/kg, s.c. of reserpine 24 hrs before the experiment. Slices of the striatum were prelabelled with ^{3}H-choline and continuously superfused with Krebs' medium.

S_1 corresponds to the percent of total tissue radioactivity released by the first period of electrical stimulation (1 Hz, 2 min) and S_2 to the second one obtained 36 min later. Drugs were added to the superfusion medium 20 min before S_2.

d-Amph : (d)-Amphetamine.

Values are mean ± S.E.M. of n experiments per group.

(a) p < 0.05 ; (b) p < 0.025 ; (c) p < 0.001, when compared with the control group.

Discussion and conclusions

The dopamine receptors involved in the modulation of the release of various neurotransmitters in the peripheral as well as in the central nervous system appear to be of the D_2 subtype. At the level of the release of noradrenaline, dopamine and acetylcholine, the presence of pre-synaptic dopamine receptors can be demonstrated through the inhibitory effects of dopamine receptor agonists on transmitter release and the selective blockade of these actions by specific D_2 dopamine receptor antagonists like S-sulpiride.

The enhancement of noradrenergic neurotransmission by high concentrations of sulpiride is not related to the blockade of dopamine or α_2-adrenoceptors nor to inhibition of neuronal uptake of noradrenaline and may reflect a direct facilitating effect of sulpiride, at high concentrations, on noradrenaline release.

The dopamine receptor modulating the release of acetylcholine in the striatum has been extensively studied in the slice preparation (Miller and Friedhoff, 1979; Hertting et al., 1980; Scatton, 1982; Lehmann et al., 1982). Since the release of ^{3}H-acetylcholine evoked by potassium depolarization in the presence of tetrodotoxin is still inhibited by dopamine receptor agonists, it is likely that the dopamine receptor modulating the stimulation-evoked release of ^{3}H-acetylcholine is localized at the terminals of the striatal cholinergic interneurons (Lehmann and Langer, 1983). The inhibition of ^{3}H-acetylcholine release by dopamine released during electrical stimulation is clearly observed when neuronal uptake of dopamine is inhibited by nomifensine (Hertting et al., 1980), suggesting that released dopamine must normally diffuse a relatively long distance before it interacts with inhibitory dopamine receptors on cholinergic nerve terminals in the striatum. In support of the view that dopamine released by electrical stimulation does not normally reach the dopamine receptors on the cholinergic nerve terminals is the fact that the release of ^{3}H-acetylcholine elicited by electrical stimulation was not enhanced after the endogenous stores of dopamine were depleted by pretreatment with reserpine (Table 4).

Amphetamine can inhibit the electrically-evoked release of ^{3}H-acetylcholine from slices of the rabbit and rat striatum in concentrations (less than 0.3 μM) which do not yet inhibit the neuronal uptake of dopamine (Kamal et al., 1983). Therefore, it appears that amphetamine can release dopamine from a strategically important pool to stimulate the dopamine receptors which inhibit acetylcholine release. Although tyramine is equipotent with amphetamine in releasing ^{3}H-dopamine from the rabbit caudate (Kamal et al., 1983), tyramine is only weakly active when compared to amphetamine in inhibiting the release of ^{3}H-acetylcholine evoked by electrical stimulation (Table 4). In addition, pretreatment with reserpine abolishes the inhibition by tyramine of ^{3}H-acetylcholine release while it does not reduce the inhibitory effects of amphetamine on the release of ^{3}H-acetylcholine elicited by electrical stimulation (Table 4).

The inhibitory effects of amphetamine on ^{3}H-acetylcholine release and their association with a special pool of recently synthetized dopamine, which is resistant to pretreatment with reserpine, is of particular interest in view of the well established ability of amphetamine to produce schizophrenic symptoms in man (Angrist and Gershon, 1970). Although direct, post-synaptic effects of amphetamine on dopamine receptors in the striatum (Feltz and De Champlain, 1973) and on amphetamine recognition sites in the hypothalamus (Paul et al., 1982) have been suggested, our results are compatible with the following hypothesis : Amphetamine can stimulate the synthesis and subsequent release of dopamine from a reserpine-resistant extragranular pool. The release of recently synthetized dopamine by amphetamine occurs at sites which can easily reach the inhibitory dopamine receptors on the nerve terminals of the cholinergic interneuron in the striatum. The possible role of this special pool of reserpine-resistant, recently synthetized dopamine in the pathogenesis of schizophrenia remains an open question. However, in view of the fact that overactivity of dopaminergic transmission appears to be involved in the pathophysiology of schizophrenia, it is tempting to speculate that the special pool of dopamine acted upon by amphetamine may be of particular importance in schizophrenia. If the latter were true, then one should predict that a drug which can selectively antagonize the effects of amphetamine in reserpine treated rats may possess a potential antischizophrenic effect through a novel mechanism of action, when compared to the classical neuroleptics which block dopamine receptors. The crucial question is whether this reserpine-resistant, recently synthetized pool of dopamine contributes to neurotransmission under normal or pathological conditions or if it is only implicated in the pharmacological actions of (d)-amphetamine. Additional work is required to further clarify the physiopathological role of the pool of recently synthetized dopamine acted upon by amphetamine.

REFERENCES

Angrist, B.M. and Gershon, S. *1970* - The phenomenology of experimentally-induced amphetamine psychosis - Preliminary observations. *Biological Psychiatry, 2* : 95-107.

Arbilla, S. and Langer, S.Z. *1981* - Stereoselectivity of presynaptic autoreceptors modulating dopamine release. *Eur. J. Pharmacol, 76* : 345-351.

Dubocovich, M.L. and Langer, S.Z. *1980* - Dopamine and alpha-adrenoceptor agonists inhibit neurotransmission in a cat spleen through different presynaptic receptors. *J. Pharmacol. Exp. Ther., 212* : 144-152.

Enero, M.A. and Langer, S.Z. *1975* - Inhibition by dopamine of ^{3}H-noradrenaline release elicited by nerve stimulation in the isolated cat's nictitating membrane. *Naunyn-Schmiedeberg's Arch. Pharmacol., 289* : 179-203.

Feltz, P. and De Champlain, J. *1973* - The postsynaptic effect of amphetamine on striatal dopamine-sensitive neurons. *In : Frontiers in Catecholamine Research*, E. Usdin and S.H. Snyder (eds) ; p. 951-956. Oxford, Pergamon Press.

Galzin, A.M., Dubocovich, M.L. and Langer, S.Z. *1982* - Presynaptic inhibition by dopamine receptor agonists of noradrenergic neurotransmission in the rabbit hypothalamus. *J. Pharmacol. Exp. Ther., 221* : 461-471.

Hertting, G., Zumstein, A., Jackish, R., Hoffmann, I. and Starke, K., *1980* - Modulation by endogenous dopamine of the release of acetylcholine in the caudate nucleus of the rabbit. *Naunyn-Schmiedeberg's Arch. Pharmacol., 315* : 111-117.

Kamal, L.A., Arbilla, S. and Langer, S.Z. *1981* - Presynaptic modulation of the release of dopamine from the rabbit caudate nucleus : Differences between electrical stimulation, amphetamine and tyramine. *J. Pharmacol. Exp. Ther., 216* : 592-598.

Kamal, L.A., Arbilla, S., Galzin, A-M. and Langer, S.Z. - Amphetamine inhibits the electrically-evoked release of ^{3}H-dopamine from slices of rabbit caudate. *J. Pharmacol. Exp. Ther.* (submitted).

Langer, S.Z. *1980* - Presynaptic regulation of the release of catecholamines. *Pharmac. Rev. ; 32* : 337-362.

Langer, S.Z., Arbilla, S., Kamal, L. and Cantrill, R. *1982* - Peripheral and central dopamine receptors modulating the release of neurotransmitters. Proceedings of the Symposium on Dopamine Receptor Agonists. Stockholm, Sweden. *Acta Pharmaceutica Suecica* : 98-107.

110

Lehmann, J. and Langer, S.Z. *1983* - Dopamine receptors modulating striatal cholinergic function : a valid model for the postsynaptic actions of dopamine ? *Neuroscience* (in press).

Lehmann, J., Arbilla, S. and Langer, S.Z. *1981* - Dopamine receptor mediated inhibition by pergolide of electrically-evoked ^{3}H-dopamine release from striatal slices of cat and rat : slight effect of ascorbate. *Naunyn-Schmiedeberg's Arch. Pharmacol., 317* : 31-35.

Lehmann, J., Smith, R.V. and Langer, S.Z. *1982* - Stereoisomers of apomorphine differ in affinity and intrinsic activity at presynaptic dopamine receptors modulating [^{3}H]-dopamine and [^{3}H]-acetylcholine release in slices of cat caudate. *Eur. J. Pharmacol.* (in press).

Massingham, R., Dubocovich, M.L. and Langer, S.Z. *1980* - The role of presynaptic receptors in the cardiovascular actions of N, N-di-n-propyldopamine in the cat and dog. *Naunyn-Schmiedeberg's Arch. Pharmacol., 314* : 17-28.

Miller, J.C. and Friedhoff, A.J. *1979* - Dopamine receptor-coupled modulation of K$^+$-depolarized overflow of ^{3}H-acetylcholine from rat striatal slices : alteration after chronic haloperidol and alpha-methyl-p-tyrosine pretreatment. *Life Sci., 25* : 1249-1256.

Paul, S.M., Huliham-Giblin, B. and Skolnick, P. *1982* - (+) Amphetamine binding to rat hypothalamus : relation to anorexic potency of phenylethylamines. *Science, 218* : 487-490.

Scatton, B. *1982* - Effect of dopamine agonists and neuroleptic agents on striatal acetylcholine transmission in the rat : evidence against dopamine receptor multiplicity. *J. Pharmacol. Exp. Ther., 220* : 197-202.

Shepperson, N.B., Duval, N., Massingham, R. and Langer, S.Z. *1982*— Differential blocking effects of several dopamine receptor antagonists for peripheral pre- and post-synaptic dopamine receptors in the anaesthetized dog. *J. Pharmacol. Exp. Ther., 221* : 753-761.

DISCUSSION

Ch. Eggers
If I understood you correctly, the supersensitivity you have noticed on dopamine autoreceptors does potentiate the dopamine post-receptor blockade after neuroleptic treatment, or not ?

S.Z. Langer
Yes, you could argue that if you have a supersensitive autoreceptor and if the function of this receptor is to inhibit dopamine release, a supersensitive receptor would reduce dopaminergic neurotransmission and therefore contribute to the anti-schizophrenic effects of neuroleptics.

Ch. Eggers
Yes, that is what I understood, and now my question : How can you now explain the tardive dyskinesia on one side and on the other side the reflux of psychotic symptoms you see in long-term treatment with neuroleptics in adult patients ?

S.Z. Langer
Why should my results explain these two questions ? I simply find a result which I think is interesting, I am not intending that this result should explain these two rather complex questions and in fact I am not able to. I think this is a rather complex situation, however I am able to say, although with a great deal of caution, that it is very likely that during chronic treatment with neuroleptics super sensitivity of the autoreceptor develops which inhibits dopaminergic neurotransmission and this is likely to result in decreased dopamine release, but this is one of the many factors involved. You could also argue that there is perhaps supersensitivity of the somatodendritic dopamine autoreceptors that regulate the firing of the dopaminergic neurons. Yet, perhaps all the relevant action occurs at the level of the post-synaptic dopamine receptor and this pre-synaptic contribution is only of minor importance. I am not able to say, even at the level of speculation, what is the degree of contribution, of supersensitivity, of pre-synaptic dopamine autoreceptors to the clinical situations you just mentioned.

N. Matussek

In this context, I would like to ask you : If you have a lower outflow of dopamine after chronic treatment, would you expect supersensitivity also of the post-synaptic dopamine receptor site ?

S.Z. Langer

This could be a contributing factor and on the other hand chronic blockade of these post-synaptic dopamine receptors, which occurs from the very beginning, is another factor that is involved.

M. Ackenheil

I have a question in the same direction. The problem is, if you compare your results with clinical and biochemical clinical research in man, how these fit together ? Therefore, I would like to ask you, firstly, you have shown that the dopamine release is dependent on the frequency of stimulation ; is the same true for the alpha-2-receptors, e.g. for noradrenaline release, meaning that with lower frequent stimulation a better effect of antagonists occurs than with higher stimulation ?

S.Z. Langer

I would like to stop you right there, because what you said is relevant when you add your exogenous dopamine agonist. What I showed is that for pergolide the potency in inhibiting dopaminergic neurotransmission depends on the frequency of stimulation. And now you are concerned with the antagonist. The reverse should be true for the antagonist, in other words, the facilitation of dopamine release by sulpiride should be more pronounced the higher the frequency of stimulation. Why ? Because if dopamine is able to auto-inhibit its own release, the more you release the more you auto-inhibit and the more blockade of this auto-inhibition should enhance release. If you look at the frequency dependence for sulpiride you get exactly the opposite ; that is an important point, it is exactly the reverse for the antagonist as for the agonist. If you look at the facilitation by sulpiride on dopaminergic neurotransmission, the effect at 1 Hz is less pronounced than that at 3 Hz and it is even more effective at 6 Hz, which is exactly what you would expect if auto-inhibition would be related to the concentration of dopamine released in the synaptic gap. In fact, you get a mirror image of what you get with pergolide, so, the frequency dependence exists, but it is exactly the reverse for the antagonist than it is for the exogenous agonist, and interestingly enough, the antagonist is blocking endogenously released dopamine acting on the autoreceptor, while the exogenous agonist like pergolide is adding exogenous inhibition on dopaminergic neurotransmission.

M. Ackenheil

May I ask another question ? Since you investigated the drugs also in an isolated system always applied together with cocaine, the question arises what does cocaine alone do in the stimulation experiments ?

S.Z. Langer

As far as the second question is concerned, we have seen that cocaine does not make any difference to the interactions that we have shown, in other words, you can demonstrate the effects of agonists or antagonists in the absence or in the presence of cocaine and this is particularly true for sulpiride where inhibition of noradrenaline re-uptake is not involved.

M. Ackenheil

Cocaine inhibits noradrenaline re-uptake and DMI too, then you get two additional effects.

S.Z. Langer

We have used both DMI and cocaine and when you use DMI (we used 0,1 micromolar concentrations) there is no difference whatsoever in inhibiting re-uptake of noradrenaline by DMI or with cocaine. We have no evidence at all that DMI at that concentration has any effect on alpha-receptors ; that is what you meant, because DMI had been reported to block alpha-receptors, but you need very high concentrations to show that effect and it is at least a 100-fold higher concentration than that required to inhibit noradrenaline uptake. Both DMI and cocaine behave in our system equally.

112

G. Groß
Have you any suggestions concerning the mechanism of action of sulpiride and the increased noradrenaline release. It does not seem that uptake is involved, neither in your opinion are alpha-2-receptors, nor a tyramine-like action. What could it be ?

S.Z. Langer
I do not know. I think it is a very interesting problem, we are trying to clarify this question and we are trying amongst others to see whether this effect is selective for the calcium-dependent release of noradrenaline for instance. We are comparing tyramine-evoked release with electrical stimulation. I do not know whether you looked at this problem yourself, but we for instance, do not know whether these concentrations of sulpiride facilitate noradrenaline release by an effect that is not necessarily specific for the calcium-dependent electrically-evoked release ; this is one of the questions we would like to clarify. We were surprised to see that the stereo-selectivity of the isomeres of sulpiride was not really very striking at the level of noradrenaline release, whilst this is quite clear at the level of dopamine release. However, to come back to your question, I honestly think that this is a very interesting problem. We do not know what the mechanism is whereby sulpiride (although in high concentrations) can enhance noradrenergic neurotransmission. I do not think that alpha-2-adrenoreceptors are involved in this effect of sulpiride.

W.H. Fennell
In your series of potency of the agonist and antagonist you claimed dipropyl dopamine as a D_1 agonist. Have you found a difference between it as a D_1 agonist, centrally or peripherally ?

S.Z. Langer
Dipropyl dopamine is active as a D_1 agonist in two preparations that we have used. The isolated splenic artery of the rabbit contracted by PGF-2-alpha, here it is only a partial agonist and of low potency, and also on the mesenteric bed in the anaesthetized dog with ganglion blockade, alpha and β-adrenoreceptor blockade. In both cases, dipropyl dopamine is less potent and has a lower intrinsic activity than the other D_1 agonists and in our hands dipropyl dopamine is definitely a preferential pre-synaptic D_2 agonist. There is no doubt about the fact that dipropyl dopamine has some D_1 activity, but it is not as potent and it does not have a fully intrinsic activity in our hands.

Effects of some neuroleptics on central dopamine neurons

H. Hallman and G. Jonsson

Department of Histology, Karolinska Institute, Stockholm, Sweden

Summary : The effect of haloperidol, sulpiride (racemic) and clozapine on dopamine (DA) turnover has been investigated, using the tyrosine hydroxylase inhibition model, in the CNS of the rat, in regions representing the main meso-telencephalic DA systems, including axonal nerve terminal fields, cell body groups, and dendrites. The noradrenaline (NA) turnover was also analyzed in these areas. The administration of the tyrosine hydroxylase inhibitor α-methyl-p-tyrosine methylester (H44/68) caused a time dependent, often multiphasic DA and NA depletion pattern that varied in different regions. The most rapid DA depletion, after H44/68 administration, was found in the cortical (frontal, cingulate, entorhinal) regions and the cell body areas A9 and A10, in particular in the cingulate cortex ($t_{1/2} \sim 20$ min) indicating a very rapid DA turnover. The NA depletion, after H44/68 administration, was slower than that of DA in most regions. Haloperidol was found to markedly enhance DA turnover in most of the regions analyzed, although the effect was relatively small in the cortical regions. Sulpiride was also observed to increase DA turnover in most regions and its most potent action was found to be in the olfactory tubercle and the frontal cortex. Clozapine was found to have its most potent action on DA turnover in the nucleus accumbens. Haloperidol and sulpiride had, in general, very little effect on the H44/68 induced reduction of NA in most regions analyzed, although sulpiride produced a significant potentiation in the cingulate cortex. Clozapine on the other hand, caused a very marked enhancement of NA turnover in several regions, especially in the cortical ones. The present results show that each neuroleptic investigated has its own pattern of action on regional DA turnover. The data do not provide any clear picture as to differential effects of classical (haloperidol) versus atypical (sulpiride, clozapine) neuroleptics on various DA systems, although the latter group appears to have a preferential action on the mesolimbic-cortical DA systems.

Introduction

The central dopamine (DA) neurons, which form several more or less distinct systems from a neuroanatomical point of view, are known to be involved in the regulation of a number of functions, for example the locomotor activity and the stereotyped behavior. The DA neurons are also considered to play an important role in higher mental functions, since the common denominator of neuroleptic drugs is their property of blocking DA receptors. In spite of extensive work conducted over the last 15-20 years, there is still an incomplete understanding of the neuroanatomical correlations between the various DA related functions. When the so called « atypical neuroleptics », like sulpiride and clozapine, were introduced some years ago, certain possibilities seemed to open up with respect to a differentiation between the various DA neuronal systems as to function. Two important effects of the neuroleptics are their extrapyramidal and antipsychotic actions. While classical neuroleptics like haloperidol are known to produce fairly frequent and severe extrapyramidal side effects, the atypical neuroleptics are considered to have a low incidence of such effects. Several studies have indicated that atypical neuroleptics affect preferentially the mesolimbic DA system (Andén and Stock,

115

1973 ; Bartholini, 1976 ; Stawarz et al., 1975 ; Zivkovic et al., 1975 ; Carlsson, 1978 ; Fuxe et al., 1976 ; Fuxe et al., 1977). However, very few systematic investigations have been carried out on this problem, and in many studies the subdivision between the various DA neuronal systems has been rather inexact. It was therefore considered that a clearer picture of the situation might be achieved by performing a more precise sampling of the striatal and of several of the mesolimbic cortical systems. For this purpose, a rapid and simple dissection technique was adopted which allows a sampling of representative areas of the nigrostriatal, mesolimbic-cortical DA systems of the rat, with respect to nerve terminal fields, cell body groups and dendrites. The aim of the present study was to investigate the acute effects of haloperidol as a classical neuroleptic and of sulpiride and clozapine as atypical neuroleptics on the DA « turnover », using the tyrosine hydroxylase inhibition model. Since the employed chemical-analytical technique also assays noradrenaline (NA), data on NA turnover will be presented.

Material and methods

Male albino rats (Sprague-Dawley, 150-175 g b.wt.) were used ; the animals were kept on a 14/10 hr light/dark schedule, with food and water *ad libitum*. The drugs were administered intraperitoneally (i.p.) in 1.5-1.75 ml of physiological saline, and the controls received an equal amount of the solvent. The rats were sacrificed by decapitation, the brains were rapidly removed and placed in ice-cold saline for a few minutes before being dissected, as schematically illustrated in Figure 1. Three 1 mm thick frontal sections (A, B, C) were made and frozen on metal plates placed on dry ice. The different brain regions were then either punched out, or dissected freehand. The following regions were sampled ; *Ac* = nucleus accumbens ; *A9* = substantia nigra, pars compacta ; *A10* = ventral tegmental area ; *C* = nucleus caudatus putamen ; *CCx* = cingulate cortex ; *ECx* = entorhinal cortex ; *EM* = median eminence ; *FCx* = frontal cortex ; *SNR* = substantia nigra, pars reticulata ; *TO* = olfactory tubercle. The dissection of each brain was completed in 8-10 min. The samples were immediately placed in tubes containing the extraction medium (0.1 M perchloric acid) containing appropriate amounts of internal standard (α-methyl—dopamine), frozen and stored at —18°C until the time of chemical-analytical analysis.

The endogenous catecholamine concentrations were determined using liquid chromatography with electrochemical detection (LCEC), as previously described (Keller et al., 1976 ; Jonsson et al., 1980). The tissue samples were homogenized with an ultrasonic cell disruptor (Branson Sonifier B30) and the homogenates subjected to an Al_2O_3 adsorption-desorption purification step. Aliquots of the purified extracts were injected in the chromatograph and dopamine (DA) and noradrenaline (NA) concentrations were evaluated. The catecholamine levels were expressed as ng/g of wet tissue weight, except for the median eminence where the values were expressed as total amount in pmol per tissue sample (unless otherwise stated). The values were corrected for the recovery value (50-85 %), evaluated by internal standard measurements using α-methyl-DA for each sample.

Drugs : α-methyl-dopamine·HCl (MSD, Rahway) ; haloperidol (Haldol[R], Leo, Helsingborg) ; α-methyl-p-tyrosine methylester·HCl (H44/68 ; Astra Läkemedel AB, Södertälje) ; sulpiride (racemic ; Lab. Delagrange International, Paris) ; clozapine (a gift from Dr. Ögren, Astra Läkemedel AB).

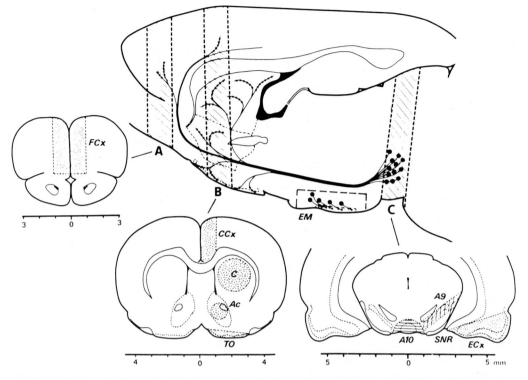

Fig. 1 — Schematic illustration of rat brain with indications of the cutting lines (- - - -) followed for sampling various brain regions to be analyzed for NA and DA content. Tree frontal slices (hatched areas A, B and C) were prepared and used for further dissection, as indicated in the insets showing frontal sections of A, B and C. The figures have been modified according to König and Kippel (1963). *FCx* = frontal cortex ; *CCx* = cingulate cortex ; *C* = nucleus caudatus putamen ; *Ac* = nucleus accumbens ; *TO* = olfactory tubercle ; *EM* = median eminence ; *A9* = substantia nigra, pars compacta ; *SNR* = substantia nigra pars reticulata ; *ECx* = entorhinal cortex ; *A10* = ventral tegmental area.

Results

General considerations

On the basis of extensive neuroanatomical mapping work it is now well established that the central DA neurons form several separate systems (Dahlström and Fuxe, 1964 ; Andén et al., 1966 ; Ungerstedt, 1971 ; Björklund and Lindvall, 1978 ; Domesick, 1981). The aim of the present study was to sample representative areas of the main meso-telencephalic DA systems, including cell body, dendritic and axonal nerve terminal regions (Fig. 1). The hypothalamic tuberoinfundibular DA system was also included in this study. The A9 cell body group in the pars compacta of the substantia nigra has projections mainly in the nucleus caudatus putamen (striatum), the classical nigro-striatal DA system. The dendrites of these cell bodies consist of long, varicose structures, which form a dense network in the pars reticulata of the substantia nigra (SNR, Fig. 1 ; Björklund and Lindvall, 1975). The DA perikarya of the A10 cell body group have also projections in the ventral

117

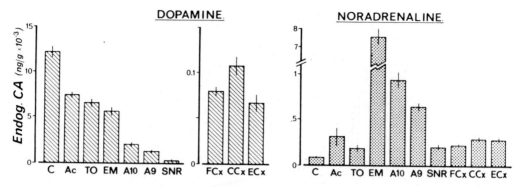

Fig. 2 — Steady state concentrations of DA and NA in various rat brain regions, expressed as ng/g of wet weight of the tissue. Each bar represents the mean ± SEM (n = 5-20). Abbreviations used as in Fig. 1.

part of the striatal complex (Domesick, 1981) as well as in the nucleus accumbens, the olfactory tubercle, and several cortical regions where we have sampled the areas with the most dense innervation, *viz.* the frontal, cingulate and entorhinal cortex. The samples of striatal tissue from the more dorsolateral side should, according to Kelley et al. (1982), represent mainly the « non limbic » part of the striatal complex. The tuberoinfundibular DA system originates in the nucleus arcuatus and periventricularis anterior (A12, according to Dahlström and Fuxe, 1964) with a main nerve terminal projection in the median eminence.

The steady-state levels of DA and NA in the various regions analyzed are shown in Figure 2. The highest DA concentration, about 12,000 ng/g, were found in the striatum, while the levels in the nucleus accumbens, olfactory tubercle and median eminence were, with the present dissection procedure, about half of the striatal DA levels (5,000 - 7,000 ng/g). The cell body regions A9 and A10 were found to contain 1,300 - 2,200 ng/g, with considerably lower values in the dendritic SNR region (about 400 ng/g). The lowest DA concentrations were observed in the cortical regions, 60-100 ng/g, with highest values in the cingulate cortex. The cortical DA constitutes about 20-25 % of the NA levels in these regions. The endogenous NA concentrations were found to range between 200 and 300 ng/g, except in the striatum where NA levels were low (about 80 ng/g), the median eminence (about 8,000 ng/g) and the cell body regions A9 and A10 (650-950 ng/g ; Fig. 2).

Since all regions analyzed contain both DA and NA in varying proportions, it is important to find out how much of the DA measured represents NA precursor in NA neurons, in particular in regions where NA is the predominating transmitter, *for example* in cortical regions. In order to solve this problem, we used the NA neurotoxin DSP4 which has been shown to produce a selective and long lasting NA depletion without affecting DA neurons (Jonsson et al., 1981). The DSP4 treatment (50 mg/kg i.p. for 4 days) was found to reduce the NA levels by 80 % or more in all cortical regions and nucleus accumbens, and by about 50 % in the A9 and A10 regions. No significant changes in DA concentration were observed in any of the regions studied. These data support, therefore, the view that most of the DA

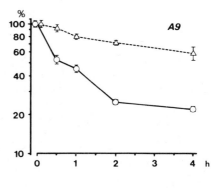

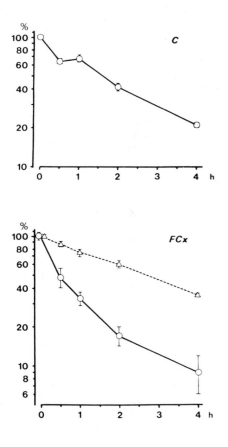

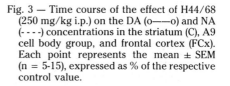

Fig. 3 — Time course of the effect of H44/68 (250 mg/kg i.p.) on the DA (o——o) and NA (- - - -) concentrations in the striatum (C), A9 cell body group, and frontal cortex (FCx). Each point represents the mean ± SEM (n = 5-15), expressed as % of the respective control value.

measured in all regions, including the cortical ones, is localized in DA neurons. These data are also in good agreement with the results recently reported by Bannon et al. (1981).

Effect of tyrosine hydroxylase inhibition by H44/68.

Tyrosine hydroxylation is the rate-limiting step in catecholamine biosynthesis (Nagatsu et al., 1964). An inhibition of this enzyme leads to a rapid depletion of the tissue catecholamine. H44/68 (α-methyl-p-tyrosine methylester) is a very efficient inhibitor of tyrosine hydroxylase (Javoy and Glowinski, 1971 ; Widerlöw and Lewander, 1978) and can be used to monitor catecholamine turnover (Andén et al., 1969). These authors have found that the rate at which NA and DA decrease following the inhibition of synthesis is related to nerve impulse activity, with an increased catecholamine depletion after activation and, conversely, a decrease after inhibition of the neuronal activity. The alterations in decline rate should, therefore, reflect changes in transmitter utilization.

An analysis of the DA and NA depletion patterns following H44/68 administration showed that they were usually multiphasic and varied between different regions. The results obtained in some representative regions are shown in Figure 3.

Although the present data do not allow an exact kinetic analysis, a tentative division into a « fast » and a « slow » decline component was made. The half-life ($t_{1/2}$) of catecholamine decline during the first half an hour was taken as an index of the « fast » component, whereas $t_{1/2}$ for the decline between one and two hours after H44/68 was considered as reflecting the « slow » component. When the half-lives were thus calculated for DA, it was found that the cortical (FCx, CCx, ECx) and the cell body regions (A9 and A10) had the most rapid 'fast' component ($t_{1/2}$ 20-40 min), in particular the cingulate cortex with a $t_{1/2}$ of about 20 min. The striatum, SNR and the median eminence displayed a somewhat slower decline rate ($t_{1/2}$ 40-50 min), while the slowest « fast » component was found in the olfactory bulb and the nucleus accumbens ($t_{1/2}$ 80-110 min). The « slow » component was found to be fairly similar in most regions ($t_{1/2}$ 60-80 min), except in the olfactory tubercle ($t_{1/2}$ about 100 min). The results indicate a predominance of the « fast » component in the cortical and the cell body regions. As for the NA decline pattern following tyrosine hydroxylase inhibition, a multiphasic NA decline pattern was also observed in most regions analyzed, although it was less evident than in the case of DA. The NA decline was most rapid in the cortical regions and considerably slower in the cell body regions. The half-lives of the two components were, in general, much longer for NA than for DA.

The multiphasic catecholamine depletion pattern had previously been observed (Javoy and Glowinski, 1971 ; Paden, 1979 ; Widerlöw, 1979) and it had been suggested that the initial « fast » phase reflected a functional compartment of newly synthetized transmitter and that the second « slow » component reflected the « main storage component » with a relatively slow transmitter turnover. However, recent studies by Paden (1979) have indicated that the multiphasic disappearance is more likely due to changes in DA synthesis and catabolism, rather than to a compartmentalization of the transmitter. Although the significance of the multiphasic disappearance pattern after H44/68 remains unclear, it was considered of interest to investigate the drug effects on the H44/68 induced catecholamine depletion at two time intervals, 30 and 120 min after H44/68 administration, in order to follow the drug effects on the « fast » and « slow » components.

Effects of haloperidol, sulpiride and clozapine on DA and NA turnover.

At the doses used, the various drugs did not show any marked and consistent effects on the steady state levels of DA and NA, although haloperidol had a tendency to lower the DA levels (15-20 %) in most regions 30 min after administration of the large dose (5 mg/kg).

Haloperidol : At a dose of 1 mg/kg, this drug was found to enhance the H44/68 (30 min) induced DA decline in several regions (Fig. 4). The enhancement was quantitatively similar in the striatum, nucleus accumbens and olfactory tubercle, while clearly less marked in the cortical regions. After the large dose of haloperidol (5 mg/kg), a marked potentiation was observed in the SNR after 2 hr, while the effects in the cortical regions were minor. However, in the latter regions there was, after 30 min, a decreased rate of DA decline as compared with H44/68 alone, which was statistically significant in the frontal and cingulate cortex. No effects of haloperidol were noticed in the A10 region. Haloperidol (5 mg/kg) was also observed to enhance the H44/68-induced depletion of DA in the median eminence.

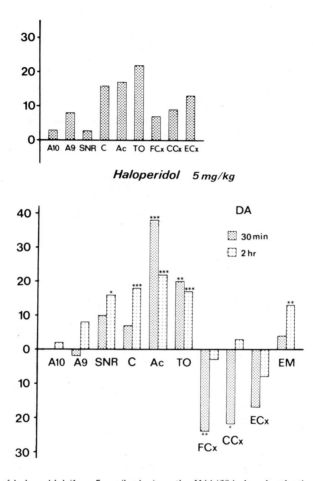

Fig. 4 — Effects of haloperidol (1 or 5 mg/kg i.p.) on the H44/68-induced reduction of DA in various regions of rat brain. The drug was administered 15 min before H44/68 (250 mg/kg, i.p., 30 or 120 min). Each bar represents the mean difference in endogenous DA levels (as % of control) after administration of H44/68 alone, or of haloperidol + H44/68. A potentiation of the H44/68-induced depletion is represented by upward bars, and a decrease by downward bars.

* = 0.05 > p > 0.001 ,
* * = 0.01 > 0.001 ,
* * * = p < 0.001 (Student's t-test).

The effect of haloperidol on NA turnover varied and a significant increase in H44/68-induced depletion was only observed in the median emincence (data not shown).

Sulpiride : The administration of sulpiride did not produce any significant effects on the H44/68-induced DA reduction in the cell body regions studied,

121

although there seemed to be a tendency for an enhanced depletion (Fig. 5). An enhanced DA reduction was observed, after both time intervals, in the striatum, nucleus accumbens and olfactory tubercle. There was a tendency for a more pronounced potentiation of DA depletion in the nucleus accumbens and the olfactory tubercle as compared with the striatum, when the analysis was performed 2 hr after H44/68 administration. In the cortical regions, sulpiride was found to potentiate the DA reduction (30 min) in the frontal and cingulate cortex, in particular in the former region. At the 2 hr interval, the effects of sulpiride were rather small in these regions, which may be due, at least in part, to the very pronounced DA reductions after H44/68 administration alone, which makes it difficult to monitor further reductions. A significant potentiation was also found in the median eminence, although only at the 2 hr interval. As to the effects of sulpiride on NA depletion, rather marked variations were observed, although there seemed to be mostly a tendency for potentiation; a significant enhancement was observed in the A10 region and the cingulate cortex.

Clozapine: The effects of clozapine were only investigated after 2 hr (Fig. 6). Rather few clear-cut changes in the DA depletion produced by H44/68 were noted, although a significant potentiation was found in the A9 perikaryal region, in the nucleus accumbens and in particular in the median eminence. Minor potentiations were also noted in the A10, SNR, striatum, olfactory and cingulate and entorhinal cortex, although they were not statistically significant. In contrast with the other two neuroleptics, clozapine caused a marked increase in the H44/68-induced NA disappearance in most regions studied, especially in the cortical regions and in the median eminence. The most pronounced potentiation was observed in the frontal cortex.

Discussion

Several methods are available to measure directly or indirectly, the turnover of monoamine neurotransmitters, *for example* by administering a radioactive precursor and measuring the disappearance of the labelled monoamine, evaluating metabolites, or, as in the present study, monitoring the transmitter depletion following the inhibition of synthesis. Most methods have limitations, although certain improvements have been indicated by Paden et al. (1980). Generally speaking, none of the methods is clearly superior to the others, the precursor technique and the synthesis inhibition method having generally shown good agreement, although it may be argued that the synthesis inhibition model is not as sensitive an indicator of turnover changes as *for example* the monitoring of a key metabolite. The present results show that the DA depletion which follows tyrosine hydroxylase inhibition leads to multiphasic DA and NA depletion patterns, which vary from region to region. The interpretation of these results is difficult and must be made with caution (Paden, 1979), although it seems unlikely that the different regional depletion rates are mainly related to varying degrees of synthesis inhibition. Rather, the data so far available indicate that the different decline rates reflect differences in turnover rates. In spite of all the complicating factors that can interfere with the interpretation of the results, certain interesting features emerge from the present data. The most rapid DA disappearance, after H44/68 administration is seen in the cortical

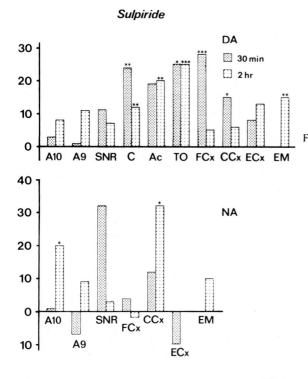

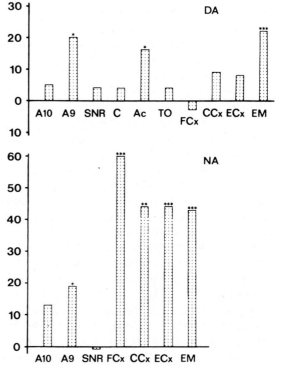

Fig. 5. — Effects of sulpiride (100 mg/kg, i.p.) on the H44/68-induced reduction of DA and NA in various rat brain regions. The drug was administered 15 min before H44/68 (250 mg/kg i.p., 30 or 120 min). The data are represented as described in Figure 4.
* = 0.05 > p > 0.01 ;
** = 0.01 > p > 0.001 ;
*** = p < 0.001 (Student's *t*-test).

Fig. 6 — Effects of clozapine (30 mg/kg, i.p.) on the H44/68-induced reduction of DA and NA in various rat brain regions. Clozapine was administered 15 min before H44/68 (250 mg, i.p., 120 min). The data are represented as in Figure 4.
* = 0.05 > p > 0.01 ;
** = 0.01 > p > 0.001 ;
*** = p < 0.001 (Student's *t*-test).

123

regions, especially in the cingulate cortex, indicating a very rapid DA turnover in these regions. This is in agreement with recent studies by Bannon et al. (1981a) who have shown that the DA turnover in the prefrontal cortex is 2-4 times faster than in the olfactory tubercle and striatum. These authors have suggested that this may be related to the lack of autoreceptors modulating synthesis in the mesocortical neurons (Bannon et al., 1981b ; Bannon et al., 1982). In this context, it seems relevant to mention that Agnati et al. (1980) have observed a very rapid DA turnover ($t_{1/2}$ about 30 min) in small size DA cell bodies localized in the medial part of the A10 region, which may be associated with cortical DA nerve terminals. From the present data it can also be seen that the DA decline pattern in the dendritic SNR region resembles more that of the striatum nerve terminal region than that of A9 and A10 cell body regions, which may reflect the more "axon-like" properties of the DA dendrites in the SNR, where dendritic DA release has been demonstrated (Korf et al., 1976 ; Geffen et al., 1976 ; Nieoullon al., 1977 ; Glowinski, 1979), although, in contrast with axon terminals, these structures have been shown not to have a vesicular DA storage compartment like the axonal nerve terminals (Wassef et al., 1981). It has been suggested that the cisterns of the smooth endoplasmatic reticulum may represent such a compartment.

In agreement with a large number of previous investigations, it was observed that all three neuroleptics investigated potentiated the H44/68 induced DA depletion in several of the DA containing regions studied, related to an increased DA turnover (Carlsson and Lindqvist, 1963 ; Andén et al., 1970 ; Tagliamonte et al., 1975 ; Fuxe et al., 1976 ; Scatton et al., 1977 ; Sedvall and Nybäck, 1973 ; Carlsson, 1978). The present data showed that there are marked regional differences as to drug action, when one considers either a single drug or compares the various neuroleptics studied. Although there is no clear-cut difference between the various drugs, some particular features with respect to the regional effects of each drug emerge from the present data. Thus, haloperidol was observed to produce approximately the same potentiation of DA decline after H44/68 administration in the striatum, the nucleus accumbens, and the olfactory tubercle, indicating that this "classic" neuroleptic is similarly effective in activating DA turnover in these regions. In contrast with the two other neuroleptics, haloperidol was also found to increase DA turnover in the dendritic SNR region at the large dose, while no effect could be observed in the A10 region. Such a differential response has also been reported by Argiolas et al. (1979) who measured DOPAC levels in the substantia nigra and the ventral tegmental area after haloperidol administration. Haloperidol was found to be less efficient in increasing DA turnover in the cortical regions than in the striatum, nucleus accumbens, and olfactory tubercle. This is in agreement with data recently reported by Bannon et al. (1982). A somewhat surprising observation was, however, that the large dose (5 mg/kg) of haloperidol decreased DA utilization in the cortical regions, in particular in the frontal cortex. The reason for this is at present unknown, but could be related to some non specific effect of haloperidol at this high dose level, or related to the findings of Bunney and Grace (1978) that DA neurons can go into an apparent depolarization block following chronic haloperidol treatment. One may speculate that these normally very active cortical DA neurons may go more rapidly into this "depolarization block" situation.

The results on the effects of sulpiride indicated that this atypical neuroleptic was rather effective in increasing DA turnover in most regions, although there was a tendency for a preferential activation of DA utilization in the nucleus accumbens and olfactory tubercle, as well as in the frontal and cingulate cortex. A preferential effect of sulpiride on mesolimbic DA neurons had previously been observed (Scatton et al., 1977 ; Carlsson, 1978 ; Waldmeier and Maître, 1976b ; Fuxe et al., 1976 ; Westerbrink et al., 1977). It should be noticed that the activation by sulpiride was particularly pronounced in the frontal cortex where the DA turnover is normally very high. This raises the possibility that sulpiride may have a preferential action on very active DA neurons, although more work is needed to substantiate this view.

The present data on the effects of clozapine on DA turnover demonstrated significant effects only in the A9 perikaryal region and in the nucleus accumbens. A preferential increase of DA turnover by clozapine in mesolimbic areas has also been reported by several authors (Andén and Stock, 1973 ; Bartholini, 1976 ; Zivkovic et al., 1975). However, it has repeatedly been reported that clozapine produces an activation of the striatal DA neurons (Wilk et al., 1975 ; Rebec et al., 1980 ; Waldmeier and Maître, 1976a), while in our study this effect was not particularly marked. This apparent discrepancy may be due at least in part to differences in dissection procedure. In the present study the striatal tissue sample was mostly from the "non-limbic" striatum, according to the subdivision of the striatal complex recently proposed by Kelley et al. (1982).

All the neuroleptics investigated were found to increase DA turnover in the median eminence, which is at variance with the data previously reported on the acute effects of neuroleptics on the tuberoinfundibular DA system (Moore and Wuerthele, 1979). The reason for this discrepancy is at present unknown, but may be due to the relatively large doses used in the present study.

The effects of the three neuroleptics investigated on the NA turnover were found to be quite different for each drug. Neuroleptics have also been previously reported to enhance NA turnover (Andén et al., 1970 ; Nybäck and Sedvall, 1970 ; Bürki et al ; 1975). In the present study it was found that haloperidol and sulpiride displayed, on the whole, rather small effects on the regional NA turnover. Haloperidol, however, was found to cause a marked enhancement of NA utilization in the median eminence, while sulpiride displayed a significant activation in the A10 region and in the cingulate cortex. The potentiating effect of sulpiride may be related to its reported weak ⍺-antagonistic effect (Kohli and Cripe, 1979 ; Le Fur et al., 1979). While the effects of haloperidol and sulpiride were generally rather small, it is clear that clozapine had a very marked enhancing effect on NA utilization in most regions, and in particular in the frontal cortex. This effect is probably related to the fact that clozapine is a potent α-adrenergic antagonist (Le Fur et al., 1979 ; Gross and Schümann, 1980, see also Arbilla et al., 1978).

The present data have demonstrated that the three neuroleptics tested have their own particular profile concerning DA turnover in the various CNS regions, which is generally consistent with studies employing other experimental models and systems used to assess DA function. While the classic neuroleptic haloperidol appears to be very potent in activating most DA neuronal systems with the exception of the mesocortical system, sulpiride appears to preferentially activate the mesolimbic cortical systems, in particular the DA nerve terminals in the frontal cortex. Clozapine is the most potent in affecting the DA nerve terminals in the nucleus accumbens and has a very marked activating effect on the NA systems, especially in cortical regions. The present data do not provide any clear-cut picture as to differential effects of classic versus atypical neuroleptics on different DA systems, in spite of the attempts to employ a rather precise, from a neuroanatomical viewpoint, sampling technique. The data do, however, bring further support to the view that atypical neuroleptics may have a preferential action on mesolimbic cortical DA systems. The reason for this differential effect is not known and there are no data pointing to different properties of the DA receptors associated with these systems (Carlsson, 1978) : This effect may rather be related to other factors, such as regional differences in biovailability, differential effects on other neuronal systems interacting with DA systems. In this context, it has been reported that the atypical neuroleptics L-sulpiride, thioridazine and clozapine preferentially reduce the *in vivo* binding of ^{3}H-spiperone (DA receptor ligand) in the meso-limbic-cortical regions, while chlorpromazine and haloperidol reduced ^{3}H-spiperone binding to the same extent in all regions studied (Köhler et al., 1981). Finally, the lack of a clear-cut differential action between classical and atypical neuroleptics on the various DA systems may indicate that the present functional grouping of the various DA systems is too simplistic and that more emphasis should be placed on how the various DA neuronal systems are related to each other and to other systems. It should be noticed that Kelley et al. (1982) found, in their mapping work, that a substantial part of the striatum, which is traditionally associated with extrapyramidal motor functions, receives afferents of limbic origin ; this led these authors to suggest a subdivision of the striatum into "limbic" and "non-limbic" compartments. Hopefully, a more precise information as to the interrelations between various DA systems and other neuronal systems may provide a better understanding of the structure-function relationships of central DA neuron systems.

Acknowledgements.

The present study was supported by grants from the Swedish MRC (04X-2295), Karolinska Institutet, and Bergvall, Wiberg and Jeansson Foundations. The skilful technical assistance of Eva Lindqvist, Birgitta Drevinger and Bodil Käller is gratefully acknowledged.

REFERENCES

Agnati, L.F., Fuxe, K., Andersson, K., Benefenati, F., Cortelli, P., D'Alessandro, R. *1980* — The mesolimbic dopamine system : evidence for a high amine turnover and for a heterogeneity of the dopamine neuron population. *Neurosci. Lett., 18* : 45-51.

Andén, N.E., Dahlström, A., Fuxe, K., Larsson, K., Olson, L., Ungerstedt, U. *1966* — Ascending monoamine neurons to the telencephalon and diencephalon. *Acta physiol. scand., 67* : 313-326.

Andén, N.E., Corrodi, H., Fuxe, K. *1969* — Turnover studies using synthesis inhibition. *In : Metabolism of amines in the brain*, G. Hooper. (ed.) pp. 38-47. London, Mac Millan.

Andén, N.E., Butcher, S.G., Corrodi, H. *1970* — Receptor activity and turnover of dopamine and noradrenaline after neuroleptics. *Eur. J. Pharmacol., 2* : 303-314.

Andén, N.E., Stock, G. *1973* — Effect of clozapine on the turnover of dopamine in the corpus striatum and in the limbic system. *J. Pharm. Pharmacol., 25* : 346-348.

Arbilla, S., Briley, M.S., Dubocovich, M.L., Langer, S.Z. *1978* — Neuroleptic bindings and their effects of the spontaneous and potassium-evoked release of ^{3}H-dopamine from the striatum and ^{3}H-noradrenaline from the cerebral cortex. *Life Sci., 23* : 1775-1780.

Argiolas, A., Fadda, F., Melis, M.R., Gessa, G.L. *1979* — Haloperidol increases DOPAC in the substantia nigra but not in the central tegmental area. *Life Sci., 24* : 2279-2284.

Bannon, M.J., Bunney, E.B., Roth, R.H. *1981a* — Mesocortical dopamine neurons : rapid transmitter turnover compared to other brain catecholamine systems. *Brain Res., 218* : 376-382.

Bannon, M.J., Michaud, R.L., Roth, R.H. *1981b* — Mesocortical dopamine neurons — lack of autoreceptors modulating dopamine synthesis. *Mol. Pharmacol., 19* : 270-275.

Bannon, M.J., Reinhard Jr., J.F., Bunney, E.B., Roth, R.H. *1982* — Unique response to antipsychotic drugs is due to absence of terminal autoreceptors in mesocortical dopamine neurons. *Nature, 296* : 444-446.

Bartholini, G. *1976* — Differential effect of neuroleptic drugs on dopamine turnover in the extrapyramidal and limbic system. *J. Pharm. Pharmacol., 46* : 736-740.

Björklund, A., Lindvall, O. *1975* — Dopamine in dendrites of substantia nigra neurons : suggestions for a role in dendritic terminals. *Brain Res., 83* : 531-537.

Björklund, A., Lindvall, O. *1978* — The meso-telencephalic dopamine neuron system : A review of its anatomy. *In : Limbic Mechanisms,* K.E. Livingston and O. Hornykiewicz (eds) pp. 307-331. NewYork, Plenum Publishing Corporation.

Bunney, B.S., Grace, A.A. *1978* — Acute and chronic haloperidol treatment : Comparison of the effects on nigral dopaminergic cell activity. *Life Sci., 23* : 1715-1727.

Bürki, H.H., Ruch, W., Asper, H. *1975* — Effect of clozapine, thioridazine, perlapine and haloperidol on the metabolism of biogenic amines in the brain of the rat. *Psychopharmacol;, 41* : 27-33.

Carlsson, A. *1978* — Antipsychotic drugs, neurotransmitters and schizophrenia. *Am. J. Psychiatry, 135* : 164-173.

Carlsson, A., Lindqvist, M. *1963* — Effect of chlorpromazine or haloperidol on formation of 3-methoxytyramine and normetanephrine in mouse brain. *Acta Pharmacol. Toxicol. (Kbh.), 20* : 140-144.

Dahlström, A., Fuxe, K. *1964* — Evidence for the existence of monoamine-containing neurons in the central nervous system. I. Demonstration of monoamines in the cell bodies of brain stem neurons. *Acta physiol. scand., 62,* Suppl. 232, 1-55.

Domesick, V.B. *1981* — The anatomical basis for feedback and feedforward in the striatonigral system. *In : Apomorphine and other dopaminomimetics. Vol. I. Basic pharmacology* G.L. Gessa and G.U. Corsini (eds) pp 27-39. New York, Raven Press.

Fuxe, K., Ögren, S.O., Fredholm, B., Agnati, L., Hökfelt, T., Perez de la Mora, M. *1976* — Possibilities of a differential blockade of central monoamine receptors. *Symposium Bel-Air V, Genève,* pp. 253-289.

Fuxe, K., Hökfelt, T., Agnati, L., Johansson, O., Ljungdahl, Å., Perez de la Mora, M. *1977* — Regulation of mesocortical dopamine neurons. In : *Advances in Biochemical Psychopharmacology, Vol.* 16, E. Costa and G.L. Gessa (eds) pp. 47-55. New York, Raven Press.

Geffen, L.B., Jessel. T.M., Cuello, A.C., Iversen, L.L. *1976* — Release of dopamine from dendrites in rat substantia nigra. Nature, 260 : 258-260.

Glowinski, J. *1979* — Some properties of the ascending dopaminergic pathways : Interactions of the nigrostriatal dopaminergic system with other neuronal pathways. *In : The Neuroscience ; Fourth study program,* F.O. Schmitt and F.G. Worden (eds) pp. 1069-1083. Cambridge, MIT Press.

Gross, G., Schümann, H.-J. *1980* — Enhancement of noradrenaline release from rat cerebral cortex by neuroleptic drugs. *Naunyn-Schmiedeberg's Arch. Pharmacol., 315* : 103-109.

Javoy, F., Glowinski, J. *1971* — Dynamic characteristics of the "functional compartment" of dopamine in dopaminergic terminals of the rat striatum. *J. Neurochem, 18* : 1305-1311.

Jonsson, G., Hallman, H., Mefford, I., Adams, R.N. *1980* — The use of liquid chromatography with electrochemical detection for the determination of adrenaline and other biogenic monoamines in the CNS. *In : Central Adrenaline Neurons,* K. Fuxe, M. Goldstein, B. Hökfelt and T. Hökfelt (eds) pp. 59-71 Oxford & New York, Pergamon Press.

Jonsson, G., Hallman, H., Ponzio, F., Ross, S. *1981* — DSP4 — (N-2-chloroethyl-N-ethyl-2-bromobenzylamine) — a useful denervation tool for central and peripheral noradrenaline neurons. *Eur. J. Pharmacol., 72* : 173-188.

Keller, R., Oke, A., Mefford, J., Adams, R.N. *1976* — Liquid chromatographic analysis of catecholamines — routine assay for regional brain mapping. *Life Sci., 19* : 995-1004.

Kelley, A.E., Domesick, V.B., Nauta, J.H. *1982* — The amygdalostriatal projection in the rat — an anatomical study by anterograde and retrograde tracing methods. *Neuroscience, 7* : 615-630.

Koenig, J.F.R., Klippel, R.R. *1963 — The rat brain : a stereotaxic atlas of the forebrain and lower parts of the brain stem.* Baltimore, Williams and Wilkins Co.

Köhler, C., Haglund, L., Ögren, S.O., Ängeby, T. *1981* — Regional blockade by neuroleptic drugs of *in vivo* ^{3}H-spiperone binding in the rat brain. Relation to blockade of apomorphine induced hyperactivity and stereotypies. *J. Neural Transm., 52* : 163-173.

Kohli, J.D., Cripe, L.D. *1979* — Sulpiride : A weak antagonist of norepinephrine and 5-hydroxytryptamine. *Eur. J. Pharmacol., 56* : 283-286.

Korf, J., Zieleman, M., Westerbrink, B.H. *1976* — Dopamine release in substantia nigra. *Nature, 260* : 257-258.

Le Fur, G., Burgevin, M.-C., Malgouris, C., Uzan, A. *1979* — Differential effects of typical and atypical neuroleptics on alpha-noradrenergic and dopaminergic postsynaptic receptors. *Neuropharmacol., 18* : 591-594.

Moore, K.E., Wuerthele, S.M. *1979* — Regulation of nigrostriatal and tubero-infundibular-hypophyseal dopaminergic neurons. *Progr. Neurobiol., 13* : 325-359.

Nagatsu, T., Levitt, M., Udenfriend, S. *1964* — Tyroxinehydroxylase, the initial step in norepinephrine biosynthesis. *J. Biol. Chem., 239* : 2910-2917.

Nieoullon, A., Chéramy, A., Glowinski, J. *1977* — Release of dopamine *in vivo* from cat substantia nigra. *Nature, 266* : 375-377.

Nybäck, H., Sedvall, G. *1970* — Further studies on the accumulation and disappearance of catecholamines formed from tyrosine — ^{14}C in the mouse brain. Effect of some phenothiazine analogues. *Eur. J. Pharmacol., 10* : 197-205.

Paden, C.M. *1979* — Disappearance of newly synthesized and total dopamine from the striatum of the rat after inhibition of synthesis : evidence for a homogenous kinetic compartment. *J. Neurochem., 33* : 471-479.

Paden, C.M., Young, S.J., Mac Gregor, R.J. *1980* — Extension of the labelled precursor method of measuring neurotransmitter kinetics to non-steady-state conditions : Application to striatal dopamine metabolism. *J. Neurochem., 34* : 1296-1303.

Rebec, G.V., Bashore, T.R., Zimmerman, K.S., Alloway, K.D. *1980* — Neostriatal and mesolimbic neurons : dose-dependent effects of clozapine. *Neuropharmacol., 19* : 281-288.

Scatton, B., Bischoff, S., Dedek, J., Korf, J. *1977* — Regional effects of neuroleptics on dopamine metabolism and dopamine-sensitive adenylate cyclase. *Eur. J. Pharmacol., 44* : 287-292.

Sedvall, G., Nybäck, H. *1973* — Effect of clozapine and some other antipsychotic agents on synthesis and turnover of dopamine formed from ^{14}C-tyrosine in mouse brain. *Isr. J. Med. Sci.,* Suppl. 9 : 24-30.

Stawarz, R.J., Hill, H., Robinson, S.E., Steler, P., Dingall, J.V., Sulser, F. *1975* — On the significance of the increase in homovanillic acid (HVA) caused by antipsychotic drugs in the corpus striatum and limbic forebrain. *Psychopharmacol., 43* : 125-130.

Tagliamonte, A., de Moutis, G., Olianas, M., Vargiu, L., Corsini, G.U., Gessa, G.L. *1975* — Selective increase of brain dopamine synthesis by sulpiride. *J. Neurochem., 24* : 707-710.

Ungerstedt, U. *1971* — Stereotaxic mapping of the monoamine pathways in the rat brain. *Acta physiol. scand.,* Suppl. 367 : 1-48.

Waldmeier, P.C., Maître, L. *1976a* — Clozapine : reduction of the initial dopamine turnover increase by repeated treatment. *Eur. J. Pharmacol., 38* : 197-203.

Waldmeier, P.C., Maître, L. *1976b* — On the relevance of preferential increases of mesolimbic versus striatal dopamine turnover for the prediction of antipsychotic activity of psychotropic drugs. *J. Neurochem., 27* : 589-597.

Wassef, M., Berod, A., Sotelo, C. *1981* — Dopaminergic dendrites in the pars reticulata of the rat substantia nigra and their striatal input. Combined immuno-cytochemical localization of tyrosine hydroxylase and anterograde degeneration. *Neuroscience, 6* : 2125-2139.

Westerbrink, B.H.C., Lejeune, B., Korf, J., van Praag, H.M. *1977* — On the significance of regional dopamine metabolism in the rat brain for the classification of centrally acting drugs. *Eur. J. Pharmacol., 42* : 179-190.

Widerlöw, E. *1979* — Dose-dependent pharmacokinetics of α-methyl-p-tyrosine (α-MT) and comparison of catecholamine turnover rates after two doses of α-MT. *J. Neural Transmission, 44* : 145-158.

Widerlöw, E., Lewander, T. *1978* — Inhibition of the *in vivo* biosynthesis and changes of catecholamine levels in rat brain after α-methyl-p-tyrosine : Time- and dose-response relationships. *Naunyn-Schmiedeberg's Arch. Pharmacol., 304* : 111-123.

Wilk, S., Watson, E., Stanley, M.E. *1975* — Differential sensitivity of two dopaminergic structures in rat brain to haloperidol and to clozapine. *J. Pharmacol. exp. Ther., 195* : 265-270.

Zivkovic, B., Guidotti, A., Revuelta, A., Costa, E. *1975* — Effect of thioridazine, clozapine and other antipsychotics on the kinetic state of tyrosine hydroxylase and on the turnover rate of dopamine in striatum and nucleus accumbens. *J. Pharmacol. exp. Ther., 194* : 37-46.

DISCUSSION

W.-H. Vogel
The methodology of your study and that of the previous papers is very elegant and scientifically in-spiring. I would like to make a general comment directed to the speaker or perhaps the audience. What do these results mean in terms of the actions of the antidepressant and antipsychotic effects of these drugs ? The rats and rabbits we use are healthy animals and are presumably free of depression or psychoses. If we administer drugs to such healthy animals and we do biochemical studies, what do we really measure ? Do we measure the antipsychotic or antidepressant effects of these drugs ? Or do we actually only measure what would happen to a mentally healthy individual who receives these drugs ? Probably, a healthy individual would show a deterioration of normal behavior.

G. Jonsson
Of course, your questions are of greatest importance, although very difficult to comment upon. As very often in basic science, it is also here very difficult to relate the data to the effects that the drugs may have in the state of disease. However, I think that they pose some interesting questions for fur-ther in-depth analyses, which hopefully can help us in the future to get a better understanding of how the drugs in question act in the human being.

S.-Z. Langer
In your studies with DSP4, if you wait until after the last administration, do you get regeneration or sprouting of your noradrenergic terminals or what happens as a function of time after the last injec-tion of DSP4 if you wait ?

G. Jonsson
There is definitely some sprouting and regeneration with time after DSP4, because this compound is mainly acting on the noradrenergic nerve terminals without affecting the cell bodies. In the occipital cortex, which is located most distant from the cell bodies, there is a very limited regeneration, whereas in the frontal cortex there is a substantial recovery within 1 — 2 months.

S.-Z. Langer
You showed very clearly that dopaminergic and adrenergic terminals remain unaffected. What about serotonin terminals, are they equally unaffected ?

G. Jonsson
That is a question of species. In mice, we have no evidence for a significant neurotoxic effect on the serotonin neurons. In rats, however, there is a minor neurotoxic effect of DSP4 on the serotonin neurons in the terminal fields (cerebral cortex, spinal cord), in the order of 20 — 30 %. This is not astonishing in view of the fact that DSP4 also has a certain affinity for the 5-HT uptake site.

N. Matussek
How is the behavior of the animal after treatment with DSP4 ?

G.Jonsson
The gross behaviour is not changed. Some studies have been performed by Dr. Archer and Dr. Ögren showing that DSP4 causes some learning deficits which would go along with the idea that the *locus coeruleus* system may have some significance with respect to learning and memory.

W.-H. Fennell
Have you done any histology of the effects of DSP4 on other organs, or has anybody else done it, I am wondering particularly what is the effect of DSP4 administration on the heart ?

G. Jonsson
DSP4 is not very effective in the peripheral nervous system and there is in general a complete rec-overy of the density of adrenergic nerves within 2 — 4 weeks after administration of a large dose. DSP4 has in our view a lower neurotoxic potency compared with 6-hydroxydopamine and therefore

does not have any obvious advantage over 6-hydroxydopamine in the periphery. One could even argue that DSP4 does not produce any terminal degeneration in the periphery, but just a transient damage.

G. Bartholini
I have just a comment which has been expressed several times since the advent of alpha-methyl-p-tyrosine (= alpha-MpT) : If you do not consider the bioavailability of alpha-MpT, you cannot conclude that in one region the turnover is more accelerated than in another. The same applies for the biphasic disappearance in dopamine : If you have a disposition of alpha-MpT which is faster in one region, you will have a second phase which is lower. So, I think that the method is very good for a single area, is very good for finding a drug action, but it is not good for comparative purposes among different regions.

G. Jonsson
In general, I would agree, but concerning the tyrosine hydroxylase inhibition model, there is no evidence that there is a preferential inhibition of the enzyme in one area compared to others. There is a very similar degree of inhibition regionally ; 90 % or more during the first couple of hours after alpha-MpT administration.

G. Bartholini
This is correct, but it refers to the activity of tyrosine hydroxylase at a given time. What we need is the measurement of the disposition of alpha-MpT over time in different areas.

G. Jonsson
Well, I agree in a way, but I do not think it is of that critical importance. Most turnover techniques have limitations and can be subjected to criticism.

S.-Z. Langer
You showed differences between sulpiride and haloperidol on the cortical dopamine neurons and the fact that sulpiride is active ; how do you reconcile it with the report by Bannon and co-workers, that dopaminergic neurons which project to the prefrontal cortex lack dopamine autoreceptors, both in the cell body and in the nerve ending ?

G. Jonsson
I cannot explain that. I think that it is perhaps a little premature at present to accept as an established fact that the dopamine nerve terminals in the frontal cortex are lacking autoreceptors.

G. Sedvall
I fail to see any discrepancy. There are post-synaptic receptors as well as regulating dopamine turn-overs, but I do not see too much reason to worry about them and of course haloperidol should produce the expected effects, which it does not.

G. Jonsson
This could be related to the fact that dopamine neurons projecting to the frontal cortex are in a more active state than the other systems.

G.U. Corsini
Have you measured other substitutes of orthomethoxy-benazmides, such as metoclopramide ?

G. Jonsson
No.

Two classes of dopamine receptors distinguishable by substituted benzamides

P. Sokoloff, M-P. Martres, M. Delandre and J-C. Schwartz[1]

P. Protais and J. Costentin[2]

1 *Research Unity of Neurobiology, INSERM U109, Paul Broca Center, Paris, France.*
2 *Pharmacodynamics and Physiology Laboratory, Medicine and Pharmacy University of Rouen, France.*

Summary : Several classes of dopaminergic binding sites can be distinguished in rat striatum according to their localization and their pharmacology. Among them, two classes of sites display a high affinity for antipsychotics, but can be differentiated by their affinity for dopamine (DA) and apomorphine (APO). Dopaminergic sites with nM affinity for DA and antipsychotics (D_2 sites) were detected as a fraction of the ^{3}H-APO and ^{3}H-domperidone bindings. Selective lesions indicate that these sites are mainly localized on intrastriatal neurons. The D_4 sites which are labelled with ^{3}H-domperidone, display a micromolar affinity for most agonists and appear to be localized in part on neurons extrinsic to the striatum. Among a large variety of antipsychotics, only some substituted benzamides recognize D_4 sites with significantly higher affinity than D_2 sites. This biochemical distinction is correlated with differences in antagonism of discrete components of apomorphine-induced stereotyped behavior. The closely parallel differences in potency of the various neuroleptics in the two sets of binding and behavioral studies, support the existence of two distinct classes of dopamine receptors responsible for various neuroleptic actions.

Introduction

Antipsychotics are agents which antagonize the various actions of dopamine (DA) and of DA-mimetic compounds in the brain ; they appear to be mediated by selective receptors. Although, during recent years, various experimental approaches have strongly suggested the existence of multiple classes of DA receptors which may constitute the targets of these drugs, no clear picture has as yet emerged on this subject. For instance, it is still difficult to classify a given dopaminergic response as being mediated by a given receptor subtype pharmacologically defined, as is the case in other fields, by the potency of agonists and the affinity constants of antagonists. As a corollary it is still difficult to compare pharmacological data obtained by various experimental approaches like biochemical, behavioral or binding studies. A solution to this problem may be to define discriminating agents, in particular antagonists, which would constitute useful tools for such a classification.

An important starting point has been the characterization of a DA-sensitive adenylate cyclase, pharmacologically well known, which permits to define the D_1 receptor (Kebabian and Calne, 1979). However, the pharmacology of the D_1 receptor does not appear to correspond to that of other responses in the brain, and the latter in turn, do not appear to be mediated by a single class of receptors, which

131

suggests that D_2 receptors (originally defined as non-D_1 receptors) may, in fact, correspond to a pharmacologically heterogeneous population of DA receptors (Seeman, 1980).

Our general approach to this problem, which will be presented here, has consisted in 1) defining with selective DA radioligands homogeneous populations of binding sites, 2) trying to find DA antagonists displaying discriminatory potencies towards these various populations of binding sites, 3) checking whether these agents show the same discriminatory potency in antagonizing various dopaminergic behavioral responses (stereotyped behaviors elicited in rats by apomorphine).

Definition and localization of two classes of binding sites (D_2 and D_4) both recognized with high affinity by dopamine antagonists

^{3}H-butyrophenones like ^{3}H-haloperidol or ^{3}H-spiperone have been used in most laboratories to study dopaminergic binding sites. However, they seem to present drawbacks such as relatively high non specific binding for the former and significant binding to non dopaminergic receptors for the latter. We have recently developed the use of ^{3}H-domperidone as a selective ligand for DA receptors, with low non specific binding (Baudry et al., 1979). These properties are obviously critical in a study aimed at distinguishing of subclasses of binding sites.

While ^{3}H-domperidone binding sites are recognized in a monophasic manner by most antipsychotics, they do not seem to be a pharmacologically homogeneous population. This is shown, in particular, by the inhibition of ^{3}H-domperidone binding to striatal membranes by either apomorphine or DA, which occurs in a somewhat biphasic manner (Fig. 1), an observation which becomes more apparent with the Scatchard analysis of the data (Sokoloff et al., 1980a). This observation has recently been repeated by the ^{3}H-domperidone binding to striatal slices, indicating that the heterogeneity holds also true for DA receptors in intact cells *in vitro* (Fig. 2). Furthermore the *in vivo* binding of ^{3}H-pimozide, another DA antagonist, is inhibited by apomorphine in a biphasic manner (Baudry et al., 1977), again showing that the process does not result from an artifact due to the alteration of receptors during membrane preparation.

Although other interpretations may be valid, we have proposed that the binding sites for ^{3}H-domperidone and other ^{3}H-antagonists, for which similar observations have been reported by other authors (Creese et al., 1979), belong to two distinct classes. The first one, that we have called D_2, is characterized by a high affinity (nM) for DA, whereas the second one (D_4) is less readily recognized by DA, which displays a μM affinity (Sokoloff et al., 1980a). The large discriminatory potencies of DA and apomorphine for D_2 and D_4 sites permits to study their properties separately, using even the same ligand, i.e. ^{3}H-domperidone. In addition D_2 sites can also be labeled with ^{3}H-apomorphine because of their high affinity for this ligand, whereas D_4 sites are not labeled due to their limited (μM) affinity for the DA agonist which induces a rapid dissociation during the washing of the membranes. All the properties of D_2 sites (capacity, pharmacology, localisation...) are quite similar when either ^{3}H-domperidone or ^{3}H-apomorphine are used as ligands. A complicating factor is that the latter also labels with high affinity a third population of sites, (D_3) which can, however, be easily separated since it is poorly recognized

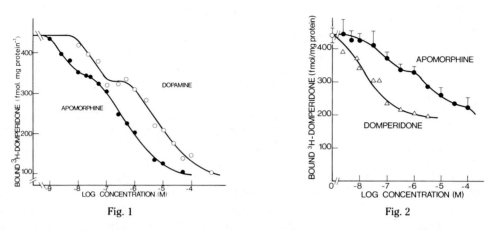

Fig. 1   Fig. 2

Fig 1 - *Inhibition of ^{3}H-domperidone binding to a particulate fraction of rat striatum*
The striata were homogenized in 50 mM Tris-HCl buffer, pH 7.4. The pellet obtained after two successive centrifugations (5.10^3 g.min and 2.10^5 g.min, respectively) was incubated 12 min at 37°C. After centrifugation, the membranes were resuspended in 50 mM Tris-HCl buffer containing 120 mM NaCl, 5 mM KCl, 1 mM CaCl$_2$, 1 mM MgCl$_2$, 0.1 % ascorbic acid and 10 μM pargyline. After a 20 min preincubation, the membranes were incubated during 30 min at 30°C with 4.5 nM ^{3}H-domperidone (24.6 Ci.mmole^{-1}, IRE, Belgium) and apomorphine, or dopamine, in increasing concentrations. The values are the mean of 6-9 determinations.

Fig 2 - *Inhibition of ^{3}H-domperidone binding to slices of rat striatum*
Pools of striatal slices (250 × 250 μm) were preincubated during 15 min at 37°C in a Krebs-Ringer medium containing 20 mM Tris-HCl and 0.1 % ascorbic acid, pH 7.4. After having been washed twice, the slices were incubated with 4 nM ^{3}H-domperidone and apomorphine or domperidone in increasing concentrations. The 30 min incubations were terminated by homogenizing the slices and filtering of aliquots through glass fiber filters whose radio-activity was measured.

by domperidone and most antipsychotics (Sokoloff et al., 1980a, b). Again the two classes of ^{3}H-apomorphine binding sites, i.e. D$_2$ and D$_3$ can be demonstrated, not only in isolated membranes (Sokoloff et al., 1980b), but also in intact cells by measuring the binding on striatal slices (data not shown). The observations leading to the definition of D$_2$, D$_3$, and D$_4$ sites are schematically summarized in Figure 3.

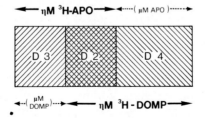

Fig 3 - *Schematic representation of three classes of dopaminergic binding sites labeled with either ^{3}H-apomorphine or ^{3}H-domperidone*
Although the three classes of binding sites are recognized by either apomorphine or domperidone, the ^{3}H-ligands label only those sites for which they display nM affinity. D$_2$ sites can, thus, be labeled with either ^{3}H-apomorphine or ^{3}H-domperidone, whereas D$_3$ sites and D$_4$ sites can only be labeled with one of the two ^{3}H-ligands.

133

It should be noticed that both D_2 and D_4 sites, which are recognized with nM affinity by domperidone, an agent almost inactive as antagonist on the DA-sensitive adenylate cyclase, clearly differ from D_1 receptors. On the other hand these two classes of sites, which are recognized by most antipsychotics with nM affinities (Baudry et al., 1979), are likely to represent the site of action of the compounds whose minimal effective concentrations in body fluids appear to be in the nM range (Seeman, 1980).

These two classes of sites are defined operationally, i.e. they are distinguished in binding studies, by their widely different apparent affinities for DA and agonists like apomorphine. However, this does not necessarily mean that they represent different molecular entities. For instance they may represent two different conformational states of the same macromolecule. There are several examples, in the literature, of a receptor molecule (nicotinic, β-adrenergic) existing in various discrete interconverting states, with different pharmacological specificities, in particular towards agonists. This possibility is of particular interest in the case of D_2 and D_4 sites in view of the action of the nucleotide GTP which decreases binding to the former while it increases binding to the latter sites (Sokoloff et al., 1980a).

Hence it is very important to establish whether they have similar localizations, a problem that we tried to solve by different approaches.

Table 1 — *A comparison of the properties of D_2 and D_4 binding sites*

	D_2	D_4
Kd or Ki of ligands (nM)		
Apomorphine	0.6	100
Domperidone	0.7	0.7
Capacity in striatum (fmol/mg protein)	126 ± 11	203 ± 11
Effect of lesions		
Kaïnate	−57 %	−17 %
6-OHDA	+39 %	+17 %
Decortication	N.S.	−30 %
Subcellular fractions	heavy	light
Effect of 25 µM GTP	−77 %	+21 %
Thermal denaturation (t1/2 at 45° C)	10 min	>30 min

The regional distributions of D_2 and D_4 sites in rat brain are restricted to dopaminergic areas and are roughly the same (Sokoloff et al., 1980a), which does not answer the question. On the other hand, studies on lesions suggest that D_2 and D_4 sites do not belong to the same cell populations in the rat striatum (Table 1). The opposite effects of two neurotoxins, 6-OHDA and kaïnate on D_2 binding sites are consistent with a main localization in intrastriatal neurons that display a high degree of denervation hypersensitivity. On the other hand, the changes elicited by these two neurotoxins are less marked on D_4 sites which, conversely, are more affected by decortication, indicating that they are present, in part, in cortico-striatal endings. These findings strongly favor the view that D_2 and D_4 sites are present in membranes of different neuronal populations.

However one should be cautious in interpreting the data of lesions because 1) in all cases the two classes of sites are affected in a similar manner, although to different extents ; 2) the changes elicited by lesions may be complex, involving adaptive mechanisms and, therefore, not always explainable by a simple disappearance of discrete neuronal populations.

Another approach has consisted in comparing the subcellular distribution of D_2 and D_4 sites in primary fractions of striatum. Whereas the relative specific binding activity is higher for D_4 sites than for D_2 sites in the microsomal fraction (P_3), the opposite holds true in the nuclear fraction (P_1) (Fig. 4). This suggests that D_4 sites may be associated with lighter particles (lighter synaptosomes ?) than D_2 sites, a finding possibly related to their presence mainly in cortico-striatal nerve endings and intrastriatal neurons, respectively.

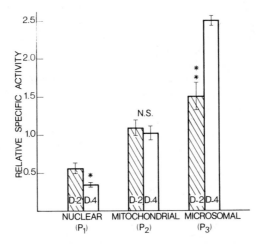

Fig 4 - *Subcellular distribution of D_2 and D_4 binding sites in the rat striatum*
Homogenates of striata (10 vol in 0.32 M sucrose) were submitted to differential centrifugation to yield the crude nuclear fraction P_1 (10^4 g.min), the crude mitochondrial fraction P_2 (2.10^5 g.min) and the microsomal fraction P_3 (6.10^6 g.min). The capacities of the D_2 and D_4 sites were determined using 4 nM ^{3}H-domperidone and a discriminating concentration of 500 nM dopamine. The relative specific activity is the ratio between the total capacity of the binding sites and the protein content of each subcellular fraction. Means ± SEM of 6 independent experiments.
*$p < 0.05$, **$p < 0.001$ in the two-tailed Student's t-test.

Taken together, these various data suggest that the two classes of sites are localized in different neuronal elements (and are, therefore, distinct molecular entities) but this conclusion must still be considered with caution in view of possible artifacts in the various experimental approaches.

Differential recognition of D_2 and D_4 binding sites by antipsychotics

There are large differences in the recognition of D_2 and D_4 sites by DA, or by DA agonists like apomorphine, as shown by the three orders of magnitude of Ki values (Table 2). This differential recognition, with a greater affinity for D_2 sites, can also be observed with other DA agonists although its amplitude is lower, for instance of only 3-fold in the case of bromocriptine. However, agonists cannot easily be used to correlate the pharmacology of binding sites and that of responses, like behavioral responses, for several reasons. Binding studies do not allow to detect easily whether a given compound is a partial or a full agonist, or even an an-

135

tagonist. In addition, the relationship between the degree of receptor occupancy by agonists and the triggering of the response may greatly differ from one response to another. Finally, agonists often display higher affinities for discrete conformational states of receptors, like the desensitized states, which may lead to wrong conclusions as to the pharmacology of the responses mediated by these receptors.

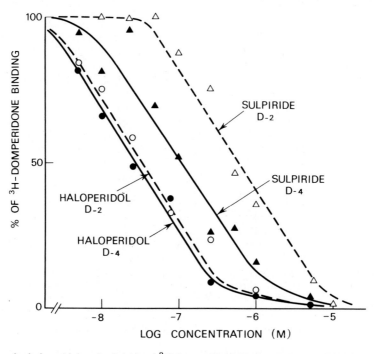

Fig 5 - *Inhibition by haloperidol and sulpiride of ^3H-domperidone binding to D_2 and D_4 sites from rat striatum*
The total specific ^3H-domperidone binding was measured in the presence of 4 nM ^3H-ligand and defined as the excess over blank values obtained in the presence of 50 μM apomorphine. The binding to D_4 sites (●, ▲) was measured in the presence of 4 nM ^3H-domperidone and 20 nM apomorphine to prevent the labeling of D_2 sites. The binding to D_2 sites (○, △) was evaluated as the difference between the binding in the absence and the presence of 20 nM apomorphine, at each concentration of competitive inhibitor. The values obtained in a typical experiment (means of triplicate determinations) are expressed as percent of specific binding to each class of site. The uninhibited binding (100 %) of 94 ± 23 fmol.mg protein^{-1} and 195 ± 15 fmol.mg protein^{-1} for D_2 and D_4 sites, respectively.

It was, therefore, thought that detection among antagonists of differential affinities for D_2 and D_4 sites might provide more useful discriminating agents for other studies, as well as reinforce the idea that D_2 and D_4 sites truly differ in their pharmacology.

The Ki values of most antipsychotics tested did not differ significantly, for D_2 and D_4 sites, as shown for haloperidol (Fig. 5). However, in the case of two benzamide derivatives, sulpiride and the recently developed compound LUR 2366, a significant difference was detected (Table 2). In both cases, the 3- to 4-fold higher af-

Table 2 : *Inhibition constants of dopamine agonists and antagonists on D_2 and D_4 site binding*

Agent	Ki Values (nM)	
	D_2 sites	D_4 sites
Dopamine agonists		
N-propylnorapomorphine	0.4 ± 0.1	3.5 ± 0.8
Apomorphine	0.6 ± 0.1	106 ± 8
ADTN	1.0 ± 0.3	80 ± 5
Bromocriptine	7.2 ± 2.3	19 ± 2
Dopamine	9.9 ± 2.8	$1,830 \pm 690$
3-PPP	41 ± 18	$2,080 \pm 430$
Dopamine antagonists		
Pimozide	2.0 ± 0.5	3.2 ± 0.4
Haloperidol	3.8 ± 1.4	3.2 ± 0.7
Chlorpromazine	19 ± 6	13 ± 1
Thioridazine	32 ± 10	29 ± 1
Clozapine	154 ± 20	225 ± 25
Metoclopramide	158 ± 81	83 ± 16
Sultopride	17 ± 5	20 ± 4
Tiapride	546 ± 113	377 ± 52
Sulpiride	$112 \pm 20*$	29 ± 11
LUR 2366	$2.9 \pm 0.6*$	1.0 ± 0.1

The binding to D_2 sites was measured using 0.8 nM ^{3}H-apomorphine and defined as the excess over the blank values obtained in the presence of 200 nM domperidone. The binding to D_4 sites was measured using 2.5 nM ^{3}H-domperidone in the presence of 20 nM apomorphine and defined as the excess over the blank values obtained in the presence of 50 μM apormorphine.
The drugs were tested at 4-6 concentrations. The Ki values were derived from the IC_{50} values, assuming a competitive inhibition and taking into account the Kd values for each ^{3}H-ligand : 0.92 nM and 0.70 nM for D_2 and D_4 sites, respectively.
LUR 2366 : N-{(1-cyclopropylmethyl 2-pyrrolidinyl) methyl} 2-methoxy 4-amino 5-ethylsulfonyl benzamide (Laboratoire Delagrange).
*p < 0.01

finity for D_4 than for D_2 sites was confirmed in a series of repeated experiments (D_2 binding sites being measured with either ^{3}H-apomorphine or ^{3}H-domperidone), which meant that the difference was highly significant, in spite of its limited amplitude.

Finally, we attempted to characterize the D_2 and D_4 sites by using directly the discriminating properties of sulpiride and LUR 2366. The inhibitions of total ^{3}H-domperidone binding by the two benzamides were compared to those obtained with two non discriminating antagonists, haloperidol and metoclopramide (Fig. 6 and 7).

As expected, haloperidol and metoclopramide did not distinguish D_2 and D_4 sites, as shown by the linear Scatchard's plots. In contrast, curvilinear Scatchard plots were obtained with sulpiride and LUR 2366, suggesting that these antagonists did indeed discriminate the two populations of binding sites.

The use of a computerized analysis, for the separation of the two components of the inhibition, permitted to determine the Ki values. The low affinity components were identical to those previously obtained for D_2 sites (85 ± 15 nM and 2.2 ± 0.1 nM for sulpiride and LUR 2366, respectively). The high affinity components, cor-

137

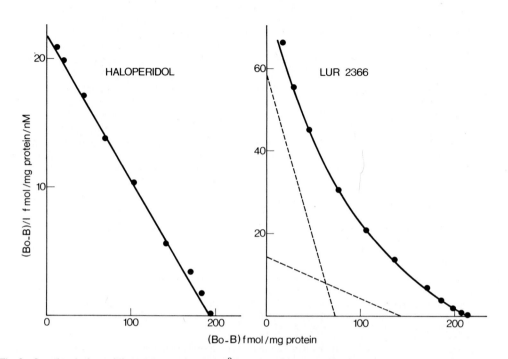

Fig 6 - *Scatchard plots of the inhibition curves of ^{3}H-domperidone binding by haloperidol and LUR 2366*
The membranes were incubated with 2.5 nM ^{3}H-domperidone and haloperidol or LUR 2366. (Bo-B) represents the inhibited binding and I the inhibitor concentration. For LUR 2366, the dashed lines were drawn after computer analysis of the data by an iterative method assuming a concomitant participation of two law of mass action components. The results represent the average of 4 independent experiments for haloperidol and 9 for LUR 2366.

responding to D_4 sites, displayed markedly higher affinities for the two benzamides : Ki values of 5.6 ± 1.4 nM and 0.28 ± 0.02 nM for sulpiride and LUR 2366, respectively. It should be noticed that the Ki value of sulpiride for D_4 sites is in rather good agreement with the Kd value of ^{3}H-sulpiride for its striatal binding sites (Freedman and Woodruff, 1981). In addition, the effects of various selective lesions on ^{3}H-sulpiride binding being very similar to those on D_4 sites (Freedman et al., 1981), it seems probable that the ^{3}H-ligand labels mostly D_4 sites.

Differential antagonism by antipsychotics of various apomorphine-induced stereotyped behaviors

It had previously been observed that sulpiride antagonizes differentially various apomorphine-induced behaviors : For instance, while it clearly blocks the climbing in mice (Protais et al., 1976 ; Puech et al., 1978), it has a low potency against head stereotypies in rats (Puech et al., 1978 ; Ljunberg and Ungerstedt, 1978). Since the climbing behavior can be elicited in selected Wistar rats (manuscript in preparation) by apomorphine at dosages which also induce head

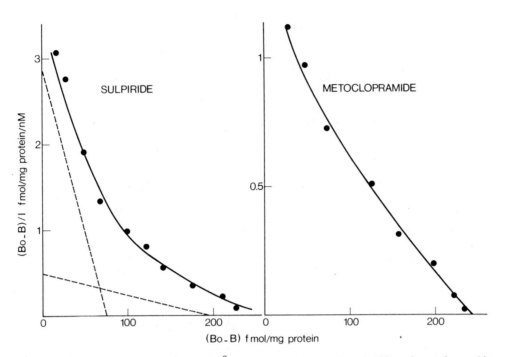

Fig 7- *Scatchard plots of the inhibition curves of* ^3H-*domperidone binding by sulpiride and metoclopramide*
The conditions were as described in the legend of Figure 6. The results represent the average of 3 independent experiments.

stereotypies, like sniffing and licking, it has been possible to compare in the same animals and under strictly identical experimental conditions the antagonist potencies of various neuroleptics towards different behaviors.

Most antipsychotics like haloperidol (Fig. 8) antagonized the climbing and sniffing behaviors at similar dosages : The ratios of ID_{50} ranged between 0.9 (clozapine) and 1.6 (sultopride) (Table 3). The exceptions were again sulpiride and LUR 2366 which antagonized the two apomorphine-induced behaviors at clearly different dosages (p < 0.001). As shown in Figure 8, the climbing behavior was almost suppressed in rats receiving 50 mg/kg of sulpiride, whereas sniffing remained almost unaffected and could not even be totally antagonized at non toxic dosages (below 150 mg/kg). It should be noticed that the comparison was made taking into account the ratios of the ID_{50} values of the drugs in the two behavioral tests, and not their absolute *in vivo* potencies, since this ensures that the pharmacokinetic parameters, such as metabolism or access to the brain, did not interfere. Under such conditions, the ratios of the ID_{50} values are more likely to reflect the selectivity of the antipsychotics towards the two classes of central DA receptors, with pharmacological

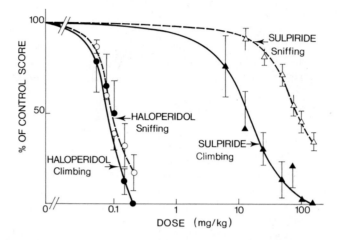

Fig 8 - *Inhibition by haloperidol and sulpiride of two apomorphine-induced stereotyped behaviors in the rat*
Male Wistar rats (200-250g) which responded to apomorphine administration (0.45 mg.kg^{-1}, s.c.) by a stereotyped climbing behavior analogous to that described in mice were selected in a preliminary experiment. On the day of the test, they received haloperidol or sulpiride (i.p.) at the indicated dosages 30 and 90 min, respectively, before the administration of apomorphine (0.6 mg.kg^{-1}, s.c.) and were immediately introduced in individual wire mesh cages (L = 25 cm, W = 18 cm, H = 30 cm). Beginning 5 min after their introduction into the cages, six animals were simultaneously scored for sniffing and climbing behavior during 1 h ; at that time both stereotyped behaviors had vanished in the controls. Sniffing was evaluated by measuring the time during which the animals displayed this behavior (52 ± 2 min in rats not pretreated with neuroleptics). Climbing was scored every 2 min and the final score of each animal was the sum of the scores attributed during the 1 h observation. Each value represents the mean ± SEM of the results obtained in experiments with 6-13 animals and is expressed as percent of the control scores (saline pretreated rats).

Table 3 : *Comparison of the discriminatory properties of various antipsychotics in relation to D_2 and D_4 sites binding and inhibition of two apomorphine-induced stereotyped behaviors*

Compounds	Ki (D_2)	ID$_{50}$ (sniffing)
	Ki (D_4)	ID$_{50}$ (climbing)
Pimozide	0.6	1.0
Haloperidol	1.2	1.3
Chlorpromazine	1.4	2.0
Thioridazine	1.1	1.2
Clozapine	0.7	0.9
Metoclopramide	1.9	1.2
Sultopride	0.9	1.6
Tiapride	1.4	1.3
Sulpiride	3.9*	3.5**
LUR 2366	2.9*	5.8**

*p < 0.01 or **p < 0.001 indicate significant differences in the Ki values for D_2 and D_4 sites, or in ID$_{50}$ values against apomorphine-induced stereotyped-sniffing as compared to stereotyped climbing.
The ratios of the Ki values were calculated from data of Table 2.
The ratios of the ID$_{50}$ values were calculated from experiments similar to those shown in Figure 8.

specificities paralleling those of the D_2 and D_4 binding sites. Thus, the ratios of the ID_{50} values regarding sniffing and climbing, in the case of sulpiride and LUR 2366, were closely similar to the ratios of the dissociation constants of these drugs for D_2 and D_4 binding sites ; the same parallelism can be observed with the other antipsychotics, in spite of ratios closer to unity (Table 3). This supports the view that these binding sites do represent true receptors and indicates that stereotyped sniffing is triggered by the stimulation of D_2 sites (or receptors), while stereotyped climbing results from the stimulation of D_4 sites (or receptors).

Conclusions

An analysis of the binding data obtained with two dopaminergic radioligands permits to distinguish two classes of binding sites, both well recognized (nM affinity) by antipsychotics ; we have previously proposed to call these two classes D_2 and D_4 sites (Sokoloff et al., 1980a). Their somewhat different localisation (according to subcellular and lesion data) suggested that these binding sites might represent different molecular entities although none of the approaches utilized allowed a complete separation. The D_2 and D_4 sites are operationally defined, not only by their large difference in affinity for DA and for some agonists, but they are also distinguished by two antagonists, the benzamide derivatives sulpiride and LUR 2366. For the latter, the discrimination factor is rather limited and such data must be interpreted with caution. However, we feel confident that this discrimination is likely to indicate the existence of two classes of DA receptors for several reasons : 1) the assays were repeated a sufficient number of times to generate significantly different affinity constants, 2) the inhibition of ^{3}H-domperidone binding (D_2 plus D_4 sites) by the two discriminating benzamides in increasing concentrations generates biphasic Scatchard representations, which is not the case with the non discriminating antipsychotics, 3) the good agreement with the behavioral data indeed supports the view that D_2 and D_4 sites are not just « binding sites in search of a function ».

It remains to be established whether the operational definition of D_2 and D_4 sites, based on discrimination by DA or apomorphine, reflects the real affinity of these sites (or receptors) for the agonists. The picture could well be even more complicated if each of the two classes existed in various interconverting forms, differing by their affinity for DA and agonists, as is the case of other aminergic receptors. The distinction between the various classes should ideally be based on the utilization of highly discriminating antagonists. Hopefully such compounds are being developed and should not only allow us to check our hypothesis of two classes of antipsychotic receptors, but also to become new interesting clinical agents.

141

REFERENCES

Baudry M., Martres, M-P., Schwartz, J.-C. *1977* - In vivo binding of ^{3}H-pimozide in mouse striatum : effects of dopamine agonists and antagonists. *Life Sci., 21* : 1163-1170.

Baudry, M., Martres, M.-P., Schwartz, J-C. *1979* - ^{3}H-Domperidone : a selective ligand for dopamine receptors. *Naunyn-Schmiedeberg's Arch. Pharmacol., 308 : 231-237.*

Creese, I., Stewart, K., Snyder S.H. *1979* - Species variations in dopamine receptors binding. *Eur. J. Pharmacol., 60 : 55-66.*

Freedman, S.B., Mustafa, A.A., Poat, J.A., Senior, K.A., Wait, C.P., Woodruff, G.N. *1981* - A study on the localization of ^{3}H-sulpiride binding sites in rat striatal membranes. *Neuropharmacol. 20* : 1151-1155

Freedman, S.B., Woodruff, G.N. *1981* - Effect of drugs on ^{3}H-sulpiride binding in rat striatal synaptic membranes. *Br. J. Pharmacol., 72 : 129 p*

Kebabian, J.W., Calne D.B. *1979* - Multiple receptors for dopamine. *Nature, 277 :* 93-96

Ljungberg, T., Ungerstedt U. *1978* - Classification of neuroleptic drugs according to their ability to inhibit apomorphine-induced locomotion and gnawing : evidence for two different mechanisms of action. *Psychopharmacol., 56 : 239-247*

Protais, P., Costentin, J., Schwartz J.-C. *1976* - Climbing behaviour induced in mice : a simple test for the study of dopamine receptors in striatum. *Psychopharmacol., 50 :* 1-6

Puech, A.J., Simon, P., Boissier, J.R. *1978* - Benzamides and classical neuroleptics : comparison of their actions using 6 apomorphine-induced effects. *Eur. J. Pharmacol., 50* : 291-300

Seeman P. *1980* - Brain dopamine receptors. *Pharmacol. Rev., 32* : 229-313

Sokoloff, P., Martres, M.-P., Schwartz, J.-C. *1980a* - Three classes of dopamine receptors (D-2, D-3, D-4) identified by binding studies with ^{3}H-apomorphine and ^{3}H-domperidone. *Naunyn-Schmiedeberg's Arch. Pharmacol., 315 :* 89-102.

Sokoloff, P., Martres M.-P., Schwartz J.-C. *1980b* - ^{3}H-Apomorphine labels both dopamine postsynaptic receptors and auto-receptors. *Nature, 288 :* 283-286.

DISCUSSION

S.Z. Langer

You did not say anything about Hill coefficients and I wonder whether they are always close to unity ? Secondly, when you express your values as K_i, that assumes that you are dealing with competitive antagonism. Is that the case for all the figures you show ? Instead of K_i you should have shown IC_{50} when it was not competitive. In the cases that you showed Ki values, does it mean that you are always dealing with a competitive interaction ?

P. Sokoloff

In our case we assume that we are dealing with competitive inhibition.

S.Z. Langer

Some of the curves that you showed at the beginning with the biphasic interaction makes me suspect that perhaps your Hill coefficient at the level of inhibition may not be unity. Consequently, you may not be dealing in all cases for all drugs with competitive interaction. Therefore, it may be perhaps preferable to use IC_{50} instead of K_i.

P. Sokoloff

When we studied the inhibition of total ³H-domperidone binding by a discriminatory agent, we have a Hill coefficient lower than unity, but when we consider the individual classes of binding sites, then we have a Hill coefficient equal to unity.

S.Z. Langer

That was a very important point that has to be clarified, because if you look at your initial slide, then your Hill coefficient should be around 0,6 to 0,5. In the second half, it is not clear why you switched to K_i and suddenly your Hill coefficients are 1.

G. Groß

Have you any indication that GTP changes agonist binding to dopamine receptors ?

P. Sokoloff

Yes, GTP marked a decrease in the binding of agonists to D_2 sites. So, it was very important to confirm our data using either the agonist or the antagonist to label the D_2 sites. The pharmacology is very similar when considering the labelling by agonist and antagonist to D_2 sites.

M. Ackenheil

Since it is known that there are great differences between stereo-isomers of sulpiride with regard to inhibiting effects on domperidone binding sites, did you use the racemate or did you use the different forms ?

P. Sokoloff

We used the racemate in binding and behavioral studies.

A.J. Puech

What is your opinion about the kind of receptor involving apomorphine-induced hypothermia and decreased locomotor activity ?

P. Sokoloff

Generally, these behaviors are antagonized by low doses of all neuroleptics including sulpiride. Therefore, it will perhaps be classified as D_4.

G. Groß

By which method did you determine K_i values when there were two different sites ?

P. Sokoloff

We used an interactive method based on the least squares, assuming a concomitant inhibition of binding to two mass action law components.

The evaluation of D_2 dopamine antagonist activity in experimental monkeys

M. Goldstein, J.M. Rabey, S. Mino and A.F. Battista

New York University Medical Center, Department of Psychiatry and Department of Neurosurgery, New York, USA

Summary :

Monkeys with surgically induced lesions in the ventromedial tegmental (VMT) region exhibit Parkinsonian like tremor and hypokinesia. The administration of DA (dopamine) agonists results in a relief of tremor and in the occurrence of abnormal involuntary movements. The ergoline derivative, pergolide, and the partial ergoline derivative, LY 141865, were found to stimulate pre- and post-synaptic DA receptors (Rabey et al., 1981). Pergolide stimulates D_1 and D_2 DA receptors, while LY 141865 selectively stimulates D_2 DA receptors. We have now investigated the effects of neuroleptics on the relief of tremor elicited by LY 141865. The administration of 0, 5 mg/kg (i.m.) of LY 141865 to monkeys with VMT lesion results in a relief of tremor for 3-4 hours. In monkeys pretreated with sulpiride (5 mg/kg, i.m.), the relief of tremor elicited by LY 141865 is abolished. These results suggest that the relief of tremor elicited by LY 141865 is due to stimulation of D_2 DA receptors. The effect of neuroleptics on the LY 141865 elicited relief of tremor in monkeys could be used for determining the *in vivo* potencies of D_2 DA antagonists.

Introduction

Monkeys with unilateral lesions in the ventromedial tegmental areas of the brain stem exhibit neurochemical and neurological deficits which are similar to those observed in Parkinson's disease (Poirier and Sourkes, 1965 ; Goldstein et al., 1969). The extrapyramidal symptomatology in human Parkinsonism is characterized by rigidity, akinesia and tremor, and in monkeys with ventromedial tegmental lesions, hypokinesia and tremor, but no rigidity develops on the extremities contralateral to the lesion side (Poirier and Sourkes, 1969). Monkeys with ventromedial tegmental lesions were found to be useful models in evaluating the antitremor efficacy of dopamine agonists (Goldstein et al., 1973). To determine whether the relief of tremor is due to stimulation of specific dopamine receptors, we have investigated the effects of dopamine antagonists on the antitremor activities of dopamine agonists. We have tested the antitremor activity of the D_1 and D_2 dopamine agonist, pergolide, and of the specific D_2 dopamine agonist, LY 141865 (partial ergoline derivative). In this presentation, we describe the effects of the D_2 dopamine antagonist, sulpiride, on the antitremor activities of pergolide and LY 141865.

Dopamine agonist activity of ergolines

Ergoline derivatives interact with various neurotransmitter receptors and only those which have high affinity for specific dopamine receptors might be of therapeutic value in disorders associated with abnormal dopaminergic functions.

145

Recently we and others have shown (Lew 1979 ; Rabey 1981) that a semisynthetic ergoline derivative, pergolide, is a potent dopamine agonist. The dopamine agonist potencies of ergoline derivatives belonging to a homologous series were tested and pergolide was found to be the most potent (Lew et al., 1979). The data in Table 1 show that pergolide more effectively displaces ^{3}H-dopamine from striatal membranes than N-ethyl ergoline or N-methyl ergoline analogue. The potencies of ergolines to displace ^{3}H-dopamine do not parallel with their potencies to displace ^{3}H-spiroperidol. Interestingly, the potencies of the ergoline derivatives to displace ^{3}H-dopamine from striatal binding sites parallel with their potency to induce rotation in rats with unilateral 6-hydroxy-dopamine lesions of the dopamine nigrostriatal neurons and with their potency to relieve tremor in monkeys with ventromedial tegmental lesions. Thus, the dopamine agonist potencies of the ergolines *in vivo* correlate with their affinities for the striatal dopamine receptors labeled by dopamine agonists, but not by dopamine antagonists.

Table 1 — *Inhibition of dopaminergic receptor binding by ergoline derivatives and their potencies to elicit rotation or to relieve tremor in monkeys*

Ergoline[c]	Ki (nM)[a]		MED[b] (mg/kg)	
	^{3}H-DA	[33]H-Spi	Rotation[d]	Tremor[e]
N-methyl ergoline	89.2 ± 5.5	171.0 ± 11.0	0.5	0.5
N-ethyl ergoline	20.4 ± 1.6	215.0 ± 14.5	0.1	0.2
N-propyl (pergolide)	12.8 ± 0.8	34.2 ± 2.4	0.05	0.1

a. The values are the means from at least three experiments ± SEM.
b. Minimum effective dose (MED).
c. N-methyl ergoline : (8β)-8-[(methylthio) methyl]-6-methylergoline.
   N-methyl ergoline : (8β)-8-[(methylthio) methyl]-6-ethylergoline.
   N-propyl (pergolide) : (8β)-8-[(methylthio) methyl]-6-propylergoline.
d. For the measurement of turning behavior, the rats were placed in a transparent plastic cage and the number of 360º turns were recorded for 3 min every 15 min by direct observation.
e. Recordings of tremors were obtained by means of a transducer attached to the extremities and were recorded on an electroencephalograph. The tremograms were quantitatively analyzed by integration of the amplitudes per unit time and by determining the frequency.

Antitremor activity of pergolide and its reversal by sulpiride

The antitremor efficacy of pergolide was investigated in monkeys with ventromedial tegmental lesions. Pergolide elicits a relief of tremor with a concomitant appearance of abnormal involuntary movements (Rabey et al., 1981). Administration of 0.1 mg/mg of pergolide results in a disappearance of tremor for 4-5 hours, while the administration of 0.5 mg/kg results in a disappearance of the tremor for almost 24 hours. The abnormal involuntary movements persist almost the entire tremor free period.

To determine whether the blockade of D_2 dopamine receptors by sulpiride abolishes the antitremor efficacy of pergolide, we have pretreated the animals with various doses of the dopamine antagonist prior to the administration of the dopamine agonist. It is evident from the results presented in Table 2 that in animals pretreated with 5 mg/kg sulpiride, the antitremor effectiveness of pergolide is decreased from 4-5 hours to 90 minutes. The occurrence of abnormal involuntary

Table 2 — *Effect of sulpiride on the antitremor activity*
of pergolide in monkeys with ventromedial tegmental lesions

Drug[a] (mg/kg)	Effect on Tremor	Drug-Induced[b] Abnormal Involuntary Movements
None	sustained postural tremor	—
Pergolide (0.1)	tremor absent for 4-5 hrs	abnormal involuntary movements, I ; 4-5 hrs
Sulpiride (5.0) and pergolide (0.1)	tremor absent for 90 min	abnormal involuntary movements, I, 90 min
Sulpiride (10.0) ± Pergolide (0.1)	tremor present all the time	no abnormal involuntary movements

a. Sulpiride was given (i.m.) 30 min prior to the administration of pergolide.
b. Abnormal involuntary movements ; I ; restlessness and aggressiveness.

movements is also apparent only for 90 minutes. Pretreatment with 10 mg/kg of sulpiride abolishes completely the antitremor efficacy of pergolide. In these animals no abnormal involuntary movements and no sedation was observed.

Dopamine agonist activity of the partial ergoline derivative, LY 141865

The phenylethylamine moiety, present in apomorphine and in some other dopamine agonists, is probably responsible for their dopamine-mimetic activity (Cannon et al., 1972). However, it has been recently questioned whether the phenylethylamine moiety of ergolines is responsible for the dopamine-mimetic activity of these compounds. It has been pointed out that the rigid pyrrolethylamine moiety of the ergolines might be the active pharmacophore (Nichols, 1976 ; Bach et al., 1980). To test this hypothesis, a number of partial ergolines which are devoid of the phenylethylamine moiety, but possess the pyrroethylamine moiety, were synthesized. We have investigated the effects of the partial ergoline derivative, LY 141865, in two behavioral animal models which measure dopamine agonist activity at the post-synaptic receptors. Thus, LY 141865 induces turning behavior in rats with 6-hydroxy-dopamine lesions of the nigro-striatal dopamine neurons and exerts antitremor activity in monkeys with ventromedial tegmental lesions. Binding studies have shown that the partial ergoline has a low affinity for striatal receptors labeled *in vitro* with ^{3}H-spiroperidol. However, the partial ergoline effectively displaces the binding of ^{3}H-N-propylapomorphine and of ^{3}H-spiroperidol *in vivo* from striatal membranes (Fuxe et al., this symposium ; G. Bartholini et al., this symposium).

Antitremor activity of LY 141865 and its reversal by sulpiride

The administration of 0.2 mg/kg of LY 141865 results in disappearance of tremor for 1-2 hours, while the administration of 0.5 mg/kg results in the disappearance of tremor for 4-5 hours. The abnormal involuntary movements persist almost the entire tremor free period. It is evident from the results presented in Table 3 that pretreatment of the animals with 5 mg/kg of sulpiride abolishes completely the antitremor efficacy of LY 141865. In sulpiride pretreated animals LY 141865 does not elicit abnormal involuntary movements.

147

Table 3 — *Effect of sulpiride on the antitremor activity of LY 141865*
in monkeys with ventromedial tegmental lesions

Drug[a] (mg/kg)	Effect on Tremor	Drug-Induced[b] Abnormal Involuntary Movements
None	sustained postural tremor	—
LY 141865 (0.5)	4-5 hrs	abnormal involuntary movements, I, 4-5 hrs abnormal involuntary movements ; II ; 1-2 hrs
Sulpiride (5.0) ± LY 141865 (0.5)	tremor present all the time	no abnormal involuntary movements

a. Sulpiride was given (i.m.) 30 min prior to the administration of LY 141865.
b. Abnormal involuntary movements I ; restlessness and aggressiveness.
   Abnormal involuntary movements II ; chorea-like movements, various types of stereotyped movements.

Stimulation of pre-synaptic dopamine receptors

To assess the activity of pergolide and of LY 141865 at the pre-synaptic dopamine receptors, we measured their potencies to reverse striatal dopa accumulation after gamma-butyrolactone administration (Walters and Roth, 1976). Both drugs were found to be potent pre-synaptic dopamine agonists (Rabey et al., 1981). The reversal of striatal dopa accumulation after gamma-butyrolactone administration by pergolide and by LY 141865 was completely abolished by sulpiride. These findings indicate that the pre-synaptic dopamine receptors have a high affinity for the D_2 dopamine antagonist sulpiride. One may therefore suggest that the pre-synaptic dopamine receptors have a similar pharmacological profile as the D_2 dopamine receptors.

Discussion

The results of our study show that the ergoline, pergolide, and the partial ergoline, LY 141865, stimulate post-synaptic and pre-synaptic dopamine receptors. The effects elicited by pergolide and by LY 141865 at the pre-synaptic and post-synaptic dopamine receptors are sulpiride sensitive. This finding indicates that both drugs stimulate D_2 dopamine receptors. However, pergolide, unlike other dopaminergic ergots, also stimulates D_1 dopamine receptors (Goldstein et al., 1980). The role of D_1 and D_2 dopamine receptors in mediating dopaminergic responses has not yet been established. Recently, it has been reported that the formation of the second messenger may be dependent on the activity states of both receptors (Stoof and Kebabian, 1981). It should be pointed out that the two drugs which seem to be most effective in treatment of Parkinson's disease, namely L-dopa and pergolide, stimulate D_1 and D_2 receptors, while drugs which stimulate D_2 dopamine receptors only seem to be less effective. Although the antitremor efficacy of dopamine agonists appears to be associated with stimulation of D_2 dopamine receptors, one cannot exclude the involvement of D_1 dopamine receptors in the control of various extrapyramidal functions.

Evidence has been obtained that pre-synaptic dopamine receptors are involved in the control of dopamine synthesis. We have shown that apomorphine inhibits synaptosomal tyrosine hydroxylase *in vitro* and that neuroleptics reverse this inhibition (Bronaugh and Goldstein, 1975). However, ergolines and the partial ergoline, LY 141865, do not effectively inhibit synaptosomal tyrosine hydroxylase *in vitro*. The discrepancy between the *in vitro* and the *in vivo* potencies of ergolines to inhibit tyrosine hydroxylase may indicate that multiple pre-synaptic dopamine receptors are involved in the regulation of synthesis of dopamine. Conversely, a single pre-synaptic dopamine receptor may regulate the synthesis of dopamine, but this receptor may be present in different conformational states. Thus, ergolines may interact with a conformational state which exists *in vivo*, but not *in vitro*.

Aknowledgement
This study was supported by NIMH grant 02717 and NINDS 06801.

REFERENCES

Bach. N.J., Kornfeld, E.C., Jones, N., Chaney, M.O., Dorman, D.E., Paschal, J.W., Clemens, J.A., Smalstig, E.B. *1980* - Bicyclic and tricyclic ergoline partial structures, rigid 3 (2-aminœthyl) pyrroles and 3- and 4-(2-aminœthyl) pyrazoles as dopamine agonists. *J. Med. Chem., 23 :* 481-491.

Bronaugh, R.L., Goldstein, M. *1975* - The effects of various chlorpromazine derivatives on the apomorphine elicited inhibition of synaptosomal tyrosine hydroxylase activity. *Psychopharmacol. Commun., 1 :* 201-208.

Cannon, J.G., Kim, J.C., Aleem, M.A., Long, J.P., *1972* - Centrally acting emetics. 6. Derivatives of β-naphthylamine and 2-indanamines, *J. Med. Chem.,* 15 : 348-350.

Goldstein, M., Anagnoste, B., Battista, A.F., Owen, W.S., Naketan, S. *1969* - Studies of amines in the striatum in monkeys with nigral lesions, *J. Neurochem., 16 :* 645-653.

Goldstein, M., Battista, A.F., Ohmoto, T., Anagnoste, B. and Fuxe, K. *1973* - Tremor and involuntary movements in monkeys : Effect of L-dopa and of a dopamine receptor stimulating agent, *Science, 179,* 816.

Goldstein, M., Lieberman, A., Lew, J.Y., Asano, T., Rosenfeld, M., Makman, M.H. *1980* - Interaction of pergolide with central dopaminergic receptors, *Proc. nat. Acad. Sci. (U.S.A.), 6 :* 3725-3728.

Lew, J.Y., Makamura, S., Battista, A.F., Goldstein, M. *1979* - Dopamine agonist potencies of ergolines, *Commun. Psychopharmacol., 3 :* 179-183.

Nichols, D.E. *1976* - Structural correlation between apomorphine and LSD : Involvement of dopamine as well as serotonin in the actions of hallucinogens. *J. Theor. Biol, 59* 167-177.

Poirier, L.J. Sourkes, T.L. *1965* - Influence of the substantia nigra on the catecholamine content of the striatum, *Brain, 88 :* 181.

Rabey, J.M., Passeltiner, P., Markey, K., Asano, T., Goldstein, M. *1981* - Stimulation of pre- and postsynaptic dopamine receptors by an ergoline and by a partial ergoline, *Brain Res.* 225 : 347-356.

Stoof, J.C., Kebabian, J.W. *1981* - Opposing roles of D-1 and D-2 dopamine receptors in efflux of cyclic AMP from rat striatum, *Nature, 284 :* 366-368.

Walters, J.R., Roth, R.H. *1976* - Dopaminergic neurons : An in vivo system for measuring drug interactions with presynaptic receptors, *Nauyn-Schmiedeberg's Arch. exp. path. Pharmak., 26 :* 5-12.

149

DISCUSSION

J.S. Kim
If I understand correctly, tremor is involved with D_2 receptors with regard to your pergolide experiment. Is this right ?

M. Goldstein
Actually, the partial ergoline derivative LY 141865 is a specific D_2 type agonist and it relieves tremor in monkey. This will indicate that the stimulation of the D_2 receptor relieves tremor. However, the SKF compound at a high dose also relieves tremor, but it is not so effective as the partial ergoline. So, it is quite conceivable that in this model the stimulation of supersensitive D_1 receptors will also produce an anti-tremor effect.

S.Z. Langer
You showed a very large difference of at least 100-fold for pergolide and the LY compound on NPA and spiroperidol binding. It is interesting that when we compare pergolide and the LY compound in our in-vitro system on the dopamine autoreceptor, they are almost equipotent. That is a dissociation that may be of great interest, because pergolide and LY are very active *in-vitro* in our system.

M. Goldstein
I think that by just homogenizing these membranes we are destroying the conformational state of the receptor.

G. Bartholini
Why do you mainly have to invoke supersensitive receptors in the SKF action and not just the fact that the compound might be unspecific ?

M. Goldstein
I cannot exclude this possibility, but I personally believe that the supersensitivity may produce some characteristic changes either in the D_2 type receptor or in the D_1 receptor, which alters to drug interaction. I would not be surprised that stimulation of the D_1 in combination with D_2 produces different effects than separate stimulation of these receptors.

K. Fuxe
In relation to this, I also wonder what really happens with the supersensitivity development. Is it a loss of selectivity, a loss of stereo-selectivity ? It may even be that SKF could hit the D_2 receptor when it becomes supersensitive, so you should really try to block the SKF action with sulpiride, because that may well happen, as you have a supersensitive receptor.

M. Goldstein
That is a possibility.

M. Ackenheil
I have a question concerning the methodology. First, you make the isolation by spiroperidol binding, in this way separating the receptors and then you make the solubilization, is that correct ? If you use the spiroperidol binding, which binds on serotonin receptors, then I would expect that you find two different receptors if you later separate by column chromatography.

M. Goldstein
We have two different procedures. One procedure is that we first solubilize the receptor and then we measure its binding affinity for ^{3}H-spiroperidol. Another procedure is to solubilize first the receptor, then ^{3}H-spiroperidol is bound to the receptor. We adsorb the ^{3}H-spiroperidol-bound receptor to concavalin A.

N. Matussek
In your monkey model, is there also rigor or only tremor ?

150

M. Goldstein
We do not observe rigidity, however, we can observe hyperkinesia.

S.Z. Langer
I wonder whether you have sodium ions in your binding studies on NPA and spiroperidol and if you know whether the LY compound may become more potent in the presence of sodium ions ?

M. Goldstein
We tried the sodium and we saw very little difference.

G.U. Corsini
Do you have any explanation for the fact that in your animal model, in which you destroyed the nigrostriatum pathway, you still have this sedative effect of dopamine agonists ? Second question : In 1976 we published that sulpiride in man does not antagonize the anti-tremor activity of apomorphine. We used a dose of 2 mg/kg at that time in humans. In your data you showed that, on the contrary, sulpiride did antagonize this effect. How do you explain this problem ?

M. Goldstein
With regard to the first question, we destroy the nigrostriatal dopaminergic system. There is some limbic dopamine left which may still have some pre-synaptic dopamine receptors and this could explain the sedation. The other question is more difficult to answer. What type of tremor did you measure, the Parkinsonian tremor ?

G.U. Corsini
Yes.

M. Goldstein
And you were not able to antagonize with sulpiride ?

G.U. Corsini
No.

M. Goldstein
This surprises me. Perhaps this is a dose-dependent situation. We gave 5 mg/kg and how much did you give ?

G.U. Corsini
2 mg/kg.

M. Goldstein
That is close. Was it injected or was it given orally ?

G.U. Corsini
In our patients we applied sulpiride intramuscularly half an hour before apomorphine.

M. Goldstein
And you did not get any antagonism ?

G.U. Corsini
No.

M. Goldstein
That is surprising. We got a very clear-cut antagonism at 5 mg/kg.

G.U. Corsini
Did you destroy 100 % of the striatum in your model ?

M. Goldstein
About 90 %.

P. Grof
Have you any experience with nomifensine, a dopaminergic agonist ? Nomifensine has some use in Parkinson's disease and it is a good, fast-acting antidepressant and I was wondering whether it fits anywhere into your scheme ?

M. Goldstein
We did not study nomifensine in the monkey model, because I understand the nomifensine action is related to the release of the dopamine from the terminals.

Interaction of substituted benzamide drugs with cerebral dopamine receptors

P. Jenner[1], B. Testa[2], H. van de Waterbeemd[2], C.D. Marsden[1]

1. *University Department of Neurology, Institute of Psychiatry,*
   & King's College Hospital Medical School, London, UK.
2. *School of Pharmacy, University of Lausanne, Lausanne, Switzerland.*

Summary : Sulpiride is a selective cerebral dopamine antagonist which interacts specifically with D_2 adenylate cyclase independent dopamine receptors. The interaction of ^{3}H-sulpiride with D_2 receptors can, however, be distinguished from that of ^{3}H-spiperone since it is entirely dependent on the presence of sodium ions in the incubation medium. The poor lipid solubility of sulpiride is not responsible for its selective interaction with D_2 receptors since newer highly lipophilic substituted benzamide drugs also fail to interact with D_1 receptors in the rat. Lipid solubility may, however, be a critical factor in determining the relative potency of substituted benzamide drugs since above and below a critical level of lipid solubility there is a marked decline in both pharmacological activity and the *in vitro* interaction of substituted benzamide drugs with D_2 dopamine receptors.

Introduction

Substituted benzamide drugs, such as sulpiride, are selective dopamine receptor antagonists (Jenner and Marsden, 1979 a, b ; 1981). These compounds differ, however, from classical neuroleptic compounds in that they exert only part of the spectrum of behavioral activity of typical neuroleptic drugs. Substituted benzamide drugs also do not interact with neuronal receptors in brain other than dopamine (Jenner and Marsden, 1981). Classical neuroleptic compounds, in contrast, act on a range of neurotransmitter receptors including noradrenaline, 5HT, histamine and, in some cases, acetylcholine (Leysen et al., 1982). Many substituted benzamide drugs also are selective antagonists of one sub-population of dopamine receptors, namely the D_2 adenylate cyclase independent dopamine receptors (Trabucchi et al., 1975 ; Elliott et al., 1977 ; Kebabian and Calne, 1979 ; Hyttel, 1980).

Recently, two series of substituted benzamide drugs, namely the piperidylbenzyl series, such as clebopride, and the pyrrolidinylbenzyl series, such as YM 09151-2, have been introduced (Prieto et al., 1977 ; Iwanami et al., 1981). These newer substituted benzamides appear to resemble classical neuroleptic drugs. Thus, clebopride and YM 09151-2 are potent in inducing catalepsy and in inhibiting apomorphine-induced stereotyped behaviour (Elliott et al., 1977 ; Usuda et al., 1979, 1981). In addition (Usuda et al., 1981) have claimed that YM 08050 and YM 09151-2 are not selective for D_2 striatal dopamine receptors, but are selective antagonists of D_1 adenylate cyclase linked dopamine receptors. This suggestion obviously throws doubt on the concept that substituted benzamides are selective D_2 antagonists.

153

The suggestion that the compounds of the pyrrolidinylbenzyl series might be selective D_1 antagonists has been taken up by Woodruff and colleagues (1980). These workers have suggested that the specificity of sulpiride on D_2 receptors is merely due to its poor lipid solubility compared to the newer lipophilic derivatives. The implication is that there is no difference in the molecular requirements for activity at D_1 and D_2 receptors. Any neuroleptic drug will act on D_1 receptors as long as it possesses sufficient lipid solubility to allow it to penetrate some lipid barrier beyond which the adenylate cyclase enzyme lies. On this basis, drugs such as sulpiride would possess no particular steric qualities which endow them with D_2 activity, when compared to other neuroleptic compounds, but merely poor lipid solubility.

Obviously such arguments are of critical importance to our understanding of the mechanism of action of neuroleptic drugs and the classification of cerebral dopamine receptors. We have investigated the role lipid solubility might play in the relative antagonism of D_1 and D_2 receptors by examining the relationship between lipid solubility and the potency of neuroleptic drugs to produce biochemical and behavioral changes associated with cerebral dopamine function.

Are the newer more potent substituted benzamide drugs selective D_1 antagonists ?

Initially we compared the ability of a range of substituted benzamide drugs with that of classical neuroleptic compounds to inhibit ³H-spiperone binding to striatal preparations, and to antagonise apomorphine-induced stereotyped behavior (Table 1). Clebopride and YM 09151-2 indeed are very potent antagonists of dopamine receptor function both *in vitro* and *in vivo*. Other drugs in the substituted benzamide series are much less potent.

Table 1. — *Comparison of the ability of substituted benzamide drugs and other neuroleptic compounds to inhibit ³H-spiperone (³H-SPI) or ³H-piflutixol (³H-PIF) binding to rat striatal preparations, to inhibit striatal dopamine-stimulated adenylate cyclase (AC) and to inhibit apomorphine-induced stereotyped behavior.*

Drug	IC₅₀ (nM)			ID₅₀(mg/kg)
	AC	³H-PIF	³H-SPI	Stereotypy
YM 09151-2	20,000	22,000	0.4	0.017
Clebopride	19,000	100,000	18	0.34
Flubepride	>100,000	>100,000	290	24
Sultopride	>100,000	>100,000	260	41
Sulpiride	>100,000	>100,000	570	>128
Metoclopramide	>100,000	>100,000	680	5.4
Tiapride	>100,000	>100,000	1,000	48
Tigan	>100,000	>100,000	8,000	>250
cis-Flupenthixol	24	3.2	23	0.25
trans-Flupenthixol	850	89	298	>128
Spiperone	3,360	1,400	0.6	0.028
Haloperidol	1,800	1,000	6	0.16
Thioridazine	7,600	40	120	10.4

Fleminger et al. (1982) unpublished observations.

We compared also the ability of substituted benzamide drugs and classical neuroleptic agents to act on D_1 receptors, as judged by their capacity to inhibit dopamine stimulation of striatal adenylate cyclase in rat tissue preparations, or to inhibit ^{3}H-piflutixol binding to rat striatal preparations (Table 1). All the substituted benzamide drugs, including YM 09151-2 and clebopride had little or no activity in either system, in contrast to the effects of a known D_1 active neuroleptic, *cis* - flupenthixol. Most substituted benzamide drugs were inactive in these systems in the highest concentrations (10^{-4}M) employed. However, YM 09151-2 and clebopride did cause some inhibition of both dopamine-stimulated adenylate cyclase activity and specific ^{3}H-piflutixol binding, nevertheless, neither of these latter compounds was a selective D_1 active drug. They both were at least 1,000 times more potent in inhibiting ^{3}H-spiperone binding to D_2 receptors than acting on the D_1 test systems.

Does lipid solubility influence the action of neuroleptic drugs on D_1 receptors ?

The data described above showed that although clebopride and YM 09151-2 are not selective D_1 antagonists, they do cause some inhibition of D_1 receptor systems. This may be correlated with their greater lipid solubility compared to other substituted benzamide drugs. To investigate this possibility we have re-organised the data to examine the effect of increasing lipid solubility, as judged by log P', on the ability of the drugs to inhibit dopamine-stimulated adenylate cyclase activity and to displace ^{3}H-piflutixol from its binding site on rat striatal preparations (Table 2).

Table 2. — *Potency order of substituted benzamide drugs and other neuroleptic compounds in inhibiting dopamine-stimulated adenylate cyclase (AC) and ^{3}H-piflutixol (^{3}H-PIF) binding in rat striatal preparations ranked according to increasing lipid solubility (log P' at pH 7.4)*

Compound	log P'	IC$_{50}$ (nM)	
		AC	^{3}H-PIF
Sulpiride	−1.15	>100,000	>100,000
Tiapride	−1.08	>100,000	>100,000
Sultopride	−0.62	>100,000	>100,000
Metoclopramide	0.46	>100,000	>100,000
Tigan	0.89	>100,000	>100,000
Flubepride	1.17	>100,000	>100,000
Spiperone	2.34*	3,360	1,400
Clebopride	2.99	19,000	100,000
Haloperidol	3.03*	1,800	1,000
Thioridazine	3.29*	7,600	40
YM 09151-2	3.51	20,000	22,000
cis-Flupenthixol	3.96*	24	3.2
trans-Flupenthixol	3.96*	850	89

*Data taken from Tollenaere et al. (1977).
van de Waterbeemd et al. (1982) unpublished observations.

For both substituted benzamide drugs and for classical neuroleptic compounds, a log P' value of less than 2.0 was associated with no activity in inhibiting dopamine sensitive adenylate cyclase or in displacing ^{3}H-piflutixol from its specific binding site. Log P' values above 2.0 were associated with inhibition of both systems. However, there was no direct correlation between lipid solubility and the extent of activity at D_1 receptors. This suggests that although lipid solubility is a limiting factor, steric factors also contribute significantly to the action of neuroleptic drugs at D_1 receptors.

In conclusion, substituted benzamide drugs are selective for D_2 receptors, an effect which is not merely a function of lipid solubility. These molecules contain inherent steric factors which dictate their activity at the D_2 site but not at the D_1 receptor site. Activity at D_1 receptors is dependent to some extent on lipid solubility, but within a wide range of lipid solubilities steric factors also dictate the interaction of neuroleptic drugs with these receptor sites.

Correlation between behavioral actions of neuroleptic drugs and their interaction with different ligand binding sites

During the course of these investigations we obtained a large amount of data on the interaction of various neuroleptic drugs in a range of models of dopamine receptor action. We examined the functional effects of these compounds *in vivo* to inhibit apomorphine-induced stereotyped behavior, and their ability to displace a range of ligands from dopamine receptors. We have described already experiments in which we have measured D_2 receptor binding using ^{3}H-spiperone but we have looked also at similar interactions with ^{3}H-sulpiride which also labels adenylate cyclase independent dopamine receptor binding sites (Theodorou et al., 1979 ; 1981). In addition we have measured the interaction of D_1 receptors using dopamine stimulated adenylate cyclase and ^{3}H-piflutixol binding. There is some evidence to suggest that there may be differences between agonist and antagonist binding sites (for example Creese and Sibley, 1979) so we have measured also ^{3}H-N, n-propylnorapomorphine binding to striatal preparations (Hall et al., 1982, unpublished observations).

Using a correlation matrix (Table 3), there was a good correlation between the ability of neuroleptic drugs to inhibit ^{3}H-spiperone binding and their ability to inhibit apomorphine-induced stereotyped behavior *in vivo*. This confirms the assertion that D_2 activity of neuroleptic drugs is associated with functional effects (Leysen, 1982 ; Seeman, 1980). There was no correlation between the ability of neuroleptics to inhibit apomorphine stereotypy and the capacity to act at D_1 receptors as indicated by their ability to inhibit adenylate cyclase activity, or to inhibit ^{3}H-piflutixol binding. There was a correlation between the ability of neuroleptics to displace ^{3}H-spiperone from D_2 sites and their actions in displacing ^{3}H-sulpiride, suggesting overlap in the sites labelled by these ligands. However, there was only marginal correlation between the ability of neuroleptics to inhibit stereotyped behavior and their ability to inhibit ^{3}H-sulpiride binding, suggesting that the functional effects of neuroleptics are not due solely to activity at D_2 receptors labelled by ^{3}H-sulpiride. Also, there was no correlation between the ability of neuroleptics to inhibit apomorphine induced stereotypy and their action at ^{3}H-N,n-propyl-

156

Table 3. — *Correlation matrix for the ability of the neuroleptic drugs examined*
to inhibit apomorphine-induced stereotypy, to inhibit striatal dopamine stimulated adenylate cyclase (AC)
and to inhibit specific binding of ^{3}H-spiperone, ^{3}H-sulpiride, ^{3}H-piflutixol
and ^{3}H-N,n-propylnorapomorphine (NPA) to rat striatal preparations.

	pIC_{50} Stereotypy	pIC_{50} (AC)	pIC_{50} (^{3}H-NPA)	pIC_{50} (^{3}H-piflutixol)	pIC_{50} (^{3}H-spiperone)
pIC_{50} (stereotypy)	-----				
pIC_{50} (AC)	—	-----			
pIC_{50} (^{3}H-NPA)	—	?	-----		
pIC_{50} (^{3}H-piflutixol)	?	?	?	-----	
pIC_{50} (^{3}H-spiperone)	+ +	—	(+)	—	-----
pIC_{50} (^{3}H-sulpiride)	(+)	—	—	?	+

+ + highly significant (p < 0.001)
 + significant (p < 0.01)
(+) marginally significant (p < 0.1)
 — no correlation (p < 0.1)
 ? insufficient data (n ≤ 3)

van de Waterbeemd et al. (1982) unpublished data.

norapomorphine binding sites. Furthermore, there was only a marginal correlation between the ability of neuroleptics to displace ^{3}H-spiperone and to displace ^{3}H-N, n-propylnorapomorphine. Neuroleptic action thus appears separable from agonist binding sites. These data show that the various dopamine receptor sites labelled by different ligands do not all correlate with neuroleptic activity. This does not mean that more than one type of dopamine receptor exists, but may simply reflect the fact that different ligands label different parts of the same receptor complex.

Correlation between lipid solubility and the interaction of neuroleptic drugs with dopamine receptor sites

To investigate the concept that lipid solubility may be the important criteria in determining the action of neuroleptic drugs at dopamine receptor sites, we compared the true partition coefficient (log P) values obtained for the range of neuroleptics examined with indices of their activity at D_2 adenylate cyclase independent receptors. Obviously, we cannot make such comparisons without also considering the steric factors which may also play a marked role in determining relative activity.

The substituted benzamide drugs can be divided into four categories (Fig. 1). These are 1) the diethylaminoethyl substituted benzamides, such as metoclopramide ; 2) the methylpyrrolidinyl substituted compounds, such as sulpiride ; 3) the benzylpyrrolidinyl compounds, such as YM 09151-2 ; and 4) the benzylpiperidinyl substituted benzamides, such as clebopride. As has been discussed previously in this volume (Testa et al., 1982), the relative involvement of the extended and folded conformers of these compounds dictates whether they are sterically favourable or unfavourable for interacting with dopamine receptors. Using this classification we have divided the substituted benzamide drugs into

157

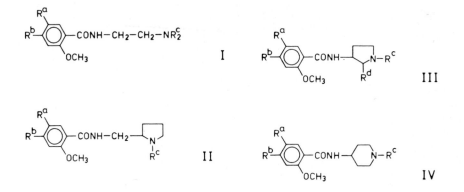

Fig. 1 — Structural classification of substituted benzamide drugs.

Table 4. — *Steric classification of the neuroleptics examined*

Drug	Steric classification	Drug	Steric classification
1. Metoclopramide	—	8. Tigan	—
2. Tiapride	—	9. *cis*-Piflutixol	+
3. Sulpiride	+	10. *trans*-Piflutixol	—
4. Sultopride	+	11. *cis*-Flupenthixol	+
5. Flubepride	+	12. *trans*-Flupenthixol	—
6. YM 09151-2	+	13. Spiperone	+
7. Clebopride	+	14. Haloperidol	+
		15. Trifluoperazine	+
		16. Thioridazine	+

+ = sterically favourable
— = sterically unfavourable
Drugs were classified according to Testa et al (1982).

favourable and unfavourable categories (Table 4). The classical neuroleptic drugs *a priori* are presumed to be sterically favourable, with the exception of the inactive geometric isomers of compounds such as piflutixol and flupenthixol.

Comparison of the ability of the neuroleptic compounds to displace ^{3}H-sulpiride binding with their partition coefficient reveals an interesting relationship (Fig. 2). There is a very limited band of lipid solubility in which maximal pharmacological activity is exerted. A log P value of approximately 4 is optimal for interaction with D_2 receptors. On either side of this value pharmacological activity falls away sharply. It is apparent also that the sterically unfavourable compounds do not fit into the same pattern as those compounds which are deemed sterically favourable. A similar relationship is apparent when we compare the ability of neuroleptics to displace ^{3}H-spiperone from striatal membranes with their partition coefficients (Fig. 3). Again, maximal pharmacological activity is associated with a log P value of approximately 4, and sterically unfavourable compounds do not fit this relationship. Surprisingly, there is a similar relationship between the ability of

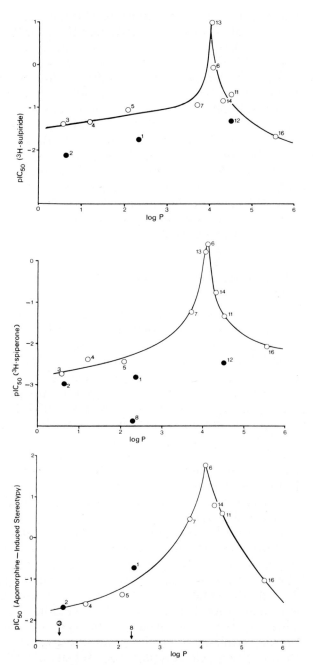

Fig. 2— Correlation between the ability of neuroleptic drugs to displace ^{3}H-sulpiride from rat striatal membranes (pIC$_{50}$) and the true partition coefficient (log P). →

Fig. 3 — Correlation between the ability of neuroleptic drugs to displace ^{3}H-spiperone from rat striatal membranes (pIC$_{50}$) and true partition coefficient (log P). →

Fig. 4 — Correlation between the ability of neuroleptic drugs to inhibit apomorphine-induced stereotyped behavior (pIC$_{50}$) and the true partition coefficient (log P). →

Fig. 2, 3, 4 — The numbers refer to the individual compounds as classified sterically in Table 4. Open circles represent sterically favourable compounds and closed circles sterically unfavourable drugs.

neuroleptic drugs to inhibit apomorphine-induced stereotyped behavior and log P (Fig. 4). In this case, some of the sterically unfavourable compounds appear to fit whereas sterically favourable compounds fall off the correlation. Obviously one must also consider the pharmacodynamic effects of *in vivo* administration when considering such a relationship. This may be responsible for the failure of a poorly lipid soluble drug such as sulpiride to fit on the *in vivo* correlation curve.

As opposed to log P' no correlation exists between the two biological activities and log P'. This suggests that the true, not the apparent, partition coefficient was a dominating factor despite a limited influence of transport phenomena in these *in vitro* systems. There was no correlation between log P and the ability of neuroleptic drugs to inhibit the binding of ^{3}H-N, n-propylnorapomorphine. Whatever sites are identified by this ligand, they are not identical to those which are labelled by ^{3}H-spiperone or ^{3}H-sulpiride or, indeed, to those involved in stereotyped behavior.

The conclusion from these correlations must be that pharmacological activity of the neuroleptic compounds is little influenced by partition coefficient, except within a small range where activity rises and then declines sharply, defining a narrow optimum in the lipophilicity. Such a well defined and narrow optimum in lipophilicity is quite unexpected ; there appear to be few other cases of biological data yielding a similar type of correlation.

Differentiation of the binding of ^{3}H-sulpiride and ^{3}H-spiperone on the basis of cation specificity

All the substituted benzamide drugs we have examined would appear to be selective D_2 dopamine receptor antagonists. However, these drugs may be further sub-divided on the basis of their behavioral actions. Most substituted benzamide drugs, such as sulpiride, do not induce catalepsy and only weakly inhibit other dopamine mediated behaviors, such as apomorphine-induced stereotypy (Jenner and Marsden, 1981). In contrast, the newer potent lipid soluble substituted benzamides, such as clebopride and YM 09151-2, induce pronounced catalepsy and potently inhibit other dopamine mediated behaviors (Elliott et al., 1977 ; Usuda et al., 1981). In this respect they exactly resemble classical neuroleptic compounds, such as spiperone or haloperidol, which also are thought to be selective D_2 antagonists. Why then do these various D_2 active compounds differ from one another in their *in vivo* functional activity ?

There are a number of possible explanations for this apparent difference in behavioral activity. The various drugs may differentially affect dopamine receptors found in different brain areas. There is evidence from the *in vivo* binding of ^{3}H-spiperone or ^{3}H-haloperidol to suggest that sulpiride differentially interacts with dopamine receptors compared to more classical compounds (Kohler et al., 1979, 1981 ; Bartholini, 1982 ; Chivers et al., 1982 unpublished observations). Alternatively, sulpiride may interact with one sub-set of adenylate cyclase independent dopamine receptors, namely D_4 receptors (Sokoloff et al., 1980 ; Sokoloff, 1982). These are believed to lie at a distinct anatomical location within the striatum, that is on the terminals of cortico-striate fibres. There is evidence from our own studies that sulpiride acts at a particular sub-set of dopamine D_2 receptors.

[3]H-sulpiride has specific requirements for interaction with its binding site to striatal membranes (Theodorou et al., 1979, 1982 ; Jenner and Marsden, 1981). The normal incubation buffer utilised in our laboratory includes sodium chloride, potassium chloride, magnesium chloride and calcium chloride. Removal of the cation content of the incubation buffer caused a complete loss of specific ^{3}H-sulpiride

160

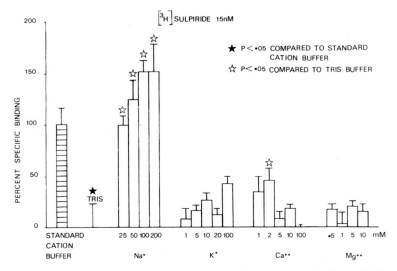

Fig. 5 — The influence of removal of the cation composition of the incubation buffer and replacement by sodium chloride, potassium chloride, calcium chloride and magnesium chloride on the specific binding of ^{3}H-sulpiride (15 nM) to dopamine receptors in rat striatal preparations.
Taken from Jenner and Marsden (1981).

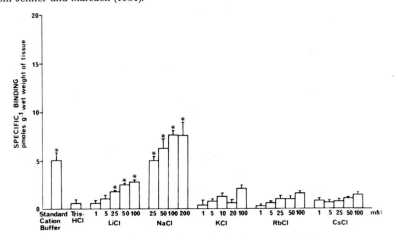

Fig. 6 — The effect of cations from Group 1A of the periodic table on the specific binding of ^{3}H-sulpiride (10 nM) to rat striatal membranes.
Statistical significance is indicated between specific binding obtained in the presence of Tris-HCL buffer alone and that obtained in the presence of the various cations.

* $p < 0.05$ Taken from Theodorou et al. (1982).

binding (Fig. 5). Inclusion of potassium chloride, calcium chloride or magnesium chloride had little or no effect in restoring ^{3}H-sulpiride binding. However, the inclusion of increasing concentrations of sodium chloride caused a concentration-dependent restoration of ^{3}H-sulpiride binding to maximal levels. More recently we have investigated the effect of a range of cations from group 1A of the periodic table. Potassium chloride, rubidum chloride and caesium chloride had no effect on the specific binding of ^{3}H-sulpiride in an otherwise cation free medium (Fig. 6). In-

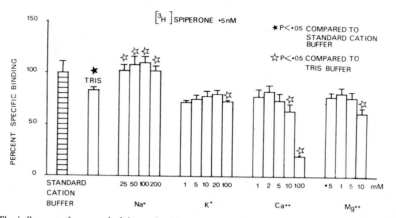

Fig. 7 — The influence of removal of the cation composition of the incubation buffer and replacement by sodium chloride, potassium chloride, calcium chloride and magnesium chloride on the specific binding of ³H-spiperone (0.5 nM) to dopamine receptors in rat striatal membranes. Taken from Jenner and Marsden (1981).

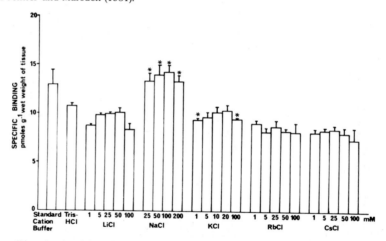

Fig. 8 — The effect of cation from Group 1A of the periodic table of the specific binding of ³H-spiperone (0.2 nM) to rat striatal membranes.
Statistical significance is indicated between specific binding obtained in the presence of Tris-HCL buffer alone and that obtained in the various cations.
* p < 0.05 Taken from Theodorou et al. (1982).

clusion of lithium chloride caused a partial but concentration-dependent increase in ³H-sulpiride binding. So, only sodium chloride can cause a maximal restoration of binding, suggesting a specific dependence upon the presence of this cation ; lithium chloride can produce a partial restoration.

In contrast, the specific binding of ³H-spiperone to striatal homogenates was only slightly reduced by the removal of the cation content of the incubation buffer (Fig. 7). Again, inclusion of potassium chloride, calcium chloride, or magnesium chloride did not restore ³H-spiperone binding, but inclusion of sodium chloride did. Of the other cations from group 1A of the periodic table, lithium chloride, potassium chloride, rubidium chloride and caesium chloride were without effect on ³H-spiperone binding to striatal homogenates (Fig. 8).

The binding of ^{3}H-sulpiride thus is critically dependent upon the presence of sodium ions suggesting an interaction with some highly sodium sensitive binding site. In contrast, the binding of ^{3}H-spiperone exhibits only partial sodium dependency; this may indicate one sodium dependent binding site which is labelled by both ^{3}H-sulpiride and ^{3}H-spiperone, and a second sodium independent site, also labelled by ^{3}H-spiperone, but not by ^{3}H-sulpiride in the concentrations used.

The effect of sodium on the binding of ^{3}H-sulpiride is not understood. It might be argued that sodium produces some conformational changes in a single dopamine receptor binding site which allows the interaction of ^{3}H-sulpiride, but which has little effect on the interaction of ^{3}H-spiperone. This should be reflected in a change in the affinity of ^{3}H-sulpiride for its binding site in the presence of increasing concentrations of sodium chloride. On the other hand, the effect of sodium may be directly involved in the interaction of ^{3}H-sulpiride with a binding site different from that labelled by ^{3}H-spiperone. This would be reflected by a change in the number of ^{3}H-sulpiride binding sites as the sodium chloride concentration was increased. To investigate these possibilities we have looked at the effect of increasing concentrations of sodium chloride and lithium chloride on the number of binding sites (Bmax) and the dissociation constant (K_D) for both ^{3}H-spiperone and ^{3}H-sulpiride to rat striatal preparations.

Increasing the sodium chloride content for the incubation buffer caused a stepwise increase in the number of ^{3}H-sulpiride binding sites (Fig. 9). Little or no change in the dissociation constant was observed. Similarly, increasing the content of lithium chloride produced an increase in Bmax, although this did not reach the level observed in the presence of sodium ions (Fig. 10). In constrast, increasing concentrations of sodium chloride or lithium chloride did not affect the Bmax for ^{3}H-spiperone binding (Fig. 11 and 12). At low salts concentrations the K_D for spiperone binding was increased compared to both cation free buffer and to buffers containing higher concentrations of these cations. The reason for this is unclear.

The conclusion from these experiments is that the sodium dependency of ^{3}H-sulpiride binding is due to a change in the number of available sites as the sodium or lithium content of the incubation buffer increases. There is other evidence to suggest that ^{3}H-spiperone and ^{3}H-sulpiride binding sites may not be identical. In older rats there is a decrease in the number of ^{3}H-spiperone binding sites compared to young rats, but no such decrease in ^{3}H-sulpiride binding is observed (Memo et al., 1980). Also, the sodium-dependent displacement of ^{3}H-spiperone by sulpiride shows a different ontogeny to the development of ^{3}H-spiperone binding sites (Nomura et al., 1981). The effect of prior neuroleptic treatment on ^{3}H-sulpiride and ^{3}H-spiperone is controversial. Trabucchi et al. (1980) have shown that pretreatment of rats with sulpiride for 3 weeks, followed by drug withdrawal, caused an increase in the binding of ^{3}H-sulpiride but not of [3]H- haloperidol. In contrast, treatment of rats with haloperidol for a similar time course produced an increase in ^{3}H-haloperidol binding but not of ^{3}H-sulpiride binding. These results are in contrast to our own data which suggest an equivalent increase in the binding of both ligands (Jenner et al., 1982). However, we employed a much higher dose of sulpiride and haloperidol than did Spano and colleagues, and it may be that the selectivity of effects is only observed at low neuroleptic dosage levels.

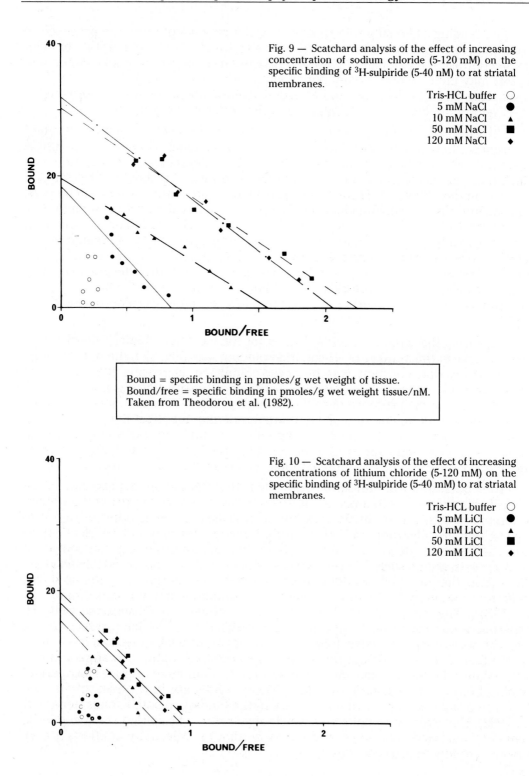

Fig. 9 — Scatchard analysis of the effect of increasing concentration of sodium chloride (5-120 mM) on the specific binding of ^{3}H-sulpiride (5-40 nM) to rat striatal membranes.

Tris-HCL buffer ○
5 mM NaCl ●
10 mM NaCl ▲
50 mM NaCl ■
120 mM NaCl ◆

Bound = specific binding in pmoles/g wet weight of tissue.
Bound/free = specific binding in pmoles/g wet weight tissue/nM.
Taken from Theodorou et al. (1982).

Fig. 10 — Scatchard analysis of the effect of increasing concentrations of lithium chloride (5-120 mM) on the specific binding of ^{3}H-sulpiride (5-40 mM) to rat striatal membranes.

Tris-HCL buffer ○
5 mM LiCl ●
10 mM LiCl ▲
50 mM LiCl ■
120 mM LiCl ◆

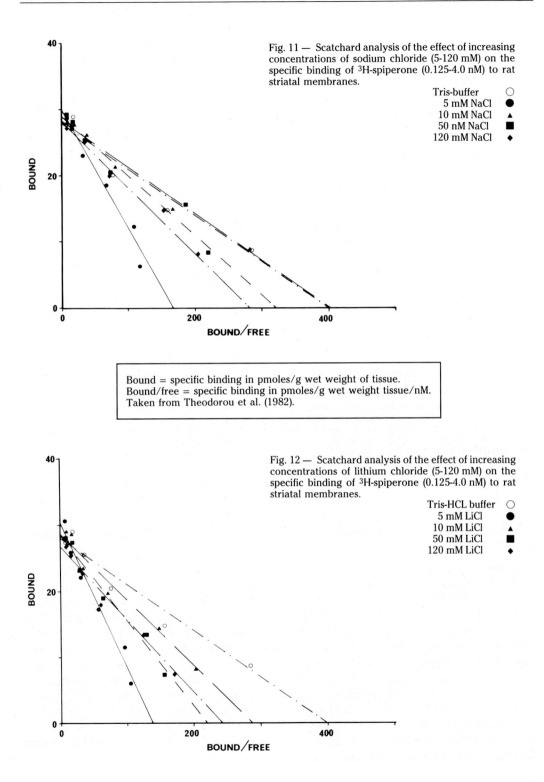

Fig. 11 — Scatchard analysis of the effect of increasing concentrations of sodium chloride (5-120 mM) on the specific binding of ^{3}H-spiperone (0.125-4.0 nM) to rat striatal membranes.

Tris-buffer ○
5 mM NaCl ●
10 mM NaCl ▲
50 nM NaCl ■
120 mM NaCl ◆

Bound = specific binding in pmoles/g wet weight of tissue.
Bound/free = specific binding in pmoles/g wet weight tissue/nM.
Taken from Theodorou et al. (1982).

Fig. 12 — Scatchard analysis of the effect of increasing concentrations of lithium chloride (5-120 mM) on the specific binding of ^{3}H-spiperone (0.125-4.0 nM) to rat striatal membranes.

Tris-HCL buffer ○
5 mM LiCl ●
10 mM LiCl ▲
50 mM LiCl ■
120 mM LiCl ◆

165

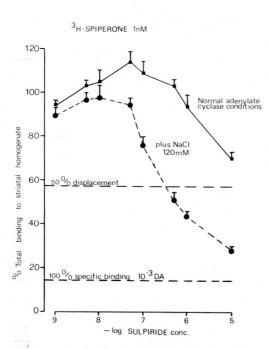

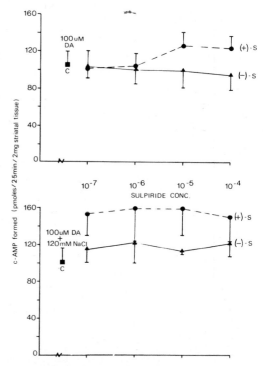

Fig. 13 — Displacement of specific binding of ³H-spiperone (1.0 nM) to rat striatal homogenates by sulpiride (10⁻⁹ — 10⁻⁵M) under conditions used for the assay of adenylate cyclase activity and in the presence and absence of 120 mM sodium chloride. Hall et al. (1982) unpublished observations.

Fig. 14 — The effect of (+)- and (—) -sulpiride (10⁻⁷ - 10⁻⁴M) on the dopamine (100 μM)-induced stimulation of cyclic AMP formation in rat striatal preparations in A) sodium free incubation buffer and in B) buffer containing 120 mM sodium chloride. Taken from Jenner and Marsden (1981).

Is sodium dependency responsible for the failure of sulpiride to inhibit dopamine stimulated adenylate cyclase activity ?

The normal adenylate cyclase system employed does not contain sodium ions. From our results on the binding of ³H-sulpiride, therefore, it is possible that the failure of sulpiride and other substituted benzamide drugs to inhibit this enzyme is due to their inability to interact with their receptor sites in this system. Examination of the specific binding of ³H-spiperone to rat striatal membranes, but using the adenylate cyclase buffer system, shows that the ability of sulpiride to displace ³H-spiperone is increased over 100 times by the inclusion of 120 mM sodium chloride (Fig. 13). However, the inability of sulpiride to inhibit the dopamine-induced stimulation of striatal adenylate cyclase activity in a sodium-free buffer was not altered by the inclusion of 120 mM sodium chloride (Rupniak et al., 1981) (Fig. 14). This again suggests that critical steric factors are involved in molecules such as sulpiride which prevent their interaction with the D_1 adenylate cyclase linked dopamine receptor binding site.

166

Conclusion

Substituted benzamide drugs as a whole are selective antagonists of the D_2 dopamine receptor binding site. The more lipophilic substituted benzamide drugs such as clebopride or YM 09151-2 did not exert a powerful action on D_1 receptors compared to their actions on D_2 receptors ; certainly they are not selective antagonists of D_1 receptors. There is, however, some correlation between lipid solubility and the ability to interact with the D_1 receptor. There appears to be a critical threshold limit above which interaction with D_1 receptors occurs. However, among the compounds showing higher lipid solubility there is no exact correlation between partition coefficient and the extent of the interaction with D_1 receptors. This suggest that considerable steric factors also dictate the interaction of neuroleptic drugs at this site. Functional neuroleptic activity is associated with an action of neuroleptics at D_2 sites. At most values of lipid solubility there is little effect on the pharmacological activity of neuroleptic drugs. However, in a critical small range of log P values, approximately 4.0, pharmacological activity is markedly increased. This would suggest a critical optimal value of lipid solubility for maximal pharmacological response in the interaction of neuroleptics with cerebral dopamine systems. It is clear, however, that neuroleptic drugs are not homogenous in their interaction with D_2 receptor sites. Our correlation matrix suggested that there may be some differences between the sites labelled by ^{3}H-sulpiride and ^{3}H-spiperone. The high sodium dependency of the interaction of ^{3}H-sulpiride with its binding site, compared to ^{3}H-spiperone, confirms this conclusion. Whether sodium independent binding sites and sodium dependent binding sites represents a true differentiation of functional dopamine receptors remains to be determined.

Acknowledgements
This study was supported by the Medical Research Council and the Research Funds of the Bethlem Royal and Maudsley Hospitals and King's College Hospital. B. Testa. and H. van de Waterbeemd are indebted to the Swiss National Science Foundation for research grants 3.448-0.79 and 3.013-0.81.

REFERENCES

Bartholini G. *1982* — Neuroleptics, dopamine receptor subtypes and functional implications. *This volume.*

Creese, I., Sibley, D.R. *1979* — Radioligand binding studies : evidence for multiple dopamine receptors. *Comm. Psychopharmacol., 3 :* 385-395.

Elliott, P.N.C., Jenner, P., Huizing, G., Marsden, C.D., Miller, R. *1977* — Substituted benzamides as cerebral dopamine antagonists in rodents. *Neuropharmacology ; 16 :* 333-342.

Hyttel, J. *1980* — Further evidence that [3]H-*cis*(Z)flupenthixol binds to adenylate cyclase — associated dopamine receptors D_1 in rat corpus striatum. *Psychopharmacology, 67 :* 107-109.

Iwanami, S., Takashima, M., Hirata, V., Hasegawa, O., Usuda, S. *1981* — Synthesis and neuroleptic activity of benzamides. *cis*-N -2-methylpyrrolidin-3-yl)-5-chloro-2-methoxy-4- (methylamino) benzamide and related compounds. *J. Med. Chem. 24 :* 1224-1230.

Jenner, P., Marsden, C.D., *1979a* — The substituted benzamides : A novel class of dopamine antagonists. *Life Sci., 25 :* 479-486.

Jenner, P., Marsden C.D., *1979b* — The mechanism of action of substituted benzamide drugs. *In : Sulpiride and other benzamides,* P.F. Spano, M. Trabucchi, G.U. Corsini and G.L. Gessa (eds) pp. 119-147. Milan, Italian Brain Research Foundation Press.

Jenner, P., Marsden C.D., *1981* — Substituted benzamide drugs as selective neuroleptic agents. *Neuropharmacology., 20 :* 1285-1293.

Jenner, P., Hall, M.D., Murugaiah, K., Rupniak, N., Theodorou, A., Marsden, C.D., *1982* — Repeated administration of sulpiride for three weeks produces behavioural and biochemical evidence for cerebral dopamine receptor supersensitivity. *Biochem. Pharmac., 31 :* 325-328.

Kebabian, J.W., Calne, D.B. *1979* — Multiple receptors for dopamine. *Nature, 227 :* 93-96.

Kohler, C., Ogren, S-O., Haglund, L., Angeby, T. *1979* — Regional displacement by sulpiride of ^{3}H-spiperone binding *in vivo*. Biochemical and behavioural evidence for a preferential action on limbic and nigral dopamine receptors. *Neurosci. Lett., 13 :* 51-56.

Kohler, C., Haglund, L., Ogren, S.-O., Angeby T. *1981* — Regional blockade by neuroleptic drugs of *in vivo* ^{3}H-spiperone binding in the rat brain. Relation to blockade of apomorphine induced hyperactivity and stereotypies. *J. Neurol. Trans., 52 :* 163-173.

Leysen, J.E. *1982* — Review on neuroleptic receptors : specificity and multiplicity of *in vitro* binding relates to pharmalogical activity. *In : Clinical Pharmacology in Psychiatry : Neuroleptic and Antidepressant Research,* E. Usdin, S. Dahl, L.F. Gram, O. Lingjaerde, (eds) Basingstoke, MacMillan.

Memo, M., Lucchi, L., Spano, P.F., Trabucchi, M. *1980* — Ageing process effects a single class of dopamine receptors. *Brain Res., 202 :* 488-492.

Nomura, Y., Oki, K., Segawa, T. *1981* — Striatal ^{3}H-spiperone binding in rats : Ontogenesis of its regulation. Abstract no. 1420, *8th International Congress of Pharmacology, Tokyo, Japan.*

Prieto, J., Moragues, J., Spickett, R.G., Vega, A., Colombo, M., Salazar, W., Roberts, D.J. *1977* — Pharmacological properties of a novel series of antidopaminergic piperidyl benzamides. *J. Pharm. Pharmacol., 29 :* 147-152.

Rupniak, N.M.J., Jenner, P., Marsden, C.D. *1981* — The absence of sodium ions does not explain the failure of sulpiride to inhibit *in vitro* rat striatal dopamine-sensitive adenylate cyclase. *J. Pharm. Pharmacol., 33 :* 602-603.

Seeman, P. *1980* — Brain dopamine receptors. *Pharmac. Rev., 82 :* 229-313.

Sokoloff, P., Martres, M.P., Schwartz, J.C. *1980* — Three classes of dopamine receptors (D-2, D-3, D-4) identified by binding studies with ^{3}H-apomorphine and ^{3}H-domperidone. *Naunyn-Schmiedebergs Arch. Pharmac., 315 :* 89-102.

Sokoloff, P. *1982* — Two classes of dopamine receptors distinguished by substituted benzamides. *This volume.*

Testa, B., van de Waterbeemd, H., Anker, L. *1982* — Structural studies of orthopramides and topological elements of the dopamine receptor. *This volume.*

Theodorou, A., Crockett, M., Jenner, P., Marsden, C.D. *1979* — Specific binding of ^{3}H-sulpiride to rat striatal preparations. *J. Pharm. Pharmacol., 31 :* 424-426.

Theodorou, A., Hall, M.D., Jenner, P., Marsden, C.D. *1980* — Cation regulation differentiates specific binding of ^{3}H-sulpiride and ^{3}H-spiperone to rat striatal preparations. *J. Pharm. Pharmacol., 32 :* 441-444.

Theodorou, A., Reavill, C., Jenner, P., Marsden, C.D. *1981* — Kainic acid lesions of striatum and decortication reduce specific ^{3}H-sulpiride binding in rats, so D-2 receptors exist post synaptically on cortico-striate afferents and striatal neurones. *J. Pharm. Pharmacol., 33 :* 439-444.

Theodorou, A., Jenner, P., Marsden, C.D. *1982* — Cation specificity of ^{3}H-sulpiride binding involves alteration in the number of striatal binding sites. *Life Sci.,* in press.

Tollenaere, J.P., Mœreels, H., Koch, M.H.J. *1977* — On the conformation of neuroleptic drugs in the three aggregation states and their conformational resemblance to dopamine. *Eur. J. Med. Chem., 12 :* 199-211.

Trabucchi, M., Longoni, R., Fresia, P., Spano, P.F. *1975* — Sulpiride : A study of the effects on dopamine receptors in rat neostriatum and limbic forebrain. *Life Sci., 17 :* 1551-1556.

Trabucchi, M., Memo, M., Battaini, F., Reggiani, A., Spano, P.F. *1980* — Effect of long-term treatment with haloperidol and sulpiride on different types of dopaminergic receptors. *In : Long-Term Effects of Neuroleptics.* F. Cattabeni, G. Racagni, P.F. Spano, and E. Costa, (ed) (Adv. Biochem. Psychopharmac. 24) pp. 275-281, New York, Raven Press.

Usuda, S., Sano, K., Maeno, H. *1979* — Pharmacological and biochemial studies on a new potential neuroleptic, N-(benzyl-3-pyrrolidinyl)-5-chloro-2-methoxy-4-methylaminobenzamide (YM-08050). *Arch. Int. Pharmacodyn. Ther., 241 :* 68-78.

Usuda, S., Nishikori, K., Noshiro, O., Maeno, H. *1981* — Neuroleptic properties of *cis*-N-(1-benzyl-2-methyl-pyrrolidin-3yl)-5-chloro-2-methoxy-4-methylamino-benzamide (YM-09151-2) with selective antidopaminergic activity. *Psychopharmacology, 73 :* 103-109.

Woodruff, G.N., Freedman, S.B., Poat, J.A. *1980* — Why does sulpiride not block the effect of dopamine on the dopamine sensitive adenylate cyclase ? *J. Pharm. Pharmacol., 32,* 802-803.

DISCUSSION

S.Z. Langer
When you look at the different concentrations of sodium, you get apparently the same K_D, but changes in the Bmax. Have you checked whether the profile of inhibition of sulpiride binding by drugs is modified at these different sodium levels, in other words, does the concentration of sodium also modify the potency of drugs to inhibit sulpiride binding ?

P. Jenner
Not that way around, but looking at ^3H-spiperone binding and the sodium dependency of sulpiride displacement of ^3H-spiperone, decreasing sodium concentration decreases the ability of sulpiride to displace the ligand.

S.Z. Langer
I think that is a sort of predictable event. What I am saying is whether it is exactly the same binding site and if it has the same profile when you are changing your Bmax as a function of increasing the sodium concentration ? For some sites there is a sodium shift in the potency of agonists and antagonists in inhibiting the high affinity binding. Do you have it for sulpiride ?

P. Jenner
We have not looked at this shift, because we think that there could be some subtle difference between the binding sites. This is the sort of experiment we want to carry out to determine if we can observe any characteristic which will distinguish between the sites, apart from the dependence on sodium ions.

W. H. Vogel
What happens to the conformation of sulpiride if you increase the sodium concentration ?

B. Testa
Within the given range of ionic strength, the conformation behavior of sulpiride is not expected to be detectably affected.

M. Goldstein
Did you check the two isomeres of sulpiride separately ?

P. Jenner
No, we did not. We have been working with racemic sulpiride. We have not determined IC_{50} values for (+) and (—) sulpiride. The major difficulty is, of course, that you cannot do anything in the absence of sodium with ^3H-sulpiride binding, because we have no specific binding at all. So, you have to look at low sodium concentrations, for example 5 or 10 mM compared to 120 mM sodium. It is very frustrating that once the sodium ions are removed you cannot observe anything at all.

K. Fuxe
You have done so much fine work here, also on the character of the action of orthomethoxybenzamides and I wonder whether you have a chance to pharmacologically characterize binding sites ? Let us say some limbic area for the striatum, to see if there is any differentiation in potency or in the Hill coefficient with regard to displacement ?

P. Jenner
From the experiments we have performed we cannot see any difference at all between binding sites for ^3H-sulpiride in nucleus accumbens or tuberculum olfactorium. Affinity appears to be similar. Although the number of sites varies, the IC_{50} values of compounds in displacing from all these areas would appear to be the same.

K. Fuxe
Obviously the conclusion from your experiments would then be that the uniqueness of this group of

compounds lies in its interaction with the different type of binding site, which is different from that of the classical neuroleptic binding sites and that is very important, because that gets you thinking in a different pattern than previously.

G. Groß

Do you only find one binding site for ^{3}H-sulpiride ? I am bearing in mind some slides in which I found no saturation of ^{3}H-sulpiride binding.

P. Jenner

It is true that if you increase the concentration of ^{3}H-sulpiride above about 40 nM, then you start to see a large number of low affinity sites ; Spano and his group say that these sites are specific for substituted benzamide drugs, while other neuroleptics do not displace from this particular site. However, we repeated those experiments and using our ligand binding technique we found that the rank order of potency of drugs in displacing from the low affinity site was the same as for the high affinity site.

Noradrenaline plasma level after sulpiride and other antidepressants during rest and ergometry

M. Ackenheil and N. Matussek

Psychiatric Clinic of the University of Munich, Federal Republic of Germany.

Summary : Sulpiride (100 mg i.v.) in healthy volunteers leads to a short, significant increase of plasma noradrenaline (NA) which is more pronounced with 50 mg i.v. under ergometric charges. It is surprising that maprotiline produces a significant increase, but desimipramine a significant decrease of NA plasma levels with 25 mg i.v. under ergometric work although both substances are powerful NA reuptake inhibitors. On the other hand, after mianserine (1 mg i.v.) there is a significant increase of NA plasma concentration under rest conditions, but not with ergometric charges. The results are discussed in relation to the mechanism of action of the different compounds and to their antidepressant properties.

Introduction

Sulpiride at higher dosage is reported as having neuroleptic and at lower dosage antidepressive properties (Borenstein et al., 1969), however, in general practice in the German Federal Republic it is prescribed more frequently as an antidepressive drug than as a neuroleptic and in spite of this, most pharmacological and biochemical investigations are almost exclusively interested in its neuroleptic effect, i.e. its influence on dopamine receptors. Only recently, it was shown (Gross and Schümann, 1980 ; see also lecture Gross from this symposium) that together with other neuroleptics also sulpiride blocks the pre-synaptic alpha-adrenoreceptors, as has been known for some time in the case of mianserine (Baumann and Maître, 1977 ; Harper and Hughes, 1979). For this reason we studied the effect of sulpiride and other antidepressants in healthy volunteers to see whether with these drugs — as found in our hospital with yohimbine, a known, presynaptic alpha-adrenergic receptor blocker (Laakmann et al., 1981) — an effect on the noradrenaline (NA) plasma level can be observed. Since significant elevations in the NA plasma levels were found with 2,5 mg yohimbine i.v. under resting conditions, we performed our investigations firstly in the same way.

Rest Conditions

With 100 mg sulpiride a short-term, significant plasma NA increase of 37 % was measured, which occurred 15 min after the beginning of the infusion (p < 0.05 ; paired Student t-test, Fig. 1 ; detailed description of the experiments see Ackenheil et al., 1982). This slight and short-term NA elevation leads to no signifi-

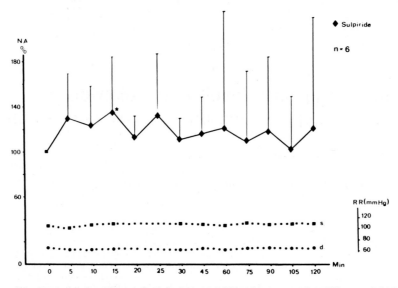

Fig. 1 — Mean NA plasma levels with standard deviation and blood pressure after 100 mg sulpiride in 6 healthy volunteers expressed in percentage of the alterations calculated against time 0 = 100 %. Infusion time between 0 and 10 minutes. *p < 0.05 compared to time 0.

cant changes in the systolic or diastolic blood pressure. On the other hand, sulpiride has no influence on the GH plasma values, but induces the well-known elevation of prolactin.

As one can expect theoretically after application of alpha-2-adrenergic antagonists and simultaneous inhibition of NA reuptake, that the NA increase in plasma should be much higher, the combination of mianserine (2 mg i.v.) and desimipramine (DMI) (0.6 mg i.v.) was investigated in healthy probands. However, in this combination only a short-lasting, non significant increase in plasma NA was found and this increase was not nearly as pronounced as in the combination of yohimbine plus tricyclic thymoleptics (Laakmann et al., 1981).

Since under rest conditions the effects of mianserine and sulpiride on the NA plasma level were not particularly clearly distinct, the studies were carried out under ergometry to see whether the theoretically postulated NA increase could be found under stimulation. In comparison to sulpiride and mianserine, the NA reuptake inhibitors maprotiline and DMI were investigated additionally, however, with the latter drugs we have not yet been able to find any significant NA elevation under rest conditions in acute experiments (unpublished results).

Ergometry

NA levels were measured during 2 successive ergometric charges (EC) in healthy male volunteers, one without medication and the other after infusion of either 50 mg sulpiride (SUL), 1 mg mianserine (MIA), 25 mg maprotiline (MAP) or 25 mg DMI in the same individuum. The ergometric charge (150 watts) was carried out and defined until a pulse rate of 120/minute was reached. The time in which

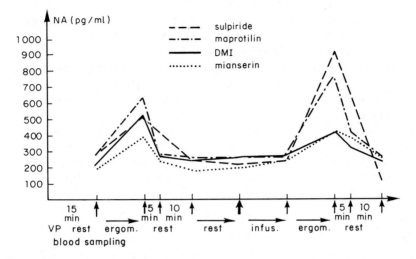

Fig. 2 — Plasma NA changes in normal volunteers during 2 ergometric charges with various antidepressants (SUL, n = 6 ; MIA, n = 8 ; MAP, n = 7 ; DMI, n = 8).
For further explanation see legends to Table I.

Table I : *NA plasma levels during ergometry*
(NA in pg/ml, mean ± SD)

	nb	1	2	3	4	5	6	7
Sulpirde 50 mg	6	285 ± 247	501 ± 217	245 ± 180	222 ± 94	247 ± 110	939 ± 797*	255 ± 109
Mianserine 1 mg	8	209 ± 73	660 ± 510	200 ± 67	206 ± 61	252 ± 52	609 ± 307n.s.	253 ± 61
Maprotiline 25 mg	7	276 ± 177	630 ± 168	259 ± 123	251 ± 63	280 ± 36	767 ± 292*	281 ± 86
Desimipramine 25 mg	8	220 ± 136	529 ± 207	248 ± 103	256 ± 95	270 ± 78	411 ± 135**	236 ± 75

1) First rest 15 min after venipuncture
2) During first ergometry
3) 15 min after first ergometry
4) After 2 hours rest
5) After end of infusion period of the drug (SUL, MAP, DMI = 15 min ; MIA = 1 hour)
6) During second ergometry
7) 15 min after second ergometry
** $p < 0.002$ Δ 2 - 1 vs. Δ 6 - 5
* $p < 0.05$ Δ 2 - 1 vs. Δ 6 - 5
* $p < 0.05$ Δ 2 - 1 vs. Δ 6 - 5

this pulse increase was reached did not differ significantly between the various drugs. Through an indwelling catheter inserted 15 min before the experiment 9 blood samples were drawn respectively before, during and after ergometric work (for details see legends Table I) for the measurement of NA. Systolic and diastolic blood pressure and pulse rate were recorded automatically throughout the whole experiment.

As expected, ergometric work led to a highly significant increase ($p < 0.0001$) of NA values and there were no statistical differences between the 4 groups, neither in basic values nor in the increase due to ergometry (Fig. 2, Table I).

173

Sulpiride (Table I and Fig. 2) administered in a small dosage of 50 mg compared to the dosage of 100 mg showed no significant effect on NA plasma levels during infusion under rest conditions, but ergometric charge-induced NA levels were markedly ($p < 0.05$) elevated, whilst pulse rate and blood pressure remained unchanged between both ergometric tasks.

In the volunteers the atypical antidepressive mianserine (1 mg i.v.) elevated slightly NA plasma levels by the infusion itself ($p < 0.01$). However, the NA elevation induced by ergometric charge was not significantly changed and systolic blood pressure was elevated.

Although the mode of action of maprotiline is considered to be similar to that of DMI, a totally different picture was given. The NA increase (Fig. 2, Table I) induced by the ergometric charge was clearly potentiated after application of maprotiline ($p < 0.05$). After the infusion of maprotiline itself a small, but not significant increase in NA plasma levels occurred. Blood pressure and pulse rate during both ergometric charges were the same.

The DMI infusion (Fig. 2, Table I) again showed a small, but not significant change in the NA secretion after 15 min infusion and surprisingly the NA increase during the second ergometric charge was considerably less ($p < 0.002$) than in the ergometric charge without DMI.

Discussion

Our investigations have shown for the first time *in vivo* on probands, that with sulpiride under rest conditions in a dosage of 100 mg i.v. a short-lasting NA increase occurred, which was even more pronounced with 50 mg i.v. under ergometric charge. This effect is caused most probably through the pre-synaptic alpha-2-adrenergic blockade, as has been demonstrated in animal experiments (Gross and Schümann, 1980). However, the pre-synaptic dopamine receptor blockade on noradrenergic neurons as postulated by Langer (1981) should also be able to induce an enhanced NA release. The NA increase after sulpiride is not as intense as with 2,5 mg or 20 mg yohimbine (Laakmann et al., 1981). The lack of mianserine, which should also influence pre-synaptic alpha-2-adrenergic receptors (Baumann and Maître, 1977 ; Harper and Hughes, 1979), to induce a potentiation of the ergometric-induced increase is most likely due to the fact that mianserine, which is not well tolerated when given i.v., was therefore only given in a low dosage. Whether such a pre-synaptic alpha-adrenergic blockade is responsible for the described antidepressive effect of sulpiride and mianserine cannot be decided according to our results or to the findings reported in the literature. In this context, it should be mentioned that 5 endogenously depressive patients, who have been treated in our clinic with a combination of yohimbine (2.5 and 20 mg i.v.) and tricyclic thymoleptics and in whom a dramatic increase in plasma NA could be measured (Laakman et al., 1981), showed no antidepressive effect. However, further investigations are necessary to prove whether antidepressants with mainly pre-synaptic alpha-adrenergic blockade such as sulpiride and mianserine, probably yohimbine as well, are therapeutically more effective in exogenous (neurotic reactive) depressions. According to neuroendocrine investigations, one could assume that in neurotic-reactive depression a more pre-synaptically induced amine deficit occurs, whereas in endogenous depression diminished post-synaptic alpha-adrenergic receptor sensitivity can be postulated (Matussek, 1982). Especially with regard to so-called « beta-down-regulation » (Sulser et al., 1980), which could be found after repeated administration of antidepressants, one has to remember, that this effect could be observed only with the classic tricyclic thymoleptics, but not with mianserine (Sulser, personal communication). As yet, nothing is known about repeated, chronic administration of sulpiride with regard to this beta-down-regulation.

The most surprising result was that the plasma NA level under ergometric charge with maprotiline increased significantly ($p < 0.05$) whereas with DMI under ergometric charge the plasma NA level was significantly decreased ($p < 0.002$). Both substances inhibit the NA uptake in the brain and the periphery, but in a series of biochemical and pharmacological tests DMI has shown still more pronounced effects on the NA uptake mechanism than maprotiline (for review see Delini-Stula, 1980).

However, on the basis of all the present knowledge about both antidepressants, it is not possible to explain the different effects found by us, therefore, further investigations are necessary.

REFERENCES

Ackenheil, M., Frank, K., Münch, U., Wahlster, U., Matussek, N. *1982* — The influence of various antidepressants on ergometric-induced NA plasma levels. (In preparation).

Baumann, P.A., Maitre, L., *1977* — Blockade of presynaptic alpha-receptors and of amine uptake in the rat brain by the antidepressant Mianserine. *Arch. Pharmacol., 300* : 31-37.

Borenstein, P., Champion, C., Cujo, P., Gekiere, F., Olivenstein, C., Kramarz, P., *1969* — Un psychotrope original : le sulpiride. *Sem. Hôp. Paris 19* : 1301-1314.

Delini-Stula, A., *1980* — Drug-induced alterations in animal behavior as a tool for the evaluation of antidepressants : correlation with biochemical effects. *In : Psychotropic Agents, Part I : Antipsychotics and Antidepressants.* Hoffmeister, F., Stille, G. (eds) Chapt. 21 c, pp 505-526. Berlin/Heidelberg/New York, Springer Verlag.

Gross, G., Schümann, H.J. *1980* — Enhancement of noradrenaline release from rat cerebral cortex by neuroleptic drugs. *Naunyn-Schmiedeberg's Arch. Pharmacol., 315* : 103-109.

Harper, B., Hughes, I.E. *1979* — Presynaptic alpha-adrenoceptor blocking properties among tri- and tetra-cyclic antidepressant drugs. *Br. J. Pharmacol., 67* : 511-517.

Laakmann, G., Dieterle, D., Weiss, L., Schmauss, M. *1981* — Therapeutic and neuroendocrine studies using yohimbine and antidepressants in depressed patients and realthy subjects. Lecture in Nagasaki, Japan, *Symposium « New Vistas in Depression ».* (In press).

Langer, S.Z. *1981* — Presynaptic regulation of the release of catecholamines. *Pharmacol., Rev., 32* : 337-361.

Matussek, N. *1982* — Drugs as tools for exploring neuroendocrine functions. Lecture at the Nobel Conference « *Frontiers in Biochemical and Pharmacological Research in Depression* », Stockholm, 18-19 June. (In press).

Sulser, F., Mobley, P.L. *1980* — Biochemical effects of antidepressants in animals. *In : Psychotropic Agents. Part I : Antipsychotics and Antidepressants.* Hoffmeister, F., Stille, G. (eds.) Chapt. 21 a, pp 471-490. Berlin/Heidelberg/New York, Springer Verlag.

This study was supported by SANDOZ-TIFTUNG for THERAPEUTIC RESEARCH.

DISCUSSION/N. MATUSSEK

J. Mendlewicz
Have you used yohimbine alone in depressed patients ?

N. Matussek
No, we have not.

J. Mendlewicz
Are you aware of such studies ?

N. Matussek
No, but I think that we should do some with untreated depressive patients, maybe first with yohimbine alone and then in combination with another antidepressant. My hypothesis would be : Both neurotic-reactive depressive patients and Prof. Vogel's animals will show a fast antidepressant or activating effect.

W.H. Vogel
When I asked for some criticism of my model, I did not ask for that much criticism — joking aside ! Your data were very interesting, but I think they differ a bit from what we do. You challenge with a drug, we do not challenge with a drug, we challenge the animal with an outside situation, with which the animal can either cope or cannot cope.

R.M. Post
Did the normal volunteers on yohimbine become more anxious ?

N. Matussek
With the dosages we used in volunteers no anxiety appeared. But when it was applied in patients in combination with tricyclics, sometimes agitation and restlessness were observed.

Y. Lecrubier
We made very similar studies, because we had the same idea about this possibility with yohimbine and effectively we did not find any potentiation of antidepressant effect of tricyclic antidepressants, but we found a quite good effect on orthostatic hypotension, which was very interesting even therapeutically for patients. We had a lot of patients with that association due to that other indication and looking at the moment when the combination was given, we can say that with most patients nothing happens really for either endogenous or reactive depressives. I am of the opinion that there is no effect. One problem is that we do not know the clinical pharmacology of yohimbine in man and I think this is a basic problem and when giving those 10 to 20 mg range doses in man you probably have no effect on the CNS. I am not sure whether this has been done before.

N. Matussek
We gave an increasing dosage up to 20 mg in the first 7 days. But I have a question : Did the reactive depressive patients in your group really not react to yohimbine ?

Y. Lecrubier
One of our group tried monotherapy, but only in some reactive depressed patients. He claimed that it was good, but I think he also claimed that this lasted some days and disappeared, so with such results in reactive patients I am not sure how you can interpret them. I think it is amazing that there is not any really up-to-date controlled study using yohimbine alone in depression.

N. Matussek
Yes, it is a pity.

G. Groß
Have you read about the bioavailability of yohimbine in the brain ? Does it pass the blood-brain barrier to a greater extent ?

N. Matussek
I think so.

S.Z. Langer
I think that from the known animal studies, yohimbine crosses the blood-brain barrier very effect-ively and studies on turnover of noradrenaline and MOPEC levels in the CNS indicate that yohimbine does indeed cross the blood-brain barrier without any problem. The question I wanted to pose con-cerns the selectivity of yohimbine for alpha-2-adrenoreceptors, which is perhaps a little bit over-estimated or exaggerated. Yohimbine does indeed block alpha-2-adrenoreceptors preferentially, but it does block alpha-1-adrenoreceptors as well and that can be demonstrated very clearly in the periphery. Therefore, if one assumes that one is blocking alpha-1-adrenoreceptors in the CNS with the doses of yohimbine used, it is not to be excluded that such blockade of the alpha-1-adrenoreceptors may influence the results. If for a moment we speculate that increasing noradrenergic neurotransmission or increasing the concentration of noradrenaline in the synaptic gap is somehow involved in the amelioration of depression by tricyclics which inhibit noradrenaline uptake, then at least 4 receptor sub-types for noradrenaline could be involved post-synaptically in this action (alpha-1, alpha-2, β-1 and β-2). If the β-1 receptor is down-regulated, one could conclude that it may be an epi-phenomenon and not the receptor directly involved in antidepressant action. The alpha-2 is unlikely, because we know that alpha-2-agonists acting centrally would produce in-hibition or depression rather than stimulation. So, although this is highly speculative, I must admit, that the alpha-1-receptor may be the important one and then if you use a compound like yohimbine, which is preferential, but not selective enough and you block simultaneously the alpha-1 and the alpha-2-receptor, you may be really blocking a receptor necessary for this effect. Perhaps, what we need is an alpha-2-antagonist acting centrally which is much more selective than yohimbine. In order to block exclusively and selectively the alpha-2-adrenoreceptor, we need a sort of equivalent of prazosin for the alpha-1-receptor. Maybe the compounds that are becoming available now, for in-stance the compound of Reckitt and Colman 781094, which is 10-times more selective than yohim-bine in blocking alpha-2-adrenoreceptors, will provide the possibility to explore this hypothesis.

N. Matussek
Laakmann et al. (1981) of our hospital showed that the DMI-induced GH response is reduced after yohimbine as with phentolamine, which could result from a post-synaptic alpha-adrenoreceptor blockade. But is the increase in blood pressure not a sign that there is also a post-synaptic adrenergic receptor stimulation ?

S.Z. Langer
I do not know. Some people say that the increase in blood pressure by yohimbine is a centrally mediated effect and that is much more complicated.

N. Matussek
I do not know either. What do you think about the mechanism of clonidine in this connection ? Together with the stimulation of post-synaptic alpha-2-receptors in the brain you find a decrease in blood pressure. Similarly, would you not expect after yohimbine together with the increase in noradrenaline in the brain a decrease in blood pressure ? However, what you find is an increase !

S.Z. Langer
You could argue that the sites of action of clonidine, which are predominantly in the medulla oblon-gata, are not the same sites where increased levels of noradrenaline in the brain would produce the same effect. The effects of clonidine are really quite selective to certain areas of the brain where you produce this cardiovascular depression which is reflected in hypotension.

K. Fuxe
I remember that when we analysed yohimbine a couple of years ago, actually many years ago, we not only saw this very powerful action on noradrenaline turnover, but we also noticed a concom-itant reduction of serotonin within approximately the same dose range, again indicating that yohim-bine is still a rather unselective drug and that may be a problem for interpretation.

N. Matussek

But with some antidepressants you also block the post-synaptic serotonin receptor, as you have demonstrated. If yohimbine had such action, it could be a more effective antidepressant.

K. Fuxe

I certainly agree with you. I just wanted to indicate that perhaps with yohimbine we should not only focus on the alpha-2 or alpha-1 receptors.

M. Goldstein

I would just like to point out that in spontaneously hypotensive rats, yohimbine actually lowers blood pressure and does not increase it. This could be the answer to your question about the noradrenaline in the brain.

K. Fuxe

It may be of interest to mention that we did some experiments with intracysternal injections of yohimbine in anaesthetized rats and similar to many other alpha-blockers it increases blood pressure upon central administration. There is a very clear-cut, rather powerful increase of the arterial blood pressure.

Y. Lecrubier

We are focusing on receptors, but perhaps we should not forget the patients ! What I mean is that we do not know why enhancing noradrenaline in the CNS could be useful for these patients. We do not know if these patients would react like normal volunteers when you give them yohimbine. What happens with the alpha-2-receptor of depressed patients, and if you block it can you really enhance the level of noradrenaline in the patient ? That is, if you do not know the mechanism of depression.

N. Matussek

This is very true. We have to consider the state of the system, where a drug develops its action. The metabolic situation of a nerve ending is certainly different in a depressed patient from that in a healthy volunteer or in a rat. Actually, some neuroendocrine studies have shown that antidepressant treatment with the same drug produces different results in endogenously depressed patients as compared to neurotic-reactively depressed patients regarding their GH responses to insulin, clonidine or DMI. Therefore, we have to be careful when interpreting the mechanism of action of antidepressant drugs found in animal experiments and then applying it to depressed patients.

DISCUSSION/M. ACKENHEIL

W.H. Vogel

These data are very interesting to me. You find that the adrenaline increases more in individuals who have to do mental arithmetic as opposed to physical activity. In our animals we find that the plasma adrenaline seems to be most responsive to the situation of which an animal has control over or has no control over. In other words, if the animal can cope, adrenaline seems to rise slightly ; if the animal cannot cope with the situation, then the adrenaline levels in the plasma rise significantly. Is it possible that the individual goes on the ergometer and says : That is a very simple task, I can cope with it. On the other hand, in the mental arithmetic task he may say : Now I have to subtract a figure from another figure and maybe I will fail, maybe I cannot do it. He is fearful that he cannot cope, therefore, the difference is a measure of the coping capability of the individual. This is the first question. Second question : As a clinician, do you feel that the depressed patient has a deficit in the coping mechanism : The depressed patients feels, « I cannot cope » and therefore he gives up more easily. A volunteer or normal person would say « I can cope with it, I can do it » and his adrenaline levels would then not rise as much ?

M. Ackenheil

It is more complicated. When considering e.g. the coping capability for this arithmetic task, of course, you do not know exactly how the volunteer or patient feels whether he will be able to cope with the situation or not. In the other situation, such as unstructured noise, it is probable that it will not be coped with, however, it depends again on how one reacts to this situation and it seems e.g. that patients do not react adequately to noise.

J. Mendlewicz

I am sure, Prof. Vogel, that you must be famil ar with Beck's hypothesis of cognitive dysfunction in depression and this may very well be relevant to these types of experiments.

P. Grof

I was wondering, were you able to look at individual volunteers as they went through different antidepressant experiments, whether they were showing similarity in the response over a period of time ? We have been conducting neuroendocrine experiments with a variety of challenges and it is striking, that when you look at individuals over a specific period of time there seems to be much more intra-individual similarity than one would expect from different challenges. Many volunteers seem to respond in a certain individual pattern, almost regardless of the pharmacological challenge, particularly in the acute experiments. I think that sometimes the results may reflect more the final composition of the sample than the challenge, i.e. how many high-reactive and how many low-reactive subjects you have. The only way to tease such reactivity out, is to look at individuals over a length of time and to go back to the data and try to identify it. Have you made such observations ?

M. Ackenheil

This problem is very complex. As it is known from the stress literature that habituation effects occur which depend on the kind of stress situation and if the same stress experiment is repeated in the same individuum. With regard to our experiments with psychiatric patients, we could not repeat the experiments. Therefore, we compared the patients' data with random samples according to age and sex. To investigate the effect of drugs, we used the ergometer challenge twice, because there should be no adaptation to this challenge.

N. Matussek

If some types of depression were related to a noradrenaline deficit, you should treat such patients with ergometer tasks, jogging or some other physical activity, in order to increase their noradrenaline output, as in your experiments. Have you or someone else experience with the antidepressant action of body activity ?

M. Ackenheil

It could be that depending on the nosology, neurotic or endogenous depressives could react with a deviation to the ergometric task, similar to our results with sleep deprivation. One can speculate that a series of events are necessary for such a therapeutic effect. At the beginning a noradrenaline increase, later on changes in receptor sensitivity, which can be measured with binding assays on peripheral blood cells. We are investigating such effects at the moment in our clinic.

J. Mendlewicz

Prof. Matussek, if the patients are able to jog, then they do not have a very severe depression !

Y. Lecrubier

The correlation between therapeutic effect and plasma levels of antidepressants was described sometimes as an inverted U-shape. For your DMI results, do you have several dosages, so that you can perhaps pick up different effects on noradrenaline with different plasma levels of that drug ?

M. Ackenheil

Until now we have not done such investigations. In volunteers only one dosage was applied. We have not done this yet with patients, but we are just beginning to make such investigations under treatment with antidepressives.

179

N. Matussek

Dr. Lecrubier, I would like to mention that Dr. Laakmann in our hospital found a quite nice dose-response curve of GH after DMI, but no differences in noradrenaline plasma levels after the various DMI dosages. On the other hand, GH response to maprotiline was similar to that after DMI.

M. Ackenheil

There is the possibility that after 3 weeks of treatment with sulpiride the increased noradrenaline release is reversed. This assumption is supported by a preliminary result.

Ch. Eggers

Prof. Matussek, I think you are right. I can only tell you about a single case : I have a colleague at the faculty in Essen, who has a mixed reactive-endogenous depression and therefore has to take antidepressants. Since he has become involved in playing tennis regularly, he has become less depressed and his subjective feeling is that he has far fewer phases.

J. Mendlewicz
Even if he loses ?

Clinical, biochemical and pharmacokinetic studies of sulpiride in schizophrenic patients

G. Sedvall, G. Alfredsson, L. Bjerkenstedt, C. Härnryd, G. Oxenstierna and F.-A. Wiesel.

Department of Psychiatry and Psychology, Karolinska Institute, Stockholm, Sweden.

Summary : The clinical, biochemical and pharmacokinetic variables were recorded in 50 schizophrenic patients participating in a double-blind comparison of the effects of sulpiride (800 mg daily) and chlorpromazine (400 mg daily). The study lasted eight weeks. Six patients in the sulpiride group and eight patients in the chlorpromazine group were removed from the study due to unsatisfactory therapeutic responses. There were marked and significant reductions in the ratings of psychotic morbidity (CPRS) in both treatment groups. One to two weeks after the beginning of the treatment, the patients treated with sulpiride had significantly lower global scores and lower scores in hallucinations and withdrawal. Side effects occurred in about the same low frequency in both treatment groups. The concentration of the major dopamine metabolite, homovanillic acid, increased during the treatment, with a maximal concentration after two weeks and a tendency towards tolerance at the end of the treatment period. The prolactin concentrations in plasma and CSF were more markedly increased in sulpiride treated patients. The prolactin levels reached a plateau after one week of treatment and remained high during the rest of the study period. The morning values of sulpiride concentration in the serum reached steady-state levels within the first week of treatment and varied between 225 and 1125 μg/ml. There was no tendency towards a reduction of sulpiride concentration in serum during the study period. The results support the view that sulpiride has a marked antipsychotic effect in schizophrenic patients and that the dose administered results in a marked blockade of the central receptors for dopamine.

Introduction

The development of benzamides with different pharmacological profiles (Justin-Besançon et al., 1967) during the last decades has been of considerable theoretical and practical interest. The claim of a rather specific D_2-receptor interaction with some of these compounds (Trabucchi et al., 1975) and their promotion for the treatment of as different clinical entities as gastrointestinal disturbances, schizophrenia and depression (Borenstein et al., 1968 ; Ishimaru et al., 1971, Burchard et al., 1972) has attracted the attention of neurobiologists, as well as of clinical psychiatrists to this class of compounds. However, the claim of a broad clinical profile of action of sulpiride calls for a critical evaluation of the therapeutic efficacy under the conditions mentioned.

The present study was performed to further evaluate the clinical potential of sulpiride in the treatment of psychotic reactions of the schizophrenic type. The clinical, biochemical and pharmacokinetic variables were recorded during the treatment of schizophrenic patients for eight weeks, using a fixed dose of sulpiride. Chlorpromazine was used as the reference compound. The present report describes the results obtained by a preliminary evaluation.

Methods

The study was performed on 50 schizophrenic patients fulfilling the Research Diagnostic Criteria (RDC) of Spitzer et al., 1977. The age range of the patients was between 18 and 45 years. After an initial period, during which the patients were kept drug free, sulpiride or chlorpromzine was administered according to a double-blind design. The protocol of the study, which was approved by the ethics committee, is presented in Figure 1. The patients received 800 mg of sulpiride or 400 mg of chlorpromazine, daily. The doses were successively increased during the first five days of treatment until the final doses were reached. These were kept constant during the rest of the study which lasted eight weeks. Before and during the course of the treatment, clinical ratings of psychotic morbidity (CPRS, Åsberg et al., 1978) and side effects (Bjerkenstedt et al., 1978) were recorded. In relation to the clinical ratings, lumbar cerebrospinal fluid and plasma samples were taken to measure monoamine metabolites, prolactin and drug concentrations. The monoamine metabolite concentrations were measured according to the GC/MS-method of Swahn et al., 1976, and the prolactin concentrations in CSF and plasma were measured using a commercial radioimmunoassay (Serono, Italy). The concentrations of sulpiride, chlorpromazine and of two of its metabolites were determined using high performance liquid chromatography (Alfredsson et al., 1979) and GC/MS (Alfredsson et al., 1976).

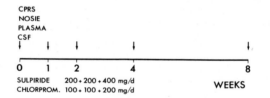

Fig. 1 - Protocol for double blind comparison between sulpiride and chlorpromazine in the treatment of 50 young schizophrenic (RDC) patients.

Results

During the early phase of the study six patients in the sulpiride group and eight patients in the chlorpromazine group were eliminated, either because they refused to follow the protocol, or because the severity of the psychosis was such as to make it impossible to complete the study for ethical reasons.

During the initial part of the study, additional medication, in the form of benzodiazepines for sedative purposes and biperiden for extrapyramidal manifestations, were administered to some patients. The sedatives were mostly administered as single doses during the early part of the study. The total amount of benzodiazepines was higher in the sulpiride treated patients than in those treated with chlorpromazine. Three patients in the sulpiride group showed extrapyramidal manifestations which required treatment with biperiden, while only one patient in the chlorpromazine group required such treatment.

Psychotic morbidity

Using several evaluations of psychotic morbidity from the CPRS variables, it was found that both treatments resulted in a significant improvement. Some examples of such effects are shown in Figures 2-4. During the early course of the treatment sulpiride treated patients often showed a significantly lower degree of morbidity than chlorpromazine treated patients.

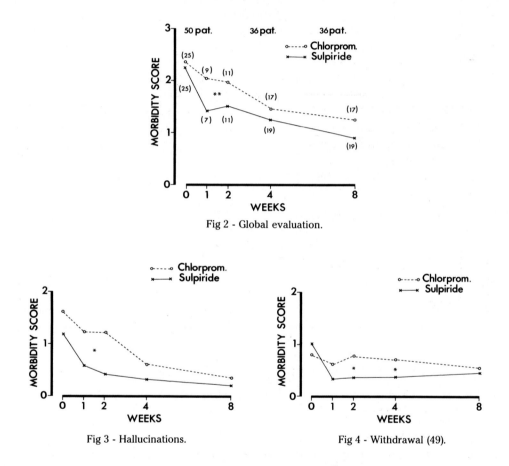

Fig 2 - Global evaluation.

Fig 3 - Hallucinations.

Fig 4 - Withdrawal (49).

Side effects

The frequencies of side effects were of about the same low order of magnitude in both groups. There were no significant differences in the degree of sedation, or of extrapyramidal manifestations in the two groups. Parkinsonian symptoms occurred in some patients in both groups.

Biochemical variables

Both treatments increased the concentration of the major dopamine metabolite, homovanillic acid (HVA), in the lumbar cerebrospinal fluid (Fig. 5). The

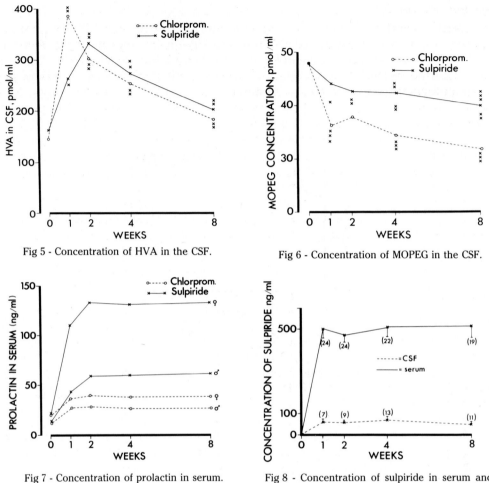

Fig 5 - Concentration of HVA in the CSF.

Fig 6 - Concentration of MOPEG in the CSF.

Fig 7 - Concentration of prolactin in serum.

Fig 8 - Concentration of sulpiride in serum and CSF of schizophrenic patients (oral dose 800 mg/day).

HVA increase did not differ between the two groups. The HVA effect was more marked during the first two weeks of treatment, decreasing subsequently. After eight weeks, HVA was still significantly high in both groups. The concentration of the major noradrenaline metabolite (MOPEG) decreased significantly in both groups (Fig. 6). The MOPEG reduction was significantly more marked in the chlorpromazine group. The prolaction concentrations in serum were much higher in sulpiride treated patients than in the chlorpromazine treated ones. In both groups prolactin concentrations were markedly sex-dependent (Fig. 7).

Pharmacokinetic variables

The concentration of sulpiride was determined in plasma, as well as in CSF (Fig. 8). Already during the first week of treatment, the concentration reached a

184

plateau, which remained approximately constant during the following part of the treatment.

Discussion

In the present study fixed doses of sulpiride and chlorpromazine were used for a comparative study in young schizophrenic patients. The doses were selected on the basis of previous clinical experience of other authors as well as of our own clinicians (Klein and Davis, 1969 ; Toru et al., 1972, Bratfos and Haug 1979, Wode-Helgodt et al., 1977 ; Bjerkenstedt et al., 1979). In previous studies, the doses selected here were found to produce a marked reduction of psychotic morbidity in patients of the same type as those examined in the present investigation. The results confirmed the marked psychotic morbidity reduction in patients submitted to either of the two treatments. During the first two weeks of treatment, the reduction of psychotic morbidity as regards global rating, hallucinations and withdrawal indicated a more rapid onset of action of the sulpiride treatment than of the chlorpromazine treatment. These findings may reflect a true difference in the rate of onset of the antipsychotic action of sulpiride and chlorpromazine. Ishimaru et al., 1971 and Cassano et al., 1975 had previously found that sulpiride had a faster action than perphenazine and haloperidol, respectively. However, sulpiride treated patients received greater amounts of benzodiazepines for sedation during the early phase of the treatment. This indicates a lower sedative effect of sulpiride, possibly also that the interaction of sulpiride and benzodiazepines may result in a more marked reduction of psychotic morbidity. Four and eight weeks after the beginning of treatment, there were no significant differences in morbidity scores between the two treatment groups. The antipsychotic effect of the reference drug, chlorpromazine, has been well documented during more than two decades. The present results, which demonstrate a similar reduction in psychotic morbidity in sulpiride and chlorpromazine treated patients, give strong support to the view that the dose of sulpiride used has an antipsychotic effect of a similar magnitude as that of the reference treatment.

Side effects occurred at low frequency in both treatment groups. Extrapyramidal manifestations of the Parkinsonian type, requiring the administration of an anticholinergic agent, occurred in three sulpiride and one chlorpromazine treated patients. This finding supports the view that both drugs interfere with dopaminergic mechanisms also in basal ganglia, and there does not appear to be any marked difference in the degree of extrapyramidal manifestations after either treatment. Side effects like sedation and salivary secretion occurred also in about the same low frequency during either treatment.

The clinical results of this study thus support the view that sulpiride has about the same potential as chlorpromazine for the treatment of psychoses of the schizophrenic type.

The biochemical results strongly support the view that sulpiride blocks central dopamine receptors in schizophrenic patients (Bjerkenstedt et al., 1979). The marked increase in HVA concentration and the effect on prolactin concentration indicate a blockade of the striatal and pituitary dopamine receptors at the dose used. The time course of these effects differed, however. Whereas the prolactin increase was maintained throughout the study period, there was a marked reduction in HVA

185

increase during the course of treatment. The reduction of the HVA elevation with time may indicate the development of tolerance to the dopamine receptor blockade in the basal ganglia, as regards the eight week treatment period. This is in agreement with the results previously obtained by Post and Goodwin (1975) in haloperidol treated patients. Since the prolactin did not decrease with time, one may think that the pituitary dopamine receptors do not develop tolerance, or that the drug concentrations produced a supramaximal effect.

The determinations of drug concentration indicated that steady state levels had already been obtained within the first week of treatment. There was no tendency towards a decrease in drug concentrations either in the plasma, or in CSF, which is against the view that sulpiride metabolism may be induced during the treatment. This maintainance of sulpiride concentration in the body fluids during the course of treatment is in conflict with the possibility that the reduction with time, of HVA levels in CSF is related to a pharmacokinetic tolerance. Rather, the finding that the prolactin increase as well as the drug concentration are maintained in spite of a reduction in HVA concentration in the CSF, strongly supports the view that a pharmocodynamic tolerance, possibly the induction of more dopamine receptors, is the cause of the decrease in HVA concentration.

It should be noticed that, as previously found for chlorpromazine, melperone and electroconvulsive treatment (Wode-Helgodt et al., 1977 ; Härnryd et al., 1979), sulpiride treatment results in a reduction of MOPEG concentration in the CSF. As regards the apparent lack of effect of sulpiride on noradrenaline receptors (Kohli and Cripe, 1979), the MOPEG reduction may be related to secondary mechanisms induced by these treatments. A further analysis of the mechanism of this effect should be valuable for the elucidation of its role in the production of the antipsychotic effect of sulpiride.

Acknowledgements
The present study was supported by the Swedish Medical Research Council (B82-21X-03560-11A), AB Essex, Stockholm, Karolinska Institutet, and the Groschinsky and Jeansson Foundations.

REFERENCES

Alfredsson, G., Wode-Helgodt, B., Sedvall, G. *1976* - A mass fragmentographic method for the determination of chlorpromazine and two of its active metabolites in human plasma and CSF. *Psychopharmacology, 48 :* 123-131.

Alfredsson, G., Sedvall, G., Wiesel, F.-A. *1979* - Quantitative analysis of sulpiride in body fluids by high performance liquid chromatography with fluorescence detection. *J. Chromatogr., 164 :* 187-193.

Asberg, M., Montgomery, S., Perris, C., Schalling, D., Sedvall, G. *1978* - CPRS - The comprehensive psychopathological rating scale. *Acta Psychiatr. Scand.,* Suppl. 271.

Bjerkenstedt, L., Härnryd, C., Grimm, V., Gullberg, B., Sedvall, G. *1978* - A double-blind comparison of melperone and thiothixene in psychotic women using a new rating scale, the CPRS. *Arch. Psychiatr. Nervenkr., 226 :* 157-172.

Bjerkenstedt, L., Härnryd, C., Sedvall, G. *1979* - Effect of sulpiride on monoaminergic mechanisms in psychotic women. *Psychopharmacology, 64 :* 135-139.

Borenstein, P., Cujo, P., Champion, C., Olivenstein, C. 1968 - Études d'un nouveau psychotrope - le sulpiride (1403 RD). Méthodes et résultats clinique. *Ann. Méd.-Psychol. (Paris), 2 :* 90-99.

Bratfos, O., Haug, J.O. *1979* - Comparison of sulpiride and chlorpromazine in psychoses : A double-blind multicentre study. *Acta Psychiatr. Scand., 60 :* 1-9.

Burchard, J.M., Gross, L., Kempe, P. *1972* - Sulpirid : Stationäre und ambulante Behandlung psychiatrischer Patienten und Doppelblinduntersuchung des Wirkungsspektrums. *Int. J. Clin. Pharmacol. Ther. Toxicol., 6 :* 266-268.

Cassano, G.B., Castrogiovanni, P., Conti, L. *1975* - Sulpiride versus haloperidol in schizophrenia : A double-blind comparative trial. *Curr. Ther. Res., 17 :* 189-201.

Härnryd, C., Bjerkenstedt, L., Grimm, V.E., Sedvall, G. *1979* - Reduction of MOPEG levels in cerebrospinal fluid of psychotic women after electroconvulsive treatment. *Psychopharmacology, 64 :* 131-134.

Ishimaru, T., Kubo, S., Ishikawa, H., Jitsuiki, S., Kawamura, T., Kimura, N., Kodama, H., Masuda, K., Miyake, Y., Nomura, S., Sasaki, T., Shimonaga, K., Tsukue, I., Asada, S. *1971* - Clinical evaluation on therapeutic effects of sulpiride, a neuroleptic drug, on schizophrenia by double-blind controlled test. *Hiroshima J. Med. Sci., 19 :* 131-154.

Justin-Besançon, L., Thominet, M., Laville, C., Margarit, J. *1967* - Constitution chimique et propriétés biologiques du sulpiride. *C.R. Acad. Sci. (Paris), 265 :* 1253-1254.

Klein, D.F., Davis, J.M. *1979 - Diagnosis and drug treatment of psychiatric disorders.* Baltimore, Williams and Wilkins.

Kohli, J.D., Cripe, L.D. *1969* - Sulpiride : A weak antagonist of norepinephrine and 5-hydroxytryptamine. *Eur. J. Pharmacol., 56 :* 283-286.

Post, R.M., Goodwin, F.K. *1975* - Time-dependent effect of phenothiazines on dopamine turnover in psychiatric patients. *Science, 190 :* 488-489.

Spitzer, R.L., Endicott, J., Robins, E. *1977 - Research diagnostic criteria for a selected group of functional disorders.* Bethesda, National Institute of Mental Health.

Swahn, C.-G., Sandgärde, B., Wiesel, F.-A., Sedvall, G. *1976* - Simultaneous determination of the three major monoamine metabolites in brain tissue and body fluids by a mass fragmentographic method. *Psychopharmacology, 48 :* 147-152.

Toru, M., Shimazono, Y., Miyasaka, M., Kokubo, T., Mori, Y., Nasu, T. *1972* - A double-blind comparison of sulpiride with chlorpromazine in chronic schizophrenia. *J. Clin. Pharmacol., 12 :* 221-229.

Trabucchi, M., Longoni, R., Freisia, P., Spano, P.F. *1975* - Sulpiride : A study of the effects on dopamine receptors in rat neostriatum and limbic forebrain. *Life Sci., 17 :* 1551-1556.

Wode-Helgodt, B., Fyrö, B., Gullberg, B., Sedvall, G. *1977* - Effect of chlorpromazine treatment on monoamine metabolite levels in cerebrospinal fluid of psychotic patients. *Acta Psychiatr. Scand., 56 :* 129-142.

Wode-Helgodt, B., Eneroth, P., Fyrö, B., Gullberg, B., Sedvall, G. *1977* - Effect of chlorpromazine treatment on prolactin levels in cerebrospinal fluid and plasma of psychotic patients. *Acta Psychiatr. Scand., 56 :* 280-293.

DISCUSSION

Ch. Eggers

I would like to ask a couple of questions. Firstly, how old was your youngest patient and are there any teenagers in your group ? The second question concerns the drug chlorpromazine. In Germany the drug chlorpromazine is a "dirty" drug, because of its side effects. Which side effects have you measured ? I am particularly interested if there are side effects on the liver function. Third question : You have seen a decrease of the HVA in the 5-hydroxyindol-acetic-acid ratio. The same was found in 10 children with a tic syndrome by Cohen et al., but inverse to your findings the HVA in these cases was relatively higher than the 5-hydroxyindol-acetic-acid.

G. Sedvall

I am not quite sure what was the lowest age range of patients, but it was certainly not below 18 years of age, so there are no pubertal conditions. The age range of these patients according to the protocol should be between 18 and 45 years, just to indicate that we do not have any really severe, chronic patients in this group. Regarding your question on side effects, we have a scale for clinical recording of a number of ratings of symptoms, which include sedation, autostatism and all the extrapyramidal manifestations put down to different symptoms. With regard to the liver function test, we have not evaluated these data yet, but I feel quite sure that in a number of these patients we have quite marked elevations of the transaminases for those treated with chlorpromazine. Of course, this is the usual finding for chlorpromazine treatment, it is a dirty drug in this respect, certainly I cannot say yet whether we have any difference between sulpiride and chlorpromazine, but according to the literature there would be a difference. What was your last question ?

Ch. Eggers
The ratio of HVA and the 5-hydroxyindol-acetic-acid is an important finding in your patient group. Similar to schizophrenia, in tic disease the dopamine hypothesis is also discussed. If I understood you correctly, you have found that the HVA was lower than the 5-hydroxyindol-acetic-acid ?

G. Sedvall
No, I think you misunderstood. In this patient group there is about a 2-fold higher HVA concentration than the 5-hydroxyindol-acetic-acid before treatment and during treatment there is a stronger elevation of the HVA and 5-hydroxyindol-acetic-acid concentration, so I think this is in line with what Cohen found. This is, of course, what we found in healthy individuals. In schizophrenic patients you have an individual variation in the ratio of the dopamine metabolite to the 5-hydroxyindol-acid metabolite. In depressed patients you actually have quite low HVA concentrations.

P. Grof
As Prof. Mendlewicz has already mentioned, I think you have a very impressive study and a very clean evidence about the advantages of sulpiride. However, should one not try some additional analyses of the data, in view of the fact that you have very impressive differences in the first 2 weeks and at the same time you had considerable difference in terms of additional benzodiazepines ? Because of benzodiazepine effects on the limbic system, one has to be inquisitive about this and I think the question could be resolved if you either re-analysed the data by removing the patients who had benzodiazepines additionally, or did the analysis of variance using benzodiazepines as one of the variables.

G. Sedvall
I think you are quite right, we cannot say very much about the action in the first 2 weeks with regard to the massive dosage of benzodiazepine. Actually, I think the effect in the later phases of treatment indicates that you have these antipsychotic effects and we must re-analyse the data with this in mind. The problem in this study is that most of the patients in the sulpiride group received benzodiazepines, so, if you remove them you do not have any patients left to make the calculations on.

N. Matussek
To this point, how high were the doses of benzodiazepines ?

G. Sedvall
Oxazepam was given in doses up to 25 mg/day and that was the maximum dose. Usually, the doses were much lower, so that they were actually more in the pattern of occasional doses in the early phase of treatment.

Y. Lecrubier
Did you find a sub-group of patients which should react better to one drug than to the other ? I ask this because you said that you had few patients with negative symptoms and still making a mean — if I understood correctly — with all patients, you have a very marked improvement with sulpiride and no change with chlorpromazine. That means that the reaction is better in these patients than in the others.

G. Sevall
I cannot answer this yet. We are going to analyse sub-groups ultimately, but I would not like to make a statement with regard to this at the moment.

J.S. Kim
I would like to know what is your opinion : Which kind of schizophrenics is better treated with sulpiride and how about the hormonal side effects with sulpiride ?

G. Sedvall
There was no case of lactation in this group of subjects, even when the prolactin concentrations were very high. Unfortunately, we did not ask about the symptom of breast-swelling in women, but in those we asked, there was no lactation. However, I am sure that quite a number of patients had

188

swelling in the breasts. It is very difficult to say which patients are best treated with sulpiride. We have to make multivaried analysis here. We have the pharmacokinetic data, which are very important when you try to make this kind of evaluation and since we have such a wide spread of drug concentrations, this is a great, complicating factor, which we actually have under control in a study like this, where we have 6 doses of the treatment. So, as I said to Dr. Lecrubier, we will come back to this question when we have analysed the data in detail.

C. Gennari

A very nice protocol, very clear results. You said at the beginning of your lecture that you have also measured prolactin in cerebrospinal fluid, although I did not see the results. My question is : Considering that you demonstrated a very great increase in circulating plasma prolactin levels, what happened in the cerebrospinal fluid ?

G. Sedvall

It is roughly the same result in the cerebrospinal fluid, the average CSF concentration in the sulpiride group was 20 ng/ml, which is actually a 10-fold elevation of the prolactin concentration in women, as found in both chlorpromazine-treated and sulpiride-treated patients. However, in this respect sulpiride is enormous, so there is possibly a transport over the blood-brain barrier of the prolactin in plasma. We have examined this after a number of compounds of different classes of neuroleptics and we found the same procentual prolactin elevation in plasma as in CSF.

C. Gennari

It is possible to demonstrate if there is a transfer across the blood-brain barrier by calculating the ratio between the plasma and cerebrospinal fluid prolactin. I have seen that when plasma prolactin increases, in some instances there is no increase in prolactin in cerebrospinal fluid.

G. Sedvall

It would be interesting to see these data, because we have no other studies than those with different types of compounds in patients and here I would say that there is a time-shift in the elevation, so, it depends also on the half-life of the compound in plasma. In some conditions after neuroleptics we can see a very short half-life, that you have an elevation in the CSF, but not in the plasma, if you take your samplings late after dosing of the drug.

M. Ackenheil

In chronic schizophrenic patients treated with 600 mg sulpiride/day we found on the whole the same biochemical finding with one exception : We did not see tolerance in HVA levels. The same HVA elevation was measured after 15 and 30 days and we found the same decrease in MOPEG levels. According to the question of Dr. Gennari, we see in plasma as well as in CSF the same elevation of prolactin secretion, however, concerning the clinical therapeutic effects we have the impression that there was a difference between the classical neuroleptics and sulpiride, in that sulpiride has more activating effects in chronic schizophrenic patients than the other classical neuroleptics. It seems to me that all the symptoms which have something to do with activation are better improved than the productive symptoms. Did you also find that the minus symptoms are improved more than the other productive symptoms ?

G. Sedvall

We have not performed any studies yet in a chronic population, but it would be worthwhile to do so.

M. Ackenheil

In your opinion, what is more important, the MHPG decrease or the HVA increase, showing this tolerance ? There are discrepancies, as we found high noradrenaline levels in plasma and the same MHPG decrease in CSF. Why does this decrease, whereas noradrenaline is elevated ? What biochemical event occurs ?

G. Sedvall

This is very difficult to evaluate. I would like to try and interpret it as follows : The MOPEG reduction was a normalization of an elevation at the beginning of the treatment. We see that in a number of our schizophrenic patients we have a slight elevation of MOPEG, which then decreases. After some neuroleptics like chlorpromazine, you have a very marked reduction, which actually relates significantly to therapeutic outcome, as we found in a previous study with chlorpromazine. We also found this with one butyrophenone we studied, where we had this reduction of MOPEG concentration, also related to therapeutic outcome. However, here anxiety is quite a consistent phenomenon in these acutely psychotic patients, so it may just be a phenomenon related to the disappearance of anxiety and then the reduction in noradrenaline release within the CNS. That is our interpretation. For the sulpiride data, there is a normalization. Then for the HVA the elevation indicates a reduction in tolerance to this. In our studies where we continued to treat patients up to 8 weeks, we found that after 8 weeks we always have an elevation of concentrations. Then you will find, as Post found in the United States as well as other authors, that you actually have a normalization of the HVA concentrations in long-term treatment. CSF sampling is a very indirect technique to study the release of transmitters within the brain and there may possibly be inductional transport systems here also, so it is very difficult to evaluate.

Neurobiological findings in children with tics and Gilles de La Tourette syndrome

Ch. Eggers, T. Olbricht, A. Rothenberger

Child Psychiatric Unit, University of Essen, Federal Republic of Germany

Summary : It is a well known fact that changes within the dopaminergic system may influence the hormonal status, the electrical brain activity, and the neuropsychological functions. It is also accepted that tiapride has a dopaminergic blocking activity (mainly on D_2 - receptors). In order to examine the dopaminergic blocking activity of tiapride, we have used the above mentioned indirect measures and investigated 10 children (average age 11,6 years) with tics and Gilles de la Tourette syndrome. Each child was treated with a daily dosage of tiapride of 5 mg/kg of body weight. The children were tested three times over a period of 6 months (a : after a 4 day baseline, followed by a 7 day placebo ; b : after another 7 days with verum, and c : after an additional 6 months of verum).

The results show that :

1) Tiapride does not influence the gonadotropins, GH, STH, TSH, and the thyroid hormones. The hyperprolactinaemia was seen only during the treatment.

2) A preliminary inspection of the EEG and Evoked Potential data does not show a significant influence of tiapride on the electrical brain activity, but a further evaluation is necessary.

3) There is no systematic variation of the neuropsychological data according to an analysis of variance.

In summary, the dopaminergic blocking activity of tiapride seems to act mainly at the level of the lactotropins and not or only slightly on higher cortical functions.

Introduction

We have used tiapride, a substituted benzamide which has been proved to have antidyskinetic properties attributable to its D_2-blocking activities, for the treatment of children suffering from tic syndromes. There are very few reports on the treatment of tic disease in children using tiapride. Usually, phenothiazines (thioridazine, fluphenazine) and butyrophenones (haloperidol, pimozide, pipamperone) or minor tranquilizers are administered. We know of only two other publications reporting on tiapride therapy in children with tics (Mathé et al, 1978 ; Pasquier and Pouplard, 1977).

Methods

Our report concerns 10 children (9 boys and 1 girl) with multiple tics. Three of them had a Gilles de La Tourette syndrome (GTS). Fifteen other children with a tic syndrome are at present taking part in a double-blind cross-over study, scheduled to last six months. The average age was 11.6 years (7-16 years). None of the patients had any other medical disorder prior to the study. Nor did they receive any medication for a period of at least 4 weeks before the study began.

The test sequence (Fig. 1) comprised 4 phases : (1) 3 days drug free (baseline) ; (2) 7 days placebo ; (3) 7 days tiapride ; (4) thereafter 6 months tiapride.

Tiapride was administered at a dosage of 5 mg per kg of body weight.

The tics were rated 3 times a day for 15 minutes during meals and at the end of each investigation period (1 - 4) during video-taped play and test situations.

At the end of each period, the following testing procedures were carried out : Critical fusion frequency ; continuous performance test (vigilance) ; simple and complex reaction times (Wiener Reaktionsgerät) ; tapping (both hands). In addition ECG, EEG, SEP, VEP and AEP.

At the end of the placebo and the different verum phases the following psychodiagnostic methods were applied : The Culture Fair Intelligence Test (Cattell Weiss), the Apprehension Span Test d2 Brickenkamp, the Göttinger form of Bender Gestalt Test and a body co-ordination test. For the objectivization of family dynamics and of child personality we used the Family Relations Test, the Hamburger Neuroticism and Extroversion Scale (HANES), the Freiburger Personality Inventory (FPI) and the Personality Inventory for Children (9 - 14). The Wilcoxon test was used for statistical evaluation.

Results

The mean tic frequency showed a reduction from the middle of the placebo phase onwards. This trend continued during the verum phase (Fig. 2). The statistical comparisons of the mean values, both between the baseline and the placebo phases and between the placebo and the verum phases, showed no significance. The graph, however, does show a decline in tic frequency.

It can be stated that tiapride does not affect negatively alertness, apprehension span, visual discrimination, motor skills or visual motor reaction speed and accuracy (Fig. 3). Likewise, there is no negative effect on intellectual performance or motor coordination. The corresponding test results were very similar during all four phases. The fact that alertness, cognitive and visual-motor functions are not impaired by tiapride is of great importance for the growing child.

All the children showed evidence of disturbed family dynamics. This is reflected in a child's drawing (Fig. 4). The child commented : « The bird is an eagle or a buzzard with claws. The mouse at the bottom is trying to hide in a hole. The buzzard will attack the mouse if it does not reach its hole quickly enough. » After seeing the drawing, the child's father said spontaneously : « Yes, that's how it is. »

Few investigations have been carried out on the effects of neuroleptic drugs on spontaneous EEG in childhood. Visual inspection of the EEG power spectra showed that, under tiapride treatment, the activity of the slow waves and α-waves did not change appreciably in 6 children (Fig. 5). In 3 children there was a slight increase of these wave activities, and one child showed decreasing values over all frequencies (Fig. 5).

The variability during the two non-verum phases (baseline and placebo) was as low as that during the two verum phases (short-term and long-term tiapride treatment) (Fig. 6). A further statistical evaluation which includes topographical aspects, is under way.

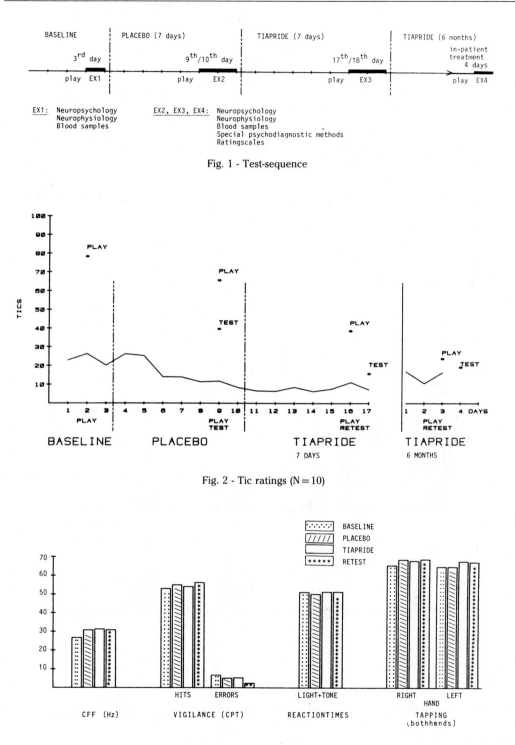

Fig. 1 - Test-sequence

Fig. 2 - Tic ratings (N = 10)

Fig. 3 - Neuropsychological tests - Mean values (n = 10)

193

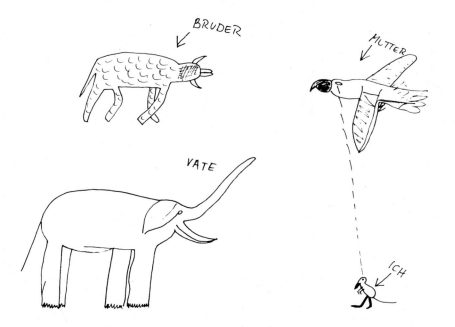

Fig. 4

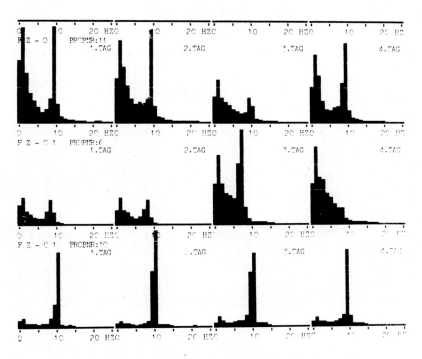

Fig. 5 - Example of power spectra for three children during phase 1-4

194

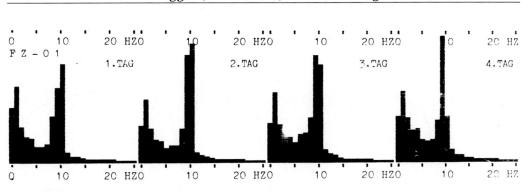

Fig. 6 - Grand average of power spectra of all 10 children during phase 1-4

The use of sophisticated power spectral techniques in psychopharmacology has given variable results among investigators (Tasman et al., 1981). This may be one of the reasons why, in recent years, the attention has shifted to the drug changes seen in Event-Related-Potentials (ERPs). We shall confine ourselves to the results of VEPs in our sample. The recording was bipolar from Fz-01, according to the 10-20 system. The stimulus was a checkerboard pattern. There were two conditions : One with stimuli of 1 s^{-1} and another with random frequencies (range 1-0.3 s^{-1}). One computed individual average consisted of 40 trials, checked for artifacts. After plotting these averages, the peak latencies, peak amplitudes, as well as the maximum-minimum amplitude were detected visually and measured manually with a scanning pattern. For statistics we used the Wilcoxon test and the ProcMeans procedure, both included in the SAS-programme.

We reliably detected 5 components (Fig. 7). P1 around 50-90 msec, N1 (100-130 msec), P2 (140-200 msec), N2 (200-300 msec) and a late positive component (LPC) around 350-500 msec.

Our investigation on the influence of tiapride on the VEPs of middle and long latency peaks did not show any appreciable changes, either in latencies or amplitudes, during placebo or tiapride. Furthermore, the maximum-minimum amplitudes of the averaged curves and the comparison between random and non random conditions likewise indicated that tiapride had no statistically significant effect on the VEPs of the 10 children tested. The ERP curves remained relatively stable with wave shapes during time and treatment. Also concerning latencies and amplitudes of SEPs (Somato-sensory Evoked Potentials) tiapride does not show any significant influence (Fig. 7).

The fact that tiapride had no significant influence on the VEPs of our children is in good agreement with our neuropsychological data, as well as with the computerized oculography results of Aschoff et al. (1980) in adults treated with tiapride. In contrast with our results on VEPs during tiapride treatment, sulpiride, a related drug, and other neuroleptics like thiothixene and fluphenazine, resulted in distinct, dose-dependent changes of VEPs in children and adults (Brosteanu and Floru, 1980 ; Saletu, 1977 ; Shagass, 1981). This might indicate that, on a neurophysiological level, tiapride has a different action than neuroleptics.

From recent publications (Chouza et al., 1982, Gennari et al., 1981, L'Hermite et al., 1978, 1979) we can conclude that in adults tiapride induces an increase in pro-

195

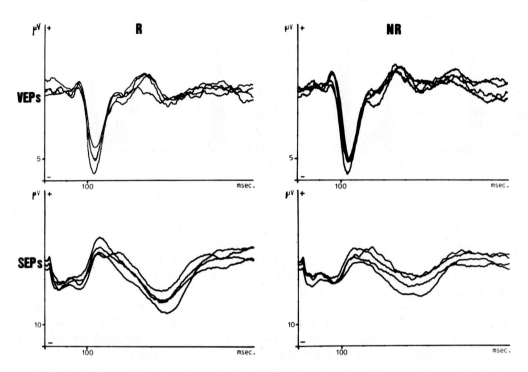

Fig. 7 - Grand average of VEPs of all 10 children during phases 1-4 (FZ-01 ; s = 40)

Table 1. : *Prolactin levels (ng/ml) in children with multiple tics before (—15 - 0 min) and after (+30 min) stimulation with 200 μg TRH, and after cessation of treatment.*

Initial	Sex	Age	Pubertal stage (Tanner)	Placebo			Tiapride 7 days			Tiapride 6 months			after cessation of tiapride
				—15 min	0 min	+30 min	—15 min	0 min	+30 min	—15 min	0 min	+30 min	
L.T.	M	9	I	5.9	8.3	19.6	87.3	65.7	68.7	53.6	59.7	51.2	6.6
W.F.	M	16	III	9.8	8.3	23.4	30.8	31.4	28.5	27.2	29.6	37.4	9.1
S.S.	M	10	II	2.1	3.1	18.2	32.1	27.2	32.8	36.9	32.2	94.4	4.5
P.T.	F	7	I	4.3	3.3	14.4	28.7	29.6	40.2	18.4	14.6	51.3	4.6
S.O.	M	13	II	4.3	3.8	24.1	42.7	28.8	47.4	37.6	33.5	50.1	—
G.G.	M	9	I	6.6	7.5	39.6	(31.0)	31.0	77.8	(17.7)	17.7	66.9	7.7
A.M.	M	11	II	5.6	4.2	12.9	31.9	28.8	40.2	(19.0)	19.0	44.4	6.8
S.J.	M	9	I	4.6	4.2	21.6	27.0	25.0	32.5	18.0	16.0	27.3	2.0
H.O.	M	11	II	10.9	9.4	21.0	34.8	42.6	53.4	195.4	148.9	144.4	10.2
G.M.	M	12	II	10.4	13.7	45.1	31.6	28.0	58.6	42.7	40.7	62.2	—
Group values				n = 10			n = 10			n = 10			n = 8
X				6.45	6.58	25.09	39.94	33.81	48.01	46.74	41.19	62.96	6.43
SD				2.80	3.28	10.14	14.83	11.54	15.59	50.91	38.22	32.17	2.50
± SEM				0.89	1.04	3.21	4.69	3.65	4.93	16.10	12.08	10.17	0.88

( ) extrapolated values ; - missing values.

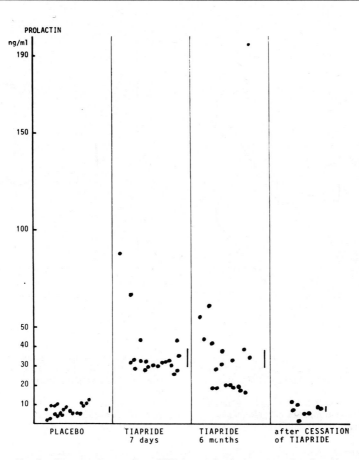

Fig. 8 - Group values and ± SEM for prolactin in serum (result without stimulation). I = ± SEM

lactin levels. There is, at present, no information on the endocrine effects of tiapride treatment in children. Therefore, we investigated the serum levels of the following hormones at the end of the different periods : Prolactin, LH, FSH, T3, T4, TSH and HGH. LH and FSH were determined before and after the administration of 100 μg of GnRH ; and TSH, HGH and prolactin before and after stimulation with 200 μg of TRH. Endocrine testing was carried out at 2 p.m., 6 hours after drug administration. We used the Wilcoxon test and Student t-test for statistical analysis. The results are shown in Table 1 and Figure 8.

At the end of the placebo period, the prolactin levels ranged between 2.1 and 13.7 ng/ml (mean : 6.5 ± 0.97 ng/ml). All levels were within the normal range. After a 7 day treatment with tiapride at a dosage of 5 mg/kg of body weight, the prolactin levels increased in all patients and ranged between 25 and 87.3 ng/ml (mean : 36.6 ± 4.63 ng/ml). After a 6 month treatment, the prolactin level was between 14.6 and 195.4 ng/ml (mean : 43.92 ± 14.27 ng/ml). In 4 patients the basal prolactin levels were only slightly above the normal range, but clearly higher than the placebo level (Fig. 8). Non-compliance was denied in these cases.

197

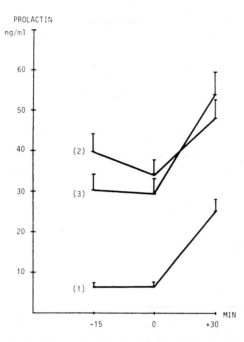
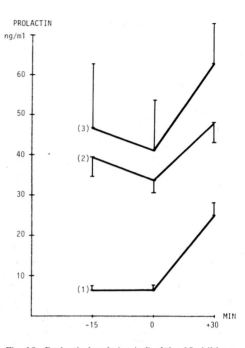

Fig. 9 - Prolactin levels (ng/ml) of the children with multiple tics before (—15 min, 0 min), and after (+30 min) stimulation with 200 μg TRH. Period (3) n = 9
(1) Placebo (n = 10) - (2) After 7 days of tiapride (n = 10) - (3) After 6 months of tiapride (n = 9).

Fig. 10 - Prolactin levels (ng/ml) of the 10 children with multiple tics before (—15 min, 0 min), and after (+30 min) stimulation with 200 μg TRH (n = 10).
(1) Placebo - (2) After 7 days of tiapride - (3) After 6 months of tiapride - Mean ± SEM.

We have tried to correlate the prolactin values with the clinical response to tiapride treatment. In 5 children, there was a good correlation between the prolactin elevation (taking levels above 30 ng/ml as indicating a good dopaminergic blockade) and the clinical response (decrease in tic rate and progress in behavior, as judged by 2 observers). One child (A.M.) had low levels of prolactin and a poor clinical response. As to the other 4 children, the prolactin level was below 30 ng/ml but, nevertheless, clinical response was good. All 10 children had elevated prolactin levels compared to those of the placebo period ; the degree of prolactin increase and the clinical response were not correlated. One month after cessation of the drug treatment, the prolactin levels returned to normal, measured after 1 month of drugs (Fig. 8).

When the excessively high prolactin levels of H.O. were omitted from evaluation, the mean prolactin was of 30 ng/ml, significantly lower than the mean prolactin after the 7 day treatment (Fig. 9). This difference was significant at the 1 % level, using the Wilcoxon test. In each case 2 basal prolactin levels (—15', 0') were measured to account for stress effects on prolactin secretion. There was, however, no significant change in the prolactin levels during this interval.

During the placebo phase, the prolactin increased in all patients after TRH stimulation (from 6.5 to 25.1 ng/ml, i.e. 4-fold). After the 7 day treatment with tiapride, this relative increase was diminished ; PRL rose from the mean value of

Table 2 : — *Mean group values and ± SEM in the periods (2), (3) and (4) of LH, FSH before and after administration of 100 μg of GnRH - TSH, STH before and after administration of 200 μg of TRH T3, T4 and TGB without stimulation.*

min	LH ng/ml	FSH ng/ml	STH ng(ml)	TSH μU/ml	T3 ng/ml	T4 μg/ml	TBG	Period
	1.03 ± 0.69	0.67 ± 0.61	2.27 ± 1.82	1.19 ± 0.70				(2)
−15	1.03 ± 0.59	0.69 ± 0.56	2.11 ± 1.41	1.0.7 ± 0.57				(3)
	0.80 ± 0.14	0.90 ± 0.02	1.46 ± 0.36	1.60 ± 0.18				(4)
	0.87 ± 0.62	0.65 ± 0.55	2.39 ± 1.83	1.01 ± 0.58	132.33 ± 5.70	8.14 ± 1.25	21.13 ± 0.15	(2)
0	0.99 ± 0.54	0.61 ± 0.52	3.65 ± 2.17	1.21 ± 0.90	130.11 ± 4.92	8.06 ± 1.30	20.99 ± 1.34	(3)
	1.00 ± 0.13	0.80 ± 0.11	1.66 ± 0.40	1.44 ± 0.15	108.00 ± 5.88	7.99 ± 0.20	29.30 ± 2.09	(4)
	3.03 ± 1.66	1.19 ± 0.90						(2)
+15	3.08 ± 1.77	1.18 ± 0.96						(3)
	3.80 ± 1.15	1.30 ± 0.27						(4)
	3.84 ± 1.85	1.61 ± 1.14	4.67 ± 2.39	8.44 ± 2.11				(2)
+30	3.92 ± 1.96	1.74 ± 1.13	1.71 ± 1.43	8.85 ± 1.94				(3)
	4.60 ± 1.20	1.60 ± 0.30	1.59 ± 0.43	8.70 ± 1.27				(4)
	3.36 ± 1.79	1.85 ± 1.20						(2)
+45	3.94 ± 1.80	2.07 ± 1.43						(3)
	4.00 ± 0.95	1.60 ± 0.30						(4)
	3.17 ± 1.57	1.79 ± 1.24						(2)
+60	3.40 ± 1.75	1.92 ± 1.41						(3)
	3.50 ± 0.80	1.60 ± 0.33						(4)

(2) placebo ; (3) after 7 days on tiapride ; (4) after 6 months on tiapride

36.6 ng/ml before stimulation to 48.0 ng/ml after stimulation (Fig. 9 and 10). After the 6 month treatment, PRL increased after TRH from 44.0 to 62.9 ng/ml ; the latter figures are influenced by the excessively high prolactin levels of patient H.O. (Table 1 and Fig. 10). Leaving aside patient H.O., the PRL increased only from 30.0 ng/ml to 54.0 ng/ml after TRH stimulation at the end of the 6 month period (Fig. 9).

Thus, the Δ PRL was 18.6 ng/ml before, 11.3 ng/ml after 7 days and 19.0 ng/ml after 6 months of treatment*. The increases in PRL values after TRH stimulation (Δ PRL) were all significant. When the absolute Δ PRLs during the different phases were compared, there was no significant difference between them. It can be stated that in our sample the reactivity of prolactin secretion is not impaired by tiapride.

The gonadotropin secretion was in line with the stage of puberty. Three children had reached puberty stage I, 6 stage II and 1 stage III, according to Tanner. The maximum increase in LH, and FSH secretion following stimulation with 100 μg of GnRH, observed during tiapride therapy was not significantly different from the increase seen in the placebo phase. This was also true for the investigation after the 6 month tiapride treatment ; after this period, the increase in LH secretion in 9 children was slightly higher than before the treatment (Table 2). We may conclude that tiapride treatment over a period of 6 months has no adverse effects on the

* Δ : difference between the value after stimulation and the mean pre-stimulus value.

pituitary gonadotropin secretory capacity and therefore no negative influence on puberty.

The T4 levels did not change during therapy. The T3 levels were 132 ± 6 ng/ml before treatment, 130 ± 5 ng/ml after one week and 108 ± 6 ng/ml after 6 months of tiapride therapy. TSH was normal in all cases. After TRH stimulation, the Δ TSH during the placebo phase was of 7.2 μU/ml, after one week of treatment 7.4 μU/ml. After 6 months, the Δ TSH was of only 5.6 μU/ml. In contrast to other antidopaminergic drugs such as sulpiride, tiapride does not seem to stimulate TSH secretion.

No significant changes in HGH values were seen between the drug free and the treatment periods.

Discussion

On the basis of our present observations, we can state that tiapride is useful in treating children with a tic syndrome. Its antidyskinetic properties may be related to its DA_2-blocking activity in the nigro-striatal system. The hyperprolactinaemia observed in our children under tiapride treatment may indicate that tiapride also acts on the pituitary lactotrophs. This is supported by in vitro and in vivo observations, that the prolactin inhibiting action of dopamine is blocked by tiapride (L'Hermite et al., 1978, 1979).

We should not disregard the unexplainably high prolactin level of one boy (H.O.) during the long-term treatment. But even if we do not take this case into account, caution is equally called in interpreting the decrease in the mean prolactin level of 30 ng/ml. The decrease in serum prolactin concentration during long-term treatment may be in line with the findings of 3 other groups on the chronic administration of neuroleptic drugs to adults (Brown and Laughren, 1981, De Rivera et al., 1976, Naber et al., 1980).

In our opinion there are four possible explanations for a decrease in prolactin secretion during a long-term administration of antidopaminergic agents such as tiapride and neuroleptics. (1) Non-compliance of the patients — they may not take their drugs regularly, causing a lesser increase in prolactin. However, the findings of Brown and Laughren (1981) indicate that prolactin concentrations can decrease during long-term treatment with neuroleptics even if the drugs are taken regularly. (2) Changes in the pharmacokinetics of the drugs applied, resulting in a decreased efficacy. (3) Development of tolerance of the tuberoinfundibular or hypothalamic-pituitary system to the prolactin-increasing effects of tiapride or neuroleptic drugs. (4) Increase in the number of dopamine receptors in this region. An increase in both D_1 and D_2 receptors, has been demonstrated in animals, using ^{3}H-haloperidol (Burt et al., 1977, Fuxe et al., 1980) and ^{3}H-sulpiride (Memo et al., 1981) respectively.

During long-term tiapride treatment, such hypersensitivity of dopaminergic receptors may develop also in the striatal system. This could explain the sudden increase in the tic rates of some patients at the cross-over point between the different phases, during the double-blind cross-over study.

In adults, the chronic elevation of prolactin interferes with the pulsatile release of LH and with the action of gonadotropins on the gonads. The clinical correlated findings, in adults, are amenorrhea, galactorrhea and impotency, which are fre-

200

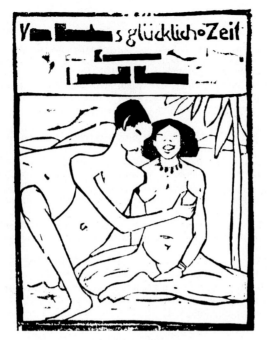

Fig. 11. (See text)

quently observed in patients with high levels of prolactin, such as patients with pituitary adenomas. We have observed no adverse effects of tiapride on gonadotropin secretion or pubertal development during the 6 month treatment. However, the effects of long-term administration of this drug on puberty have so far not been investigated in detail. Since, in most of our children on long-term tiapride treatment, prolactin was only slightly increased, such adverse effects on gonadotropin secretion or activity would seem rather unlikely, even if treatment was continued for a longer period.

We did not observe any effect of tiapride on TSH levels before or after TRH, or on circulating thyroid hormones. Nevertheless, other dopamine antagonists may influence TSH secretion, which is physiologically regulated by dopamine (Scanlon et al., 1979). In this context it is interesting to notice that, in adults, sulpiride, a drug related to tiapride, enhances the increase in TSH after TRH stimulation (Portioli et al., 1976).

In summary, tiapride appears to have no adverse effects on neuropsychological, neurophysiological or endocrinological functions in children, other than on prolactin secretion during drug intake.

Even if there remains some uncertainty as to the interaction between tiapride and prolactin, we may state that the strongest stimulus for a sudden release of PRL is induced by touching the female breast (Fig. 11). The nervous impulses act via the hypothalamus by counteracting the prolactin inhibiting factor (PIF). This is shown by Otto Müller's illustration of L. Bruun's « Van Zanten's happy time »: « If a man desireth a woman, he curveth his hand around her breast. If she is willing, she placeth her hand around his neck. »

201

REFERENCES

Aschoff, J.C., Becker, W., Jürgens, R. *1980* - Eine computerokulographische und elektroenzephalographische Doppelblindstudie unter Einbeziehung der Befindlichkeit zur Erfassung von Vigilanzänderungen unter einer Tiaprid-Medikation. *Arzneim.-Forsch. (Drug Res.), 30 :* 509-512.

Brosteanu, E.R., Floru, L. *1980* - Untersuchung der visuell evozierten Potentiale bei schizophrenen Patienten unter einer Behandlung mit Sulpirid. *Arneim.-Forsch. (Drug Res.), 30 :* 1306-1309

Brown, W.A., Laughren, T.P. *1981* - Tolerance to the prolactin-elevating effect of neuroleptics. *Psychiat. Res., 5 :* 317-322

Burt, D.R., Creese, J., Snyder, S.H. *1977* - Antischizophrenic drugs : chronic treatment elevates dopamine receptor binding in brain. *Science, 196 :* 326-328

Chouza, C., Romero, S., Lorenzo, J., Camano, J.L., Fontana, A.P., Alterwain, P., Cibils, D., Gaudiano, J., Feres, S., Solana, J. *1982* - Traitement des dyskinésies par le tiapride. *Sem. Hôp. (Paris), 58 :* 725-733.

Fuxe, K., Ögren, S.-O., Hall, H., Agnati, L.F., Andersson. K., Köhler, C., Schwarcz, R. *1980* - Effects of chronic treatment with l-sulpiride and haloperidol on central monoaminergic mechanisms - *In : long-term effects of neuroleptics*, Cattabani F. (ed.). New York, Raven Press.

Gennari, C., Nami, R., Pizzuti, M., D'Ascenzo, G., Bianchini, C. *1981* - Effets du tiapride en perfusion sur le taux plasmatique de bêta-endorphine, prolactine et dopamine chez des patients souffrant d'algies cancéreuses. *Sem. Hôp. (Paris), 57 :* 795-800

Hierholzer, K., Neubert, D. *1977* - : Endokrinologie I. *In : Gauer, O.H., Kramer, K., Jung, R. (Eds.) : Physiologie des Menschen, Bd. 18.* München-Wien-Baltimore, Urban u. Schwarzenberg 1977

L'Hermite, M., MacLeod, R.M., Robyn, C. *1978* - Effects of two substituted benzamides, tiapride and sultopride, on gonadotrophins and prolactin. *Acta endocrinol., 89 :* 29-36

L'Hermite, M., Michaux-Duchêne, A., Robyn, C. *1979* - Tiapride-induced chronic hyperprolactinaemia : interference with the human menstrual cycle. *Acta endocrinol., 92 :* 214-227

Mathé, J.F., Cler, J.M., Venisse, J.L. *1978* - Utilisation du tiapride dans le traitement de certains mouvements anormaux. *Sem. Hôp. (Paris), 54 :* 15-16.

Memo, M., Battaini, F., Spano, P.F., Trabucchi, M. *1981* - Sulpiride and the role of dopaminergic receptor blockade in the antipsychotic activity of neuroleptics. *Acta psychiat. scand., 63 :* 314-324

Naber, D., Finkbeiner, C., Fischer, B., Zander, K.-J., Ackenheil, M. *1980* - Effect of long-term neuroleptic treatment on prolactin and norepinephrine levels in serum of chronic schizophrenics : relations to psychopathology and extrapyramidal symptoms. *Neuropsychobiology, 6 :* 181-189

Pasquier, C., Pouplard, F. *1977* - Quelques réflexions sur les tics de l'enfant. A propos d'un essai thérapeutique. *Rev. neuropsychiat. infant., 25 :* 645-651.

Portioli, I., Modena, G., Fantesini, C., Bellefelli, A., Dotti, C. *1976* - Interelations TRH - sulpiride sur la sécrétion de prolactine. *Nouvelle Presse méd., 5 :* 931.

Rivera, J.L. de, Lal, S., Ettigi, P., Hontela, S., Muller, H.F., Friesen, H.G. *1976* - Effect of acute and chronic neuroleptic therapy on serum prolactin levels in men and women of different age groups. *Clin. Endocrinol., 5 :* 273-282

Saletu, B. *1977* - Cerebral evoked potentials in psychopharmacology. *In : Auditory evoked potentials in man. Psychopharmacology correlates of EPs.* Desmedt, J.E. (ed.) pp. 175-207 - (Progr. clin. Neurophysiol., Vol. 2.) Basel, Karger

Scanlon, M.F., Weightman, D.R., Shale, D.J., Mora, B., Heath, M., Snow, M.H., Lewis, M., Hall, R. *1979* - Dopamine is a physiological regulator of thyrotrophin (TSH) secretion in normal man. *Clin. Endocrinol, 11 :* 7-15

Shagass, C. *1981* - Psychotropic drugs and evoked potentials, paper presented at the *Xth International Congress of Electroencephalography and Clinical Neurophysiology, Kyoto, Japan 1981*.

Tasman, A., Hale, M.S., Simon, R.H. *1981* - Neuroleptics drug effects on average evoked response augmentation - reduction in rats. *Neuropsychol, 7 :* 292-296

DISCUSSION

D. Lefaucheur
Are you sure that tiapride has no effect on puberty, as the onset of puberty is marked by nocturnal peaks of LH, which should be investigated through a circadian rhythm?

Ch. Eggers
We have thought of this, therefore, we made regular examinations at 2 p.m., six hours after administration. This was the reason for always doing it at the same time. Our patients were mainly at the age before puberty and one patient was in stage III of Tanner and this may influence our endocrinological findings.

D. Lefaucheur
I wanted to ask you whether you have measured the steroids, because this is another way that prolactin could interfere with puberty : As Mac Natty has shown in-vitro, hyperprolactinaemia can prevent granulosa cells from responding to gonadotropins.

Ch. Eggers
No, we did not measure steroids.

N. Matussek
The improvement in your symptomatology started during the placebo period?

Ch. Eggers
Yes.

N. Matussek
Are you convinced that tiapride is really a good drug?

Ch. Eggers
I cannot answer this until the double blind cross-over study is completed. You have seen from my slide that the decrease in tics is in middle of the placebo phase. We wanted to find where there was a decline in the tic rate and therefore we used the Wilcoxon test to evaluate the mean tic rate in the last two days of baseline, the first two days and the last two days of the seven day tiapride treatment. The same procedure was repeated six months later. We have seen a statistically significant decrease in the tic rate in the middle of the placebo phase. I am sorry to have to say that, it is not a happy discovery for Schürholz, but it is good news for my clinic ! Perhaps you remember from the second slide, a few days or one day before the patients leave the tic rates are slightly elevated. To be sure of the beneficial effects of tiapride on tics, a double blind cross-over study is necessary and is going on at the present. It seems that tiapride has good effects on Gilles de la Tourette syndrome respectively polymorphous tics in children. All 3 children with the GTS syndrome have been very well remitted by tiapride.

M. Ackenheil
You mentioned the influence on evoked potentials. Was this influence on the latency or on the height of the potentials?

Ch. Eggers
We did not see any influence of tiapride either on the latency or on the amplitudes of VEPs.

M. Ackenheil
That does not fit in with neuroleptics.

Ch. Eggers
That does not fit with neuroleptics, but it is in agreement that tiapride is not a neuroleptic drug. I am familiar with the discoveries of Saletu, but tiapride has no influence on the latencies or amplitudes,

neither on visual, auditory nor somatosensorically evoked potentials in our children and this is in good agreement with our neuropsychological data.

W.H. Vogel
Coming back to what Prof. Matussek said about the placebo period and what you said about the family dynamics, that in certain children the tic is produced by the stressful situation at home. Is it an anxiety reaction and would perhaps valium or librium be effective in these children?

Ch. Eggers
I refuse to give benzodiazepines or any tranquilizing drugs in my psychotherapy, and therefore I cannot answer this question. I only know that other publications report on positive effects of haloperidol and pimozide. We have seen some patients who have recovered with tiapride after being worsened by haloperidol or by floropipamide and who have been cured by tiapride. I hope that the double blind cross-over study will show a positive result, proving the beneficial effects of tiapride on children with tic syndrome.

W.H. Vogel
Does tiapride have an anti-anxiety effect?

Ch. Eggers
I do not know. However, I would like to mention that some patients did have headaches and there is a recent paper by Gennari et al. describing that tiapride has an analgesic effect. Perhaps this will be discussed later.

Regression of cerebellar syndrome with long-term administration of 5-HTP** or the combination 5-HTP-benserazide**

26 cases with quantified symptomatology and computerized data processing

P. Trouillas, A. Garde, J.M. Robert, B. Renaud, P. Adeleine, J. Bard and F. Brudon

Neurology Unit of Antiquaille Hospital, Alexis Carrel University, and Biochemical Neuropharmacology Laboratory, Neurologic Hospital, Lyons, France.

Summary : A quantitative evaluation of cerebellar ataxia, with an ataxia score (total, static, kinetic) and the measurement of objective values related to the major symptoms, was proposed. 21 patients with heredo-ataxias were treated for 12 months with high doses (16 mg/kg/day) of d-l-5-HTP, l-5-HTP or the combination d-l-5-HTP (16 mg/kg/day) - benserazide (6 mg/kg/day). The data obtained from regular examination were processed by computer. The ataxia showed a significant regression at the 12th month, mainly in the static forms and speed of speech. *l-5-HTP appeared to be more effective than d-l-5-HTP.* Regression of the cerebellar ataxia was also observed in non-degenerative conditions such as multiple sclerosis and surgical lesion of the anterior lobe vermis, showing that 5-HTP was active on the cerebellar syndrome in general. The regression of the cerebellar ataxia was very slow in inherited diseases and continued for 2 or 4 months after the treatment stopped. A serotoninergic cerebellar control of motoricity is discussed.

Introduction

The essential clinical features of cerebellar ataxia, whether experimental or human — deficient postural equilibrium, hypermetria, adiodochokinesia, dyschronometria — have not been significantly influenced by drugs so far. We considered it logical to examine the pharmacology of human cerebellar ataxia by manipulating the principle mediators found at the level of the nerve terminals of the cerebellum or of the inferior olive : GABA (Schon and Iverson, 1972), noradrenaline (Hoffer et al., 1978 ; Fuxe, 1965 ; Hökfelt and Fuxe, 1969 ; Hoffman and Sladek, 1973 ; Sladek and Bowman, 1975 ; Bloom et al., 1971), dopamine (Thierry et al., 1974 ; Burkard et al., 1976) and serotonin (Hökfelt and Fuxe, 1969).

---

* Quietim. Nativelle Laboratories.
** Benserazide, non-commercialised product, Roche Laboratories.

Table 1 — *Quantitative evaluation of cerebellar syndrome.*
Ataxia score

Static functions		Kinetic functions	
1. Quality of walking	0 - 4	9. Oscillating movements of heel on knee : right-left	0 - 4
2. Quality of standing upright naturally	0 - 4	10. Quality test heel-tibia : right-left	0 - 6
3. Oscillating movements in natural position	0 - 4	11. Quality test finger-nose : right-left	0 - 6
4. Leg muscle movement in natural position	0 - 4	12. Quality test finger-finger : right-left	0 - 6
5. Quality of standing upright with feet together	0 - 4	13. Oscillating movements extended arm : right-left	0 - 3
6. Oscillating movements with feet together	0 - 4	14. Nystagmus	0 - 3
7. Leg muscle movement with feet together	0 - 4		
8. Quality of sitting position	0 - 4		

19 measurements. Maximum score : 100 %

Table 2 — *Example of assessing kinetic measurements from 0 to 6.*
Heel-knee-tibia test (measurement no. 10).

0	No trouble
1	Test subnormal
2	Lowering of heel in continuous axis, abnormally slow or abnormally abrupt
3	Lowering jerkily in the axis
4	Lowering jerkily with weak lateral clonic cramps
5	Lowering jerkily with strong lateral clonic cramps
6	Test impossible

A modification of serotonin metabolism seemed to appear primarily in experimental data. The harmaline-induced tremor which corresponds to a rhythmic electric activity in the olivary nucleus and the cerebellar cortex (Lamarre et al., 1971) can in fact be interrupted by the administration of serotonin at the level of the olive (Headly et al., 1976) and in certain cases by the administration of 5-hydroxytryptophan (5-HTP) (Bowman and Osuide, 1968). Chan-Palay has demonstrated, that rats with thiamine deficiency and ataxia show specific degeneration of various serotoninergic structures of the central nervous system, particularly of the serotoninergic cerebellar raphe system (Chan-Palay, 1979).

On this basis, we proposed a high dose treatment with 5-HTP for patients with stereotype degenerative cerebellar ataxias, usually combined with benserazide, a known inhibitor of peripheral 5-HTP decarboxylase (Lhermitte et al., 1975). Preliminary results were encouraging (Trouillas et al., 1981).

The following report presents the final long-term results observed in 26 patients.

Table 3 — *Example of assessing kinetic measurements from 0 to 6.*
Finger-nose test (measurement no. 11)

Finger-nose test	Cerebellar syndrome without tremor	Cerebellar syndrome with tremor
0	No trouble	No trouble
1	Oscillating movements without segmentation	Simple swerve at the end of the movement
2	Segmented movement in two phases	Tremor stopping immediately at the end of the movement
3	Segmented movement in three phases and final dysmetria	Tremor stopping in less than 10 seconds after reaching the nose
4	Segmented movement in four phases and considerable dysmetria	Tremor continuing more than 10 seconds after reaching the nose
5	Dysmetria preventing the patient from reaching his/her nose	Uninterrupted clonic cramps after completing the movement
6	Finger-nose movement impossible	Finger-nose movement impossible

Table 4 — *Percentage distribution of the 26 cerebellar*
patients of the study according to the severity
of their condition on the two main kinetic tests

Percentage of patients with the score :					Total
Score of the tests	0	1 or 2	3 or 4	5 or 6	
Finger-nose test before treatment	15.5	61.5	15.5	7.5	100
12th month of treatment	46.2	46.1	7.7	0	100
Heel-knee-tibia test before treatment	3.9	23	53.8	19.3	100
12th month of treatment	19.3	38.4	23	19.3	100

The score corresponds to the average score of the two limbs.
The proportion of patients with a less severe condition increased significantly at the end of treatment with 5-HTP (d-l-5-HTP-benserazide, d-l-5-HTP, l-5-HTP).
The degree of significance for the two tests, studied according to Wilcoxon's method of paired data, is $p < 0.01$.

Methods and patients

Quantitative evaluation of the cerebellar syndrome

Determination of an ataxia score

14 tests (Table 1) were quantified progressively from O (no disorder) to a maximum score in order to establish a total ataxia score expressed as a percentage.

The kinetic tests are difficult to assess. Tables 2 and 3 show the criteria used for the two main tests, the heel-knee tibia test and the finger-nose test. Table 4 shows the distribution of the 26 cerebellar patients according to the severity of the kinetic condition in these two tests.

The 8 static and 6 kinetic tests also make it possible to establish a static and a kinetic score, each calculated as a percentage of its own maximum. Example : patient no. 1 (Holmes' olivo-cerebellar atrophy) : total score : 50 %, static score : 88 %, kinetic score : 23,5 %.

Table 5 — *Quantitative evaluation of cerebellar syndrome.*
Objective measures

1. *Maximum time of standing in natural position (of 6 tests)**	7. *Rhythm of alternate movements right hand/left hand cycles/20 seconds*
2. *Maximum time of standing with feet together (of 6 tests)**	8. *Average time to pronounce arbitrary phrase (8 tests)*
3. *Average spread of feet (of 3 tests)*	9. *Time to write : first and family name*
4. *Time to walk a distance (of 12 meters) and back again*	10. *Time to write : I have come to the hospital*
5. *Distance of heel-knee hypermetria, right, left*	11. *Time to draw 3 rungs of a ladder*
6. *Rhythm of tapping foot right foot/left foot cycles/ 20 seconds*	12. *Time to draw a garland shape*
	13. *Average time to draw an Archimedes' spiral (3 tests)*

* The measurement is taken up to a maximum of 5 minutes ; this amount of time is considered indicative of standing upright for an unlimited time.

Determination of 13 objective measurements

For the sake of more exact analysis we measured 13 completely objective parameters listed in Table 5 and corresponding to 37 measurements in all. For each of these measurements there is a highly significant difference between the average observed in the 20 patients of the reference group of the study (see below) and the 25 control subjects in the same age group (van der Meersch, 1981).

Amongst the static functions, an essential symptom of cerebellar ataxia proved to be the reduction of maximum time standing upright without aid, either in a natural position or with the feet together. The average spread of the feet is increased very significantly (van der Meersch, 1981).

Amongst the kinetic functions, 9 measurements examine in greater detail the *speed of performing various movements* (Table 5). Measurements of the time required to walk a given distance (measurement 4), to write a name or a simple phrase (measurements 9 and 10) and to draw set shapes (measurements 11, 12, 13) make it possible to establish the relationship between distance and time, i.e. the speed in performing a movement. Measurement of the time required to pronounce an arbitrary sentence (measurement 8) indicates the speed of the movements involved in the spoken word. Measurement of the number of cycles in a given time for tests on hand and foot movements (measurements 6 and 7) provides the frequency of alternate movements and thus their speed of performance.

Comparison of these tests on patients and control subjects showed that cerebellar symptoms are characterized by a generalised and extremely significant slowing down of all these performance speeds (van der Meersch, 1981).

Frequency of examinations

The score and objective values were determined regularly every month or every two months at the same time of day. The patients were observed during the 12 months of treatment and then for six months after treatment was stopped.

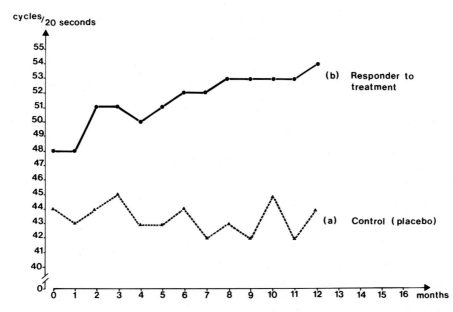

Fig 1 — The change in the frequency of alternate movements of the right hand over a period of 12 months. In case (a) with placebo (slowly developing cerebellar atrophy with predominant cortical involvement) statistical analysis by means of the Kendall method showed no signs of habituation. In case (b) (patient no. 1 : Holmes' olivo-cerebellar atrophy) a response to treatment can be confirmed (p < 0.001).

Data processing

The amount of coded data was considerable and could not be processed by hand. Thus, they were transcribed, collected on punch cards and stored in a computer, type HP-45. Thanks to « ataxia » software, this computer makes it possible to calculate all numerical variables (scores and means) and to plot the curves.

The method adopted to give a significant result over the 12 months of treatment was a method of tendency determination by means of the coefficient of rank correlation by Kendall (1970). This method was applied to the ataxia score, the kinetic scores and the various objective measurements.

Reliability of the score and the measurements. Study on habituation

A considerable problem arises from repeated examinations, in that the patients may become accustomed to the tests, thus influencing the accuracy of their results. 3 adult patients with hereditary ataxia were included in a double blind study for 12 months and given a placebo. They were examined every month.

The Kendall method showed that there was no significant variation in the level of the scores and objective measurements over this period.

By way of documentation, Figure 1 shows that the monthly examinations had no habit-forming effects on the speed of alternate movements of the right hand over a period of 12 months in a case of slowly developing cerebellar atrophy with predominant cortical involvement.

The role of habituation of movement throughout monthly examinations therefore seems negligible. Moreover, the total score variations for the 3 cases of hereditary ataxia were less than 10 % over 12 months. Thus, adult patients with hereditary ataxia constitute a reference group.

Variations in score greater than 10 % were recorded for 2 cases of arrested multiple sclerosis (see below) over 6 months which meant that these patients had to be excluded from the reference group.

Cinematography

6 patients were filmed 3-monthly over the 12 months period of treatment.

Selection of patients

The reference group

The reference group comprises 21 patients with hereditary ataxia, selected according to both genetic and clinical criteria with the aid of the CT scan.

1) Cerebellar atrophy (3 cases)*

Two cases corresponded to Holmes' original description (1907) and may be considered as having olivo-cerebellar atrophy. Aged 35 and 58 respectively, these two patients both had confirmed cases of cerebellar ataxia in their respective families with a dominant autosomal type of transmission. The cerebellar syndrome had started before the age of 30 and took the form of an isolated cerebellar ataxia, essentially static, slowly progressive, sparing the upper limbs, with dysarthria. One of the patients had lost the ability to walk and stand upright unaided.

One case corresponded to the original description of Marie et al. (1922) of slowly developing cerebellar atrophy with predominant cortical involvement. This was a sporadic case of static cerebellar syndrome with kinetic involvement predominating clearly in the lower limbs, occuring late in life (at the age of 55) and developing progressively in the absence of alcoholism. This patient was incapable of walking without aid or standing with his feet together.

2) Olivo-ponto-cerebellar atrophy (1 case)

The case studied was part of a family with dominant autosomal inherited disease (mother and grandmother affected). This female patient, aged 20, had a pronounced static and kinetic cerebellar syndrome with severe dysarthria, loss of reflexes and discrete sensory lemniscal disorders in the lower limbs. There was a bilateral positive Babinski's sign. The mother presented a similar picture, but without a positive Babinski's sign. CT scan showed both in the patient and in her mother considerable ponto-cerebellar atrophy with hollowing of the base of the pons, enlargement of the cerebellar hemispherical sulci and atrophy of the superior part of the vermis.

This case differs from the classic case of olivo-ponto-cerebellar atrophy described by Dejerine and Thomas (1900), but corresponds well with olivo-ponto-cerebellar atrophies with dominant autosomal transmission and variable symptomatology in the genealogy described by Schut and Haymaker (1951). This group

---

* All 3 cases have cerebellar cortical atrophy predominantly at the level of the superior part of the vermis on CT Scan.

210

is called « olivo-ponto-cerebellar atrophy of the Schut — Haymaker type » (Konigsmark and Weiner 1970). This unusual nomenclature is accepted by Refsum and Skre (1978).

3) Friedreich's ataxia (17 cases)

These cases were selected on the purely clinical and genetic criteria of Geoffroy et al. (1976). All the cases studied here had the following characteristics : Genealogically a recessive autosomal type of transmission ; age of onset of the illness before the end of puberty ; progressive ataxia ; premature dysarthria ; distal muscular weakness of the lower limbs ; impairment of lemniscal sensation in the lower limbs on epicritic, arthro-kinesthetic and pallesthesic testing ; loss of deep tendon reflexes, bilateral positive Babinski's sign ; pes cavus and/or scoliosis ; cardiomyopathy on electrocardiogram or echocardiogram. CT scan used in 7 cases was normal (in 4 cases) or showed a minimum atrophy of the vermis (in 3 cases). 15 of these patients were over the age of 21. Five were bedridden and had lost the ability to sit up without aid. Only one other patient was able to walk without aid at the beginning of the series of tests (a child aged 12).

4) Other cases

— One case of a cerebellar syndrome, static and developing slowly postoperatively, lasting 5 years after surgical injury to the vermis from excision of a medulloblastoma (adult aged 40) ;

— Three cases of « fixed » disseminated multiple sclerosis ;

— One case of peduncular infarction with intention dyskinesia in the upper left limb.

The criteria for selecting the cases of multiple sclerosis were as follows :

(1) predominantly cerebellar symptomatology ;

(2) entire symptomatology present for at least one year, without modification of functional indices according to Kurtzke (1961) during this period. These patients had had azathioprine therapy (2.5 mg/kg) for several years.

Therapy

After numerous preliminary studies identical long-term treatment with a fixed dose was chosen for all patients over a period of 12 months. These doses were determined by trial and error in the course of the preliminary tests.

Thus :

— One case received : 16 mg/kg/day of d-l-5-HTP for 12 months,

— One case received : 16 mg/kg/day of l-5-HTP for 12 months,

— 24 adult patients received : 16 mg/kg/day of d-l-5-HTP with 6 mg/kg/day of benserazide for 12 months.

We adhered strictly to monotherapy. The daily dose was divided into 3 portions. Overall, there was good tolerance of these high doses of l-5-HTP and d-l-5-HTP with or without benserazide association. Vomiting, however, was noted in the first week of treatment necessitating *progressive administration of the drug* ; chronic diarrhoea occurred in 2 patients and there was one case who developed an annoying habit of falling asleep during the day. It is important to note that benserazide must not be administered to patients below the age of 21, because of the risk of affecting the epiphyses. Abrupt curtailment of treatment may be marked by intense neuro-vegetative decompensation (5 cases).

Biochemical studies

These were conducted in order to assess the effects of long-term administration of 5-HTP on the cerebral metabolism and the peripheral metabolism of serotonin.

Before treatment 5-hydroxy-indol-acetic acid (5-HIAA) and homovanillic acid (HVA) were tested 17 times — 13 times in cases of Friedreich's ataxia — before and after the probenecid test. This was performed following the intravenous administration of 75 mg/kg probenecid for 5 hours. The second lumbar puncture was taken 8 hours after the beginning of the perfusion (Renaud et al., 1980). HVA and 5-HIAA were examined by means of high-performance liquid chromatography with ultraviolet amperometric detection (Menouni et al., in press). The essentials of the results of the probenecid test have already been described by one of us (Cramer et al., in press).

The study of the metabolism of serotonin before treatment also involves measuring the elimination of 5-HIAA in urine and the blood serotonin level (Matray and Moreau, 1964).

After 12 months of treatment with combined d-l-5-HTP-benserazide we had 7 cases (including 5 cases of Friedreich's ataxia) on which all these tests had been carried out. Lumbar punctures were performed 18 hours after the last dose of 5-HTP, the blood sample was taken 12 hours after the last dose ; the urine specimens were taken during the period of treatment.

Results : Effects observed during administration of treatment

Effect of d-l-5-HTP (16 mg/kg/day) in association with benserazide (24 patients)

Hereditary degenerative diseases (reference group)
Detailed results are shown in Tables 6 and 7.

1) Cerebellar cortical atrophy
— Holmes' olivo-cerebellar atrophy : In patients with a predominantly static syndrome, there was a significant effect in the two cases. The patient who could not stand up, not only progressively regained his ability to stand upright unaided (Fig. 2, case no.1) after a brief period of aggravation of the disease, but also to walk without aid. There was less marked improvement of kinetic performance both quantitatively and qualitatively. The heel-knee tests in particular hardly changed.
— Cerebellar atrophy with cortical predominance (1 case) : In this patient, who was incapable of standing with his feet together and of walking without aid, both functions were regained slowly and progressively. The speed of alternate hand movements clearly improved ($p = 0.005$ on right, $p < 0.025$ on left).

2) Friedreich's ataxia (15 adults — average age : 29 years — 5 bedridden cases)

212

Table 6 — *Study of the statistical value of the decrease*
in the ataxia score registered
over 12 months in degenerative cerebellar ataxia

Treatment	Type of ataxia	Static score	Statistical value* Kinetic score	Total score	No.
	Holmes	$p < 0.001$	$p < 0.005$	$p < 0.001$	1
	Cerebellar atrophy	$p < 0.025$	N S	N S	2
	Marie, Foix, Alajouanine	$p = 0.05$	N S	N S	3
		$p < 0.001$	N S	$p < 0.001$	4
		$p < 0.005$	$p = 0.05$	$p < 0.005$	5
		$p < 0.01$	$p < 0.025$	$p = 0.05$	6
		$p = 0.05$	N S	$p < 0.01$	7
		N S	$p < 0.005$	$p = 0.05$	8
Association		N S	N S	$p = 0.05$	9
d-l-5-HTP	Friedreich's	N S	N S	N S	10
(16 mg/kg/day)	ataxia	$p < 0.05$	N S	$p = 0.05$	11
benserazide		$p = 0.05$	N S	$p = 0.05$	12
		N S	$p = 0.05$	$p = 0.05$	13
		$p < 0.05$	N S	$p < 0.05$	14
		$p < 0.01$	N S	$p < 0.05$	15
		$p < 0.05$	$p = 0.05$	N S	16
		N S	N S	N S	17
		N S	N S	N S	18
	Olivo-ponto- cerebellar atrophy Schut-Haymaker type	$p = 0.005$	N S	N S	19
d-l-5-HTP (16 mg/kg/day)	Friedreich's ataxia	N S	$p < 0.025$	N S	20
l-5-HTP	Friedreich's ataxia	$p < 0.005$	$p < 0.01$	$p < 0.01$	21

* Study of the tendency by means of the cœfficient of rank correlation by Kendall.
NS : not significantly different.

213

Table 7 — *Degenerative ataxia (reference group).*
Effect of the combination d-l-5-HTP (16 mg/kg/day) -
benserazide (6 mg/kg/day) in the long term (12 months) on
the main measurements of ataxia.

Measurement**	Number of patients with a significant variation of measurements over 12 months*				
	Holmes' atrophy	Marie-Foix-Al. atrophy	Friedreich's ataxia	OPC atrophy Schut/ Haymaker	All degenerative ataxias
	n = 2	n = 1	n = 15	n = 1	n = 19
Total ataxia score	1/2	0/1	5/15	0/1	6/19
Static score***	2/2	0/1	6/15	1/1	9/19
Kinetic score	1/2	0/1	2/15	0/1	3/19
Time standing upright naturally***	1/1	0/1	6/9	0/1	7/12
Time standing upright, feet together	1/2	1/1	4/10	0/1	6/14
Time walking without aid	1/2	1/1	—	1/1	3/4
Average spread of feet	0/2	0/1	1/10	0/1	1/14
Frequency of alternate movements :					
right hand	1/2	1/1	7/15	0/1	9/19
left hand	1/2	1/1	5/15	0/1	7/19
right foot***	2/2	1/1	8/15	1/1	12/19
left foot	1/2	1/1	8/15	1/1	11/19
Speed of pronunciation of arbitrary sentence***	1/2	0/1	12/15	0/1	13/19
Speed of writing arbitrary sentence	0/2	0/1	7/12	0/1	7/16
Speed of drawing an Archimedes' spiral :					
increase	2/2	0/1	9/14	0/1	11/18
decrease			1/14		1/18

* Study of tendency by means of the cœfficient of correlation by Kendall. Criterion of significance p < 0.05.
** Only those measurements are taken into account corresponding to a possible test. Patients with a normal time standing upright (more than 300 sec.) before treatment are also excluded from this test as no variation can be studied.
*** Measurements influenced most frequently.

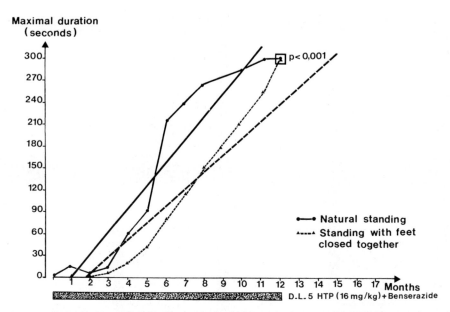

Fig. 2 — The change in the maximum time of standing upright without aid. Olivo-cerebellar atrophy of the Holmes type (patient no. 1, aged 58). Slow improvement (3 months) and then progressive improvement of standing upright without aid, in natural position and with feet together, upon administration of d-l-5-HTP (16 mg/kg/day) and benserazide (6 mg/kg/day). In the 11th month the patient was able to walk again without aid.

An overall effect was observed as 5 out of 15 cases responded significantly ($p < 0.05$) and 6 cases responded slightly ($p = 0.05$). The average score decreased from 52 % at $t = 0$ to 29.7 % at $t = 12$ months. The static score improved (6/15) more often than the kinetic score (2/15). One patient left his wheelchair to take up walking with sticks again. Dysarthria almost always improved leading to a better quality of elocution (12/15). Patients were frequently able to draw Archimedes' spiral more quickly without a great improvement in quality, apart from certain cases (Fig. 3).

The frequency of these responses must not conceal their quantitative limits. Although their static score improved, the 10 patients able to stand did not regain their ability to walk without aid. Of the bedridden patients incapable of sitting up (5 cases), only the ability to sit up consistently improved. The score curves make it possible to compare the rare « good responders » (3/15) (Fig. 4) with a steep slope, with the « poor responders », one of whom deteriorated under treatment after a brief improvement. These poor responders are patients with a long history of the disease or young patients with a high score.

3) Olivo-ponto-cerebellar atrophy, Schut-Haymaker type.

In a young 20 year old woman the ataxia regressed slightly (total score : NS* ; static score : $p = 0.005$; kinetic score : NS*). The ability to stand upright hardly changed and alternate movements were not modified at all.

---

* NS = not significantly different.

215

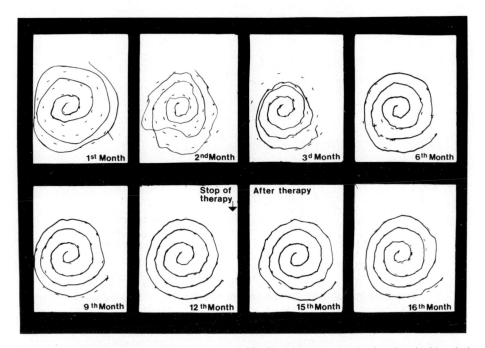

Fig. 3 — Friedreich's ataxia (patient no. 4, aged 28). Slow improvement in drawing Archimedes' spiral, extremely modified at beginning by hypermetria. Normalization was accompanied by a significant slowing down over 12 months (p < 0.05). It is interesting to note that qualitative improvement continued up to 4 months after termination of treatment.

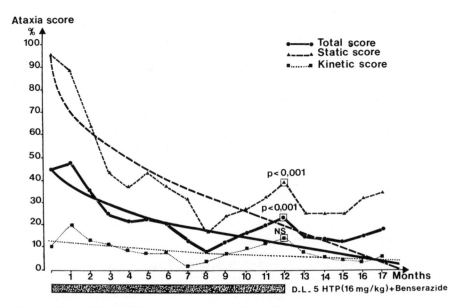

Fig. 4 — Case of Friedreich's ataxia, good responder (patient no. 4).
It is interesting to note the persistence of the effect of treatment (d-l-5-HTP, 16 mg/kg/day — benserazide, 6 mg/kg/day) with continuation of improvement over a period of 5 months after termination of treatment.

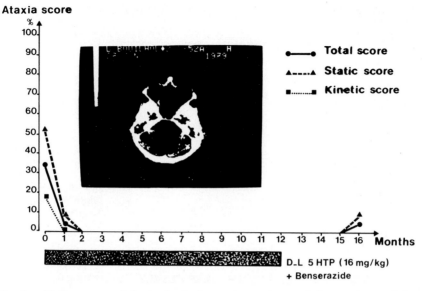

Fig. 5 — Disappearance of slowly developing post-operative cerebellar syndrome of the essentially static type upon treatment with d-l-5-HTP (16 mg/kg/day) and benserazide (6 mg). CT scan shows localization of the lesion to the vermis.

In all of 19 degenerative ataxias treatment modified the total score significantly in 6 out of 19 cases, but the static score in 9 out of 19 cases.

Non-degenerative diseases

1) Injury of the vermis developing slowly after surgery

In a patient with ataxia for 5 years, the essentially static cerebellar symptomatology disappeared within 2 months (Fig. 5).

2) Multiple sclerosis (3 cases)

In these 3 cases a highly significant improvement in the ataxia score was observed ($p < 0.001$; $p = 0.01$; $p = 0.005$ respectively). The intention dyskinesia in the right hand of one patient disappeared in the 10th month. In another patient, marked intention dyskinesia hardly changed. Dysarthria improved in all 3 cases.

3) Peduncular infarction

In one patient with dyskinesia of intention of the left arm and a discrete kinetic syndrome of the lower homolateral limb little effect on the total score ($p = 0.05$) and on the kinetic score ($p = 0.05$) was observed and the dyskinesia remained strictly unchanged.

Effect of d-l-5-HTP used alone (16 mg/kg) (Table 6 : case no. 20)

In an adolescent patient of 17 years with Friedreich's ataxia d-l-5-HTP alone brought about an improvement in the static score after 3 months, with an interruption and even aggravation up to the 12th month. The kinetic score itself improved slightly. The dysarthria improved markedly.

217

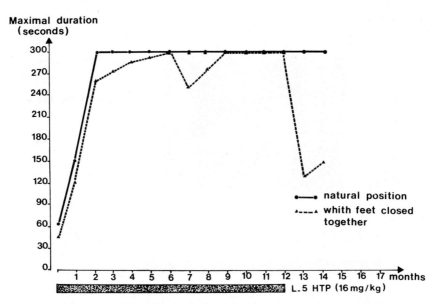

Fig. 6 — Effect of l-5-HTP (16 mg/kg/day) on static cerebellar syndrome in a case of Friedreich's ataxia (case no. 21, aged 12). A highly significant prolongation of the time of standing upright in a natural position and with feet together was observed.

Effect of l-5-HTP used alone (16 mg/kg) (Table 6 : case no. 21).

In a child of 12 years with Friedreich's ataxia l-5-HTP quickly and spectacularly influenced static performance. After one month, the child was able to keep his feet together (Fig. 6). Adiadochokinesis and more particularly elocution (p < 0.005) were improved.

Effects observed after termination of treatment

Amongst the cases of cortical atrophy, termination of treatment brought about a severe relapse in one patient after 10 days (case no. 1). Regression of ataxia continued in 2 other patients for 3 months ; they then suffered a relapse in the 6th and 7th months respectively. In the 3 cases of « good responders » with Friedreich's ataxia, regression continued for 3 months and in one case up to 5 months (Fig. 3 and 4).

In multiple sclerosis regression can also continue for 1 to 5 months. The case of surgical ataxia which had disappeared did not reappear befor the 4th month (Fig. 5).

Biochemical study

Examination of serotonin and dopamine metabolism using the probenecid test

We decided to concentrate our statistical study on the homogeneous group of patients with Friedreich's ataxia. The 13 tests carried out before treatment revealed only one abnormality : A decrease in the basal concentration of HVA without a

Table 8 — *Results of probenecid tests on 5 patients with Friedreich's ataxia carried out before treatment with d-l-5-HTP - benserazide and after 12 months of treatment*

Group of patients	Probenecid (nmol/l)	HVA (nmol/l)				5-HIAA (nmol/l)			
		Before	After	Δ	Δ/Prob	Before	After	Δ	Δ/Prob
Before treatment	24.2	127	537	310	13.0	114	228	111	4.69
(n=5)	±4.8	±11	±88	±104	±2.0	±30	±41	±36	±0.75
		(n=3)		(n=3)	(n=3)	(n=3)		(n=3)	(n=3)
During treatment	34.2	132	650	518	13.8	199	1007	808	21.62
(n=5) (12th month)	±4.4	±11	±166	±165	±3.4	±63	±220	±256	±4.64
Degree of significance of differences (NS: not significantly different)	N S	N S	N S	N S	N S	N S	$p<0.01$	N S	$p<0.05$

The results are expressed as the mean ± the standard error of the mean and the degree of significance of the differences is estimated by means of Student's t-test.
Account of the difference in probenecid concentration in the group before and after has been taken by calculating the cœfficient of the increase of concentration of the monoamine (Δ) compared with the probenecid concentration (Δ/Prob.) Treatment does not modify this quotient for the HVA while it multiplies it by more than 4 for the 5-HIAA.

decrease in the replacement rate of HVA after probenecid. The basal and replacement rates of 5-HIAA were normal. These results will be the subject of a later publication.

A probenecid test was performed on 5 of these patients after 12 months of treatment. The results obtained are presented in Table 8. They show that treatment with the combination d-l-5-HTP-benserazide modifies neither the basal rate nor the replacement rate of HVA in the cerebro-spinal fluid whilst it raises the basal rate of 5-HIAA and increases very significantly its rate after probenecid ($p < 0.01$) as well as its replacement rate ($p < 0.05$), even taking into account the raised cerebro-spinal fluid probenecid concentration « during treatment » compared with the level « before treatment ».

These results suggest that long-term treatment with d-l-5-HTP produces selective increase in the central production of serotonin with repercussions on the 5-HIAA of the cerebro-spinal fluid whilst the metabolism of dopamine and HVA does not seem to be modified.

Examination of the general metabolism of serotonin

In the 13 patients with Friedreich's ataxia the average 24 hour urinary excretion of 5-HIAA (21.89 μmol/24 hours) was at the lower limit of normal, but was not very different from that of the control subjects (20 μmol/24 hours). The average concentration of serotonin in blood was strictly normal (1.4 μmol/1).

In the 12th month of treatment of the 5 patients mentioned above, the average level of 5-HIAA excretion in urine rose considerably (1238 μmol/24 hours), while the average concentration of serotonin in blood increased significantly (2.78 micromol./1). This rise is evidence of the imperfect blockage of peripheral serotonin biosynthesis from 5-HTP by benserazide.

219

Discussion

Effect of 5-HTP on human cerebellar syndrome

We have shown that in the pure cerebellar syndrome of cortical cerebellar atrophy of the vermis long-term administration of high doses of d-l-5-HTP with benserazide can bring about a progressive and significant improvement of cerebellar ataxia. The cerebellar syndrome of Friedreich's ataxia, though complicated by other symptoms, is also affected by this treatment.

An identical result in the cerebellar syndrome, developing slowly after surgical injury to the vermis and in the cerebellar syndrome of multiple sclerosis, shows that the drug affects cerebellar ataxia in general and not hereditary degenerative diseases specifically.

d-l-5-HTP alone is minimally active ; therefore benserazide was also necessary to produce a definite effect.

Moreover, we have proven that the levorotatory form of 5-HTP is active. At the same dose (16 mg/kg) l-5-HTP alone seems equally effective as d-l-5-HTP combined with benserazide and is also better tolerated.

The response to treatment varies according to the aetiology. Cortical atrophies of the vermis responded slowly, but significantly and in a clinically interesting way. The cerebellar syndrome of Friedreich's ataxia responded poorly, apart from the dysarthria. The effect was specific : Neither sensory, nor pyramidal disorders were affected. The clinical effect on « good » responders was interesting and these patients asked for treatment to be resumed.

It can be said that olivo-ponto-cerebellar atrophy of the Schut-Haymaker type responds poorly.

Amongst the non-degenerative aetiologies the cerebellar syndrome after surgical injury to the vermis responded spectacularly. The cerebellar ataxia of multiple sclerosis was regularly sensitive with a clinically interesting result.

Effect of 5-HTP on the different features of cerebellar ataxia

From the point of view of symptoms the dominant effect of 5-HTP in the reference groups was on the static cerebellar syndrome, which was more frequently and more significantly affected than the kinetic syndrome. This effect was found for both degenerative and non-degenerative aetiologies.

Thus, 5-HTP seems to be a drug that can sometimes enable the patient to stand upright again without aid, decreases oscillating body movements and twitching of leg muscles, and helps the patient to put his feet together or even to walk again without aid.

Dysarthria seemed to be the symptom most frequently affected after improvement of static symptoms. The effect occurs particularly early, indeed usually on the 15th day of treatment.

The effect of 5-HTP on kinetic performance is irregular, slower and less pronounced. 5-HTP sometimes proves effective in adiadochokinesia, making alternate movements of the hands more rapid and more regular. It can reduce hypermetria in the finger-nose and heel-knee tests and especially in drawing the rungs of a ladder or Archimedes' spiral.

The effect of 5-HTP on tremor or on intention dyskinesias is slight or non-existent : out of 3 cases one improved, two cases were resistant.

Kinetics of the action of 5-HTP in cerebellar ataxia

The effect of 5-HTP is slow in hereditary degenerative ataxias. The best mathematical model for demonstrating the drop in score is a decreasing function of the square root of the time. It is much quicker in cerebellar syndromes due to surgical injury and multiple sclerosis.

Another essential feature is the persistence of the effect for a period of 2 to 6 months after termination of treatment ; this was observed in all the various aetiologies of ataxia.

In general, the mechanisms involved in the regression of the cerebellar syndrome following long-term 5-HTP administration cannot be correlated with the classical neuro-mediation mechanism. The slowness and the persistence of the effect suggest that the final mechanism is largely independent of the immediate effects of 5-HTP or serotonin. There is no neuro-mediation, but more likely « neuro-induction » or « neuro-modulation ».

An attempt to interpret the effects observed : Serotonin and cerebellum

At the present state of knowledge, it is too early to interpret these results precisely. It is our impression that regression of cerebellar ataxia is linked with the high level of « impregnation » of the nervous system by l-5-HTP and with an isolated increase of the cerebral biosynthesis of serotonin. This is shown by the (high) increases in the basal and replacement rates of 5-HIAA in the cerebro-spinal fluid in the probenecid test, while the metabolism of the HVA is unchanged. The process is thus serotonin-dependent but, not specifically serotoninergic.

However, it cannot be excluded that the observed phenomena are linked to specific serotoninergic structures present in the cerebellum or in anatomically connected structures such as the inferior olive. In 1969 Hökfelt and Fuxe discovered serotoninergic afferents with terminals in the cerebellar cortex. Chan-Palay (1975, 1977) describes such terminals in the grey cerebellar nuclei. The origin of these axons is in the serotoninergic cell bodies of the raphe magnus, raphe pontis and raphe centralis superior nuclei (Shinnar et al., 1975 ; Bobillier et al., 1976 ; Taber-Pierce et al., 1976 ; Batini et al., 1977) which project preferentially to the cerebellar vermis (Shinnar et al., 1975 ; Batini et al. 1977 ; Frankfurter et al., 1977).

Such serotoninergic terminals also exist in the inferior olive and are particularly dense in the dorsal accessory and medial accessory nuclei (Fuxe, 1965 ; Nobin et al., 1973). In a remarkable way these olivary zones project selectively onto the anterior lobe of the vermis (Wiklund et al., 1977) and converge with the zones receiving direct spinal afferents (Boesten and Voogd, 1975).

Finally, at the medullary level there are anatomical and functional links between the serotoninergic axons coming from bulbospinal and spino-cerebellar tracts. It is particularly interesting to note their contiguity at the bulbar and spinal level (Bobillier et al., 1976 ; Nobin et al., 1973). From a functional point of view, we recall that following degeneration of bulbospinal serotoninergic axons due to 5,

221

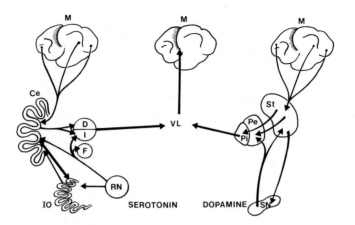

Fig. 7 — Comparison of the serotoninergic cerebellar system and the striatal dopaminergic system.
M : motor cortex ; Ce : cerebellar cortex ; IO : inferior olive ; RN : raphe nuclei ; D,I : dentate nucleus and nucleus interpositus ; F : nucleus fastigii ; St : striatum ; Pe : putamen ; Pi : pallidum ; SN : substantia nigra ; VL : thalamic ventrolateral nucleus.

6-dihydroxytryptamine treatment one finds signs of aberrant regeneration of the serotoninergic axons in the spino-cerebellar tract (Nobin et al., 1973).

The serotoninergic structures seem to develop special links with the cerebellum in general and the spino-olivo-vermis system in particular. The implication of this system on the control of postural equilibrium and walking can be compared to the specific effectiveness of 5-HTP on the static components of cerebellar ataxia.

The hypothesis of cerebellar and olivary serotoninergic receptors was formulated on the basis of neurophysiological experiments (Tsang and Lal, 1978 ; Headley and Lodge, 1976) and anatomical studies (Chan-Palay, 1975). Synaptic receptors act rapidly and cannot produce the effects observed in our study. By contrast, non-synaptic receptors with « humoral neuro-dispersion », as postulated by Chan-Palay (1975), provide an anatomical and functional basis for the slow effect observed in the study.

If such cerebellar serotoninergic receptors do exist, there would be a structural analogy between the cerebellar system innervated by non-medullated fibres from the raphe nuclei and the striatal system receiving non-medullated fibres from the substantia nigra (Fig. 7). While l-dopamine has a regulatory effect on the striatal system, l-serotonin could — according to the data presented here — prove an important biochemical regulator of the cerebellar system. As the two systems converge remarkably at the level of the ventrolateral nucleus of the thalamus, l-serotonin and l-dopamine could constitute two sides, both antagonistic and complementary, of the biochemical control of movement.

Conclusion

The clinical benefits presented in this study justify prescribing d-l-5-HTP, or better still l-5-HTP with benserazide, to patients with certain aetiological causes of cerebellar syndrome. At present, the best indications seem to be cortical cerebellar atrophies, slowly developing cerebellar syndromes after surgical injury and multiple sclerosis. Nevertheless, it is important to stress that the response may be slow and irregular.

REFERENCES

Batini, C., Corvisier, J., Hardy, O. *1977* — Projections des noyaux réticulaires bulbaires et des noyaux du raphé sur les lobules VI et VII du cortex cérébelleux du chat. *C.R. Acad. Sci., Paris, Sec. D., 284* : 1805-1806.

Bloom, F.E., Hoffer, B.V., Siggins, G.R. *1971* — Studies on norepinephrine containing afferents to Purkinje cells of rat cerebellum. I. Localization of the fibres and their synapses. *Brain Res., 25* : 501-521.

Bobillier, P., Seguin, S., Petitjean, F., Salvert, D., Touret, M., Jouvet, M. *1976* — The raphe nuclei of the cat brain stem : a topographical atlas of their afferent projections as revealed by autoradiography. *Brain Res., 113* : 449-486.

Boesten, A.J.P., Voogd, J. *1975* — Projections of the dorsal column nuclei and the spinal cord on the inferior olive in the cat, *J. comp. Neurol, 161* : 215-238.

Bowman, N.C., Osuide, G. *1968* — Interaction between the effects of tremorin and harmine and other drugs in chicks. *Eur. J. Pharmacol., 3* : 106-111.

Burkard, W.P., Pieri, L., Haefely, W. *1976* — Changes of rat cerebellar guanosin 3'5' — cyclic phosphate by dopaminergic mechanism *in vivo. Adv. Biochem. Psychopharmacol., 15* : 315-324.

Chan-Palay, V. *1975* — Fine structure of labelled axons in the cerebellar cortex and nuclei of rodents and primates after intraventricular infusions with tritiated serotonin. *Anat. Embryol. 148* : 235-265.

Chan-Palay, V. *1977* — *Cerebellar dentate nucleus organization, cytology and transmitters, 548 p.* Berlin, Springer-Verlag.

Chan-Palay, V. *1979* — Indoleamine neurons and their processes in the normal rat brain and in chronic diet-induced thiamine deficiency, demonstrated by ^{3}H-Serotonin. *J. comp. Neurol., 176* : 467-494.

Cramer, H., Warter, J.M., Renaud, B., Krieger J., Marescaux C., Hammers R. — Cerebrospinal fluid adenosine 3, 5-monophosphate, 5-hydroxyindoleacetic acid and homovanillic acid in patients with sleep *J. Neurol., Neurosurg. Psychiat. (in press).*

Dejerine, J., Thomas, A. *1900* — L'atrophie olivo-ponto-cérébelleuse. *Nouv. Iconogr. Salpêt., 13* : 330-370.

Dreux, C., Delaudeux, B. *1964* — Étude critique des méthodes biochimiques d'exploration du métabolisme de la sérotonine. *Presse méd., 72* : 2925-2929.

Frankfurter, A., Weber, J.T., Harting, J.K. *1977* — Brain stem projections to lobule VII of posterior vermis in the squirrel monkey : as demonstrated by the retrograde axonal transport of tritiated horseradish peroxidase. *Brain Res., 124* : 135-139.

Fuxe, K. *1965* — Evidence for the existence of monoamine neurons in the central nervous system. IV. Distribution of monoamine nerve terminals in the central nervous system. *Acta Physiol. Scand., 64,* Suppl. 247, 39-85.

Geoffroy, G., Barbeau, A., Breton, G., Lemieux, G., Aube, M., Léger, C. *1976* — Clinical description and roentgenologic evaluation of patients with Friedreich's ataxia. *J. Can. Sci. Neurol., 3* : 279-286.

Headley, P.M., Lodge, D., Duggan, A.N. *1976* — Drug induced rhythmical activity in the inferior olivary complex of the rat. *Brain Res., 101* : 461-478.

Headley, P.M., Lodge D. *1976* — Studies on field potentials and on single cells in the inferior olivary complex of the rat. *Brain Res., 101* : 445-459.

Hoffer, B.J., Freedman, R., Woodward, D.J., Puro, D., Moises, H. *1978* — A functional role for adrenergic input to the cerebellar cortex : interaction of norepinephrine with mossy and climbing fiber excitation and GABA-mediated inhibition. In : *Interactions between putative neurotransmitters in the brain.* S. Garattini et al. (ed.) pp. 231-243. New-York, Raven Press.

Hoffman, D.G., Sladek J.R. Jr. *1973* — The distribution of catecholamines within the inferior olivary complex of the gerbil and rabbit. *J. comp. Neurol., 151* : 101-112.

Hökfelt, T., Fuxe, K. *1969* — Cerebellum monoamine nerve terminals, a new type of afferent fibers to the cortex cerebelli. *Exp. Brain Res., 9* : 63-72.

Holmes, G. *1907* — A form of familial degeneration of the cerebellar. *Brain, 30* : 466-489.

Kendall, M. G. *1970* — *Rank correlation methods.* pp. 165-166. London, C. Griffin and Co.

Konigsmark, B.W., Weiner L.T. *1970* — The olivo ponto cerebellar atrophies : a review. *Medicine, 49* : 227-241.

Kurtzke, J.F. *1961* — On the evaluation of disability in multiple sclerosis. *Neurology, 11* : 686-694.

Lamarre, Y., de Montigny, C., Dumont, M., Weiss, M. *1971* — Harmaline-induced rhythmic activity of cerebellar and lower brain stem neurones. *Brain Res., 32* : 246-250.

Lhermitte, F., Degos, C.F., Marteau, R. *1975* — Association d'un inhibiteur de la dopadécarboxylase aux traitements par le 5-hydroxytryptophane. *Nouv. Presse Méd., 4* : 31.

Marie, P., Foix, C., Alajouanine, T. *1922* — De l'atrophie cérébelleuse tardive à prédominance corticale (Atrophie parenchymateuse primitive des lamelles du cervelet, atrophie paléo-cérébelleuse primitive). *Rev. Neurol.,* 849-885 and 1082-1111.

Matray, F., Moreau, J. *1964* — Technique du dosage de la sérotonine. *Pathol. et Biol., 12* : 1137-1140.

Menouni, V., Guardiola, P., Renaud, B., Quincy, Cl. — Liquid chromatographic determination of homovanillic acid, 5-hydroxyindoleacetic acid and probenecid levels in human cerebrospinal fluid during probenecid test. *J. Chromatography* (in press).

Nobin, A., Baumgarten, H.G., Pjorklund, A., Lachnemayer, L., Stenevi, U. *1973* — Axonal degeneration and regeneration of the bulbo spinal indolamine neurons after 5, 6-dihydroxytryptamine treatment. *Brain Res., 56* : 1-24.

Refsum, S., Skre, H. *1978* — *Neurological approaches to the inherited ataxia.* (Advances in Neurology, vol. 21) Kark R.A., Rosenberg R.N. and Schut L.J. (eds), New York, Raven Press.

Renaud, B., Mouret, J., Michel, D., Chazot, G., Laurent, B., Quincy, Cl. *1980* — Exploration pharmacologique du métabolisme des monoamines cérébrales par le test au probénécide : intérêt et limites. In : *Les neuromédiateurs du tronc cérébral,* B. Schott, G. Chazot (eds), pp. 217-231. Paris, Editions Sandoz.

Schon, F., Iverson, L.L. *1972* — Selective accumulation of ^{3}H-GABA by stellate cells in rat cerebellar cortex in vivo. *Brain Res.,* 503-507.

Schut, J.W., Haymaker, W. *1951* — Hereditary ataxia : a pathologic study of five cases with common ancestry *J. Neuropath. Clin. Neurol., 1* : 183-213.

Shinnar, S., Maciewicz, R.J., Shofer, R.J. *1975* — A raphe projection to cat cerebellar cortex. *Brain Res., 97* : 139-143.

Sladek, J.R. Jr., Bowman, J.P. *1975* — The distribution of catecholamines within the inferior olivary complex of the cat and rhesus monkey. *J. comp. Neurol., 163* : 203-214.

Taber-Pierce, E., Walberg, F., Hoddevik, G.H. *1976* — Projections from raphe nuclei to cerebellar cortex in cats. *Soc. Neurosci. Abstr., 2* : 501.

Tamarkin, N.R., Goodwin, F.K., Axelrod, J. *1970* — Rapid elevation of biogenic amine metabolites in human C S F following probenecid. *Life Sci., (Part.I), 9* : 1297-1408.

Thierry, A.M., Hirsch, J.C., Tassin, J.P. *1974* — Presence of dopaminergic terminals and absence of dopaminergic cell bodies in the cerebral cortex of the cat. *Brain Res., 79* : 77-88.

Trouillas, P., Garde, A., Robert, J.M., Adeleine, P. *1981* — Régression de l'ataxie cérébelleuse humaine sous administration à long terme de 5-hydroxytryptophane. *C.R. Acad. Sci., Paris, 292* : 119-122.

Tsang, D., Lal, G. *1978* — Accumulation of cyclic adenosine 3'5'-monophosphate in human cerebellar cortex slices : effect of monoamine receptor agonists and antagonists. *Brain Res., 140* : 307-313.

Van der Meersch, M. *1981* — *Essai de quantification du syndrome cérébelleux.* Thèse Méd. ; Lyon, 1981.

Wiklund, L., Björklund, A., Sjölund, B. *1977* — The indolaminergic innervation of the inferior olive. I. Convergence with direct spinal afferents in the areas projecting to the cerebellar anterior lobe. *Brain Res., 131* : 1-21.

*

* *

A film is projected showing a child with ataxia. 5-HTP improves significantly the ataxis disorders.

224

DISCUSSION

Ch. Eggers
How many children have you treated and do you know of any complications after treatment of cerebrellar ataxia with 5-HTP ?

P. Trouillas
In children ? I think this is the only child who has been treated. We have now more than 55 patients in the protocol, but this is the only child of the series.

Ch. Eggers
And do you know other publications about 5-HTP treatment in children ?

P. Trouillas
This is an original work and there have not been any publications about 5-HTP in cerebellar ataxia except for a note by Dr. Rascol at the end of last year, which duplicated these results, but gave no details about the age of the patients.

Ch. Eggers
Then you must publish it in our Journal of Neuropediatrics in English. I would like to publish this case.

N. Matussek
I would like to ask you, since this is quite a high dosage of 5-HTP, have you seen any side effects ? And how is sleep influenced by such treatment ?

P. Trouillas
There are some drawbacks, particularly in the gastrointestinal sphere there is diarrhoea and vomiting mainly during the first week. I observed drowsiness in 10 % of the cases. With levo-5-HTP drowsiness seems to be more frequent : We had one patient who was drowsy during the day and had insomnia during the night. From a thymic point of view, the treatment is excellent. The patients are euphoric and the depressed ones recover. I think that what has been published about 5-HTP in depression should be taken again to see whether or not the dosage was not too low. If you use the 5-HTP plus decarboxylase inhibitor you also get a better antidepressant effect. Levo-5-HTP should be an even better treatment for cerebellar ataxia and depression.

J.S. Kim
I would like to know about the multiple sclerosis patient with 5-HTP treatment. Does it have any effect ?

P. Trouillas
This series contains several patients with multiple sclerosis. Here we are dealing with the cerebellar ataxia of these patients and not the general evolution of the disease. In our protocol, the MS patients were selected as having a steady period before the treatment for 6 months at least according to the Kurtzke's scale. They were all under immunosuppressive treatment. They were also considered as having a steady clinical formula and a steady ataxia. The treatment with 5-HTP induced a very clear improvement in the ataxia. In « active » patients, 5-HTP seems to have no clear influence whatsoever on the evolution of MS.

J.S. Kim
You mean a MS patient also responds ?

P. Trouillas
Yes, very well, as far as that the evolution of the disease is controlled.

J.S. Kim
How about cerebellar speech ?

P. Trouillas
Dysarthria was one of the best influenced parameters, better than adiadochokinesia and it was not rare to find, when measuring the time for spelling of an arbitrary sentence, an achieved a shortening of 30 % to 40 %.

Immunological approach of interrelationships between the pituitary gland and some degenerative diseases of the central nervous system : Presence of autoantibodies against prolactin cells in Alzheimer's disease

A. Pouplard[1], J. Emile[2], F. Vincent-Pineau[1].

(1) Neuroimmunology Unit and (2) Department of Neurology, University Hospital, Angers, France.

Summary : For several years extensive work has been carried out on autoimmunity against pituitary cells, using mainly the indirect immunofluroescence technique. If the positive results obtained correlate well with the clinical state in some cases of pituitary insufficiency, the significance is not so clear in several other conditions, for example diabetes mellitus. One hypothesis was made that the positive reactivity could be directed against some membranous structures. Bearing this in mind, and taking into account the presence of various neurotransmitter receptors on pituitary cell membranes, we decided to look for such a reactivity in sera of patients with chronic central nervous system diseases, mainly Alzheimer's dementia and Parkinson's disease. The positive results obtained and their possible significance in relation to the pathophysiology of the disease are discussed.

Introduction

Nothing is known about the factors responsible for the brain changes in Alzheimer's disease. Among numerous hypotheses, cerebral autoimmunity has been the focus of number of reports over the past 15 years. For this reason and on the basis of our previous results on Parkinson's disease (Pouplard et al., 1979, Emile et al., 1980), we decided to look for the presence in Alzheimer's sera of specific antibodies that would react with structures of neuroectodermal origin. The most impressive results so far come from human pituitary, mostly prolactin cells.

Population studied

For this study 45 demented patients were selected after exclusion of a brain mass lesion, normopressive hydrocephaly or metabolic dementia and on the basis of history, clinical examination and routine laboratory tests especially computerized tomodensitometry scan (CT). Nine of them were seen in the Psychiatric Department. From these 45 patients, 3 clinical groups were distinguished. Age was not taken into account and Alzheimer's disease was mixed with senile dementia Alzheimer type.

227

Group I - Alzheimer type dementia.

34 patients were included (23 females, 11 males). The mean age was 68. In 14 cases, first signs had appeared before the age of 65. A clear family history was found in 3 cases. All patients had a suggestive history with no neurological abnormality except dementia. Focal signs such as spatial and temporal disorientation, impairment of speech and dyspraxia were often present. In all cases which had a CT, cortical and subcortical atrophy was demonstrated.

Group II - Multi-infarct dementia.

8 patients were included (4 females, 4 males). The mean age was 75. A suggestive history of strokes and hypertensive illness was present in all cases. Diabetes mellitus was noted in two cases. All these patients presented neurological signs especially pyramidal. The CT demonstrated one or more low density zone.

Group III - Presumed mixed Alzheimer type dementia.

3 patients (all females) were investigated. The mean age was 74. The course and the nature of the intellectual impairment and the presence of cortico-subcortical atrophy on CT without low density zones were strongly suggestive of Alzheimer type dementia. Nevertheless these 3 patients were not included in group I because of neurological abnormalities ; resulting from ischemic attacks in 2 cases and in the third case, disturbances of equilibrium secondary to previous alcoholic encephalopathy.

Methods

The technique employed was classical indirect immunofluorescence on unfixed 5 μm sections of fresh frozen post mortem pituitary (mostly human). Calf and guinea-pig pituitary were also tested. The antisera used were specific antihuman immunoglobulins (anti IgC, IgA, IgM).

Identification of positive cells was carried out using a four layer immunofluorescence technique, with specific antihormone anti-sera as described by Bottazzo et al. 1975. Antibodies were also detected in cerebrospinal fluid.

Results

By this technique we were able to demonstrate the presence of prolactin cell antibodies in the serum of 30 of the 34 patients in group I (88 per cent) 3 of the 8 cases in group II (1 or 2 females) and all the cases investigated in group III.

Results are summarized in Table I.

Table 1 : *Autoantibodies against prolactin cells in senile dementia*

Diagnosis	Nb tested	Positive	Negative
Alzheimer type	34	30	4 (88 percent)
Multi infarct	8	3	5
Mixed / A.D	3	3	0
Total	45	36	9

228

It appears that 80 per cent of the demented patients investigated had autoantibodies against prolactin cells in their sera. It is interesting that the 4 negative cases in group I were Psychiatric Department patients. Reassessment of the clinical history in these four cases did not exclude an episode of senile psychosis. Of the 3 positive cases from group II, 2 were insulin-dependent diabetic women.

Characteristics of the autoantibodies to prolactin cells in demented patients sera.

In the sera tested the antibody titre varied from 1/20 up to 1/250. The most important findings were the uniformity of the staining pattern and the homogeneity of the antibody type. The staining pattern was consistently cytoplasmic and granular. In all cases the antibodies belonged to IgA class. Occasionally, IgG was also present, but always at lower titre than that of IgA. These autoantibodies are not species-specific, although a higher titre was present to human pituitary than to guinea-pig or calf pituitary sections. Such antibodies were also detected in non concentrated cerebrospinal fluid. The presence of these antibodies was not correlated with neuroleptic therapy.

Discussion

The pathogenesis of Alzheimer's disease is not clearly understood. Humoral autoantibodies against neuronal tissues have been demonstrated in various pathological conditions, but the highest titre is commonly found in senile dementia patients ; the role played by these autoantibodies is still unclear and similar antibodies are also detected with increasing age in healthy humans and experimental animals (Nandy, 1978).

Autoimmunity increases with advancing age. Numerous factors are thought to play a role in the appearance of autoimmune reactions. The most important is probably an underlying immunodeficiency state, in conjunction with several initiating events such as a viral infection. The role of viruses has long been suspected in Alzheimer's disease with no real evidence, neither do we understand the primary events leading to chromatin abnormalities and neurofibrillary degeneration.

The possibility that an autoimmune mechanism could account for the appearance of senile dementia is supported by several other lines of evidence :
— the higher incidence in females ;
— the late age of onset ;
— the familial incidence ;
— the presence of amyloid frequently surrounded by reactive cells in the core of plaques thought to be of immunological origin ;
— immunological disturbances including oligoclonal bands in the cerebrospinal fluid with increased IgA level (personal data) and disturbances of lymphocyte subclasses.

Human autoantibodies to prolactin cells were first described by Bottazzo et al. (1975) in the sera of some autoimmune polyendocrine deficiencies. Specific autoantibodies directed against different types of pituitary cells were then described in anterior pituitary deficiencies, especially partial deficiencies (Pouplard et al. 1980).

The presence of these antibodies in the normal control population is however rare, being less than 2 percent in a sample of more than 400 sera tested. The only exception to date is the finding of such antibodies with a relatively high frequency in type I juvenile diabetes mellitus patients and their genetically predisposed relatives (Mirakian, 1982, Pouplard, 1983). The connection with an autoimmune lymphocytic hypophysitis or with the disturbances that have been already described in diabetes mellitus is still unknown. Results in diabetes are however quite different from those in senile dementia. Not only prolactin cells but also other cell types appear to be involved. Antibodies are generally of low titre and mostly of IgG class.

Considering the uniformity of the patterns and the antibody class and bearing in mind the very low incidence of these antibodies in control sera, the first question to be raised is whether prolactin cell antibodies can be considered as markers of Alzheimer type dementia ? The best proof would be the correlation with the defined histopathological features of Alzheimer type dementia. Nevertheless there is good positive correlation between the presence of these antibodies and the clinical and CT presumptive diagnosis of Alzheimer disease (88 per cent). This correlation is even higher in female cases (27/29, 93 per cent), than in male cases (9/16, 56 per cent), in good agreement with the sex ratio observed. Their presence in one third of patients classified as multi-infarct dementia fits with the histopathological data concerning these two associations. Their frequency is the expected one as vascular dementia is thought to represent 10-20 per cent of dementia. Finally their presence in 2 young patients (aged 40 and 58) with only a slight memory loss, but a family history of senile dementia, appears highly significant. However, if prolactin cell autoantibodies can be considered as a marker of Alzheimer dementia, their significance in relation to the onset of the disease needs to be clarified.

Many questions remain to be answered by further clinical and biochemical work. The nature of the antigen involved should be investigated. The hormone itself does not seem to be implicated. Absorption experiments carried out with polyendocrine patients' sera gave negative results. This point should be checked again in senile dementia, however, it shoud be noted that there was no inhibition of staining in the double immunofluorescence experiments and no inhibition in the radioimmunoassay. This agrees with the earlier finding that cytoplasmic autoantibodies are generally directed towards the intracellular membranes and not towards the hormone itself. Significant changes in the cerebral concentration of several neurotransmitters have been observed in senile and presenile dementia. Among these, the cholinergic deficiency appeared marked and specific (Roth, 1980). Other putative neurotransmitters, including peptides like somatostatin (Davies et al., 1980), appeared to be decreased but the significance of such deficiency is still unknown. Prolactin has now been found in some neurons but its functional role in the nervous system has not been clarified.

The detection of specific autoantibodies against prolactin pituitary cells in central nervous system disorders raises the question of a common antigen being present both in pituitary cells and some brain neurons. If so, it will be interesting to know the role played by these antibodies in prolactin synthesis and/or excretion.

Even if the antibodies detected are only an indirect marker of a still unknown mechanism, their high correlation with the clinical state seems to offer the possibility of recognizing patients at high risk, moreover they can add new insight into the pathogenesis of the disease.

230

Aknowledgement

We thank Professor Wartel for his collaboration and Mrs. Brouillard for technical assistance.

REFERENCES

Bottazzo G.F., Pouplard A., Florin-Christensen A., Doniach D. *1975.* — Autoantibodies to prolactin secreting cells of human pituitary. *Lancet, 2 :* 97-101.

Davies P., Katzman R., Terry R.D., *1980.* — Reduced somatostatin-like immunoreactivity in cerebral cortex from cases of Alzheimer disease and Alzheimer senile dementia. *Nature, 288 :* 279-280.

Emile J., Pouplard A., Bossu van Nieuwenhuyse C., Bernat-Viallet Ch. *1980.* — Maladie de Parkinson, dysautonomie et auto-anticorps dirigés contre les neurones sympathiques. *Rev. Neurol., 136 :* 221-233.

Mirakian R., *1982.* — Autoimmunity to anterior pituitary cells and the pathogenesis of type I (insulin-dependent) diabetes mellitus *(submitted).*

Nandy K., *1978.* — *In : Alzheimer's disease senile dementia and related disorders.* K.L. Blick (ed), New York, Raven Press.

Pouplard A., Emile J., Pouplard F., Hurez D., *1979.* — Parkinsonism and autoimmunity : antibody against human sympathetic ganglion cells in Parkinson's disease. *Adv. Neurol., 24 :* 321-326. Poirier, Sourkes, Bedard (eds). New York, Raven Press.

Pouplard A., Bigorgne J.C., Fressinaud Ph., *1980.* — Insuffisance anté-hypophysaire et auto-immunité. *Rev. Méd. interne, 12 :* 157-161.

Pouplard A., *1982.* — Autoimmunity to anterior pituitary cells and diabetes mellitus. (to be published)

Rot M., *1980.* — *In : Aging of the brain and dementia, vol. 13,* L. Amaducci et al. (ed), New York, Raven Press.

DISCUSSION

Cl. Hagen
I would like to know how old your controls are in these studies ?

A. Pouplard
With our test system we controlled all patients who came to the laboratory at our hospital. Amongst this population there were many myxoedematous patients, generally women at the age of 60 years in the mean. In this study, we have some other patients over 80 years of age and they were negative. Of course, we have to test more patients with normal mental function.

J. Mendlewicz
Were you able to study other genetic markers, such as the HLA system ?

A. Pouplard
No, but I think that this would be very important, because we had two quite young people in the study. One was a woman of 45 or 47, who came to the neurological department only due to a small loss of memory ; she was very strongly positive and according to the family history her mother died of senile dementia disease. The other one also had a loss of memory and her mother died of Alzheimer disease. I think this is one of the most important points, because they were young patients and this antibody is very rare in the normal population at this age.

Preclinical evaluation of neuroendocrine effects of psychotropic drugs : *In vitro* and *in vivo* methods

M. Valli[1], H. Dufour[2], B. Brugherolle[1], G. Jadot[1], P. Bouyard[1].

(1) Department of Clinical Pharmacology and (2) Department of Psychiatry, University Hospital La Timone, Marseille, France.

Summary : Within the group of psychotropic drugs, some neuroleptics may induce unwanted neuroendocrine effects such as hyperprolactinemia, galactorrhea or amenorrhea. Thus, it is important in the evaluation of new psychotropic drugs to elucidate their influence on the hypothalamo-pituitary-gonadal axis.
There are many methods of preclinical evaluation of neuroendocrine effects. The following are the principal ones :
1 - *In vitro* methods : Study of changes of prolactin, FSH, LH release in anterior pituitary cells in culture ; study of the drug affinities for pituitary dopamine receptors.
2 - *In vivo* methods : Monitoring of female rats oestrus cycles during acute and/or chronic treatment ; study of serum and pituitary levels of the main anterior pituitary hormones (e. g. PRL, FSH, and LH).
In order to evaluate the ability of new molecules to induce neuroendocrine effects, the monitoring of oestrous cycles and the study of serum pituitary hormones are sufficient as *screening* tests, whereas more sophisticated methods, may be used to clarify their molecular sites and mechanisms of action at the hypothalamic or pituitary level.

Introduction

Some psychotropic drugs, like the neuroleptics chlorpromazine, haloperidol, pimozide or sulpiride may induce neuroendocrine side effects such as hyperprolactinemia, which causes galactorrhea or amenorrhea, an unpleasant symptom even if the drug is effective against psychiatric symptoms (for review Simpson et al., 1981).

Thus, it is important in the evaluation of new psychotropic drugs - especially neuroleptic drugs — to elucidate their possible influence on the hypothalamo-hypophyso-gonadal axis.

It is well known that the secretion of anterior pituitary hormones is controlled by a mechanism involving the interaction of brain neurotransmitters with hypophysiotropic factors selectively secreted from hypothalamic neurons (for review, see Kordon et al., 1980, Meites and Sonntag, 1981).

Therefore, such studies are of growing clinical importance in view of the wide use of drugs in neurology and psychiatry and the need for better understanding of possible neuroendocrine side effects of these treatments. This type of investigation is also of great theoretical importance. Since these molecules act specifically on the biosynthesis or release of monoamines, they are still the best available tool for investigating the mechanisms by which aminergic or peptidergic fibers can affect the neuroendocrine control system (Kordon et al., 1980).

In this article, we will present not so much a review as an overview of the different methods which may be used to predict the ability of new drugs to modify gonadotropin secretion. There are many methods of preclinical evaluation of neuroendocrine effects, however, it seems that the following are the principal ones :

— *In vitro* methods : Study of changes of hormones release in anterior pituitary cells, study of the drug affinities for pituitary dopamine receptors.

— *In vivo* methods : Monitoring of female rats oestrus cycles during long term treatment, study of serum and pituitary levels of the major anterior pituitary hormones (prolactin, FSH and LH).

Basically, we will summarize these different methods and present some examples to illustrate characteristic data.

In vitro methods

Changes of hormone release in anterior pituitary cells

The *in vivo* secretion of prolactin by the anterior pituitary gland is normally inhibited by the hypothalamus. When the pituitary gland is transplanted to organs remote from the hypothalamus, when it is incubated *in vitro* or when lesions are placed in the median eminence region of the hypothalamus, the pituitary gland secretes large amounts of prolactin.

It has been clearly demonstrated that catecholamines can directly inhibit the *in vitro* secretion of prolactin. Pharmacological agents which deplete the hypothalamus of catecholamines or interfere with their biological action are known to stimulate prolactin secretion.

McLeod and Lehmeyer (1974) investigated the ability of these drugs to block the *in vitro* inhibitory action of dopamine.

The results of incubating anterior pituitary glands of female rats with ^{3}H-leucine in the presence of 5×10^{-7}M dopamine is illustrated in Figure 1. Four daily injections of 1 mg perphenazine or 0.1 mg haloperidol significantly increased the amount of newly synthetized prolactin found in the gland ($p < 0.01$). The drug had a slight but not significant stimulatory effect on total synthesis. When the gland of rats treated with these drugs were incubated in the presence of dopamine, it was found that these glands were extremely resistant to the inhibitory action of the catecholamine.

Figure 2 illustrates the ability of *in vitro* perphenazine to antagonize the dopamine effect. Addition of 1.25×10^{-5}M perphenazine to culture medium had no significant effect by itself, but it completely blocked the inhibition of prolactin secretion produced by 5×10^{-7} dopamine.

When 5×10^{-9}M haloperidol was co-incubated with dopamine it produced a 50 % recovery from the effect of the catecholamine (Fig. 3).

In the rat, sulpiride modifies serum gonadotropins and prolactin levels. The aim of the study by Debeljuk et al. (1974) was to demonstrate whether sulpiride can act directly on the pituitary gland. This possibility was investigated by incubating pituitary glands *in vitro* in the presence of sulpiride.

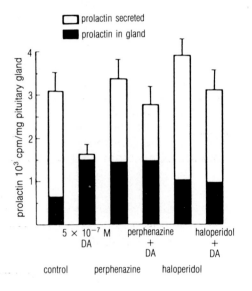

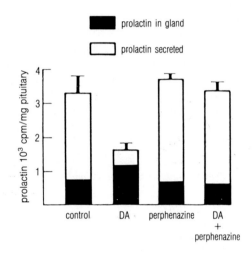

Fig. 1

Fig. 2

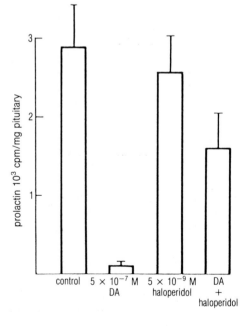

Fig. 1 A study of the inhibition of prolactin release by the *in vitro* addition of dopamine (DA) to pituitary glands of control rats and those injected with perphenazine and haloperidol. Perphenazine (1 mg) or haloperidol (0.1 mg) was administered subcutaneously daily for 4 days. Hemipituitary glands from 4 rats were incubated in 1 ml T.C. medium 199 containing 10 μCI of 4,5—3H-leucine and incubated for 6 hr. Each group contained at least 3 flasks. (From McLeod and Lehmeyer, 1974)

Fig. 2 *In vitro* blockade by perphenazine of the dopamine-induced inhibition of prolactin secretion. Four hemipituitary glands were incubated with 5 × 10−7M dopamine (DA), 1.25 × 10−5M perphenazine, or both substances. The values presented are the mean ± SEM of 3 incubation flasks per group. (From McLeod and Lehmeyer, 1974)

Fig. 3 Blockade of the dopamine-mediated inhibition of prolactin secretion with haloperidol. Each of 3 flasks per group contained hemipituitary glands from 4 rats and was incubated with the indicated concentration of dopamine (DA), haloperidol, or both. (From McLeod and Lehmeyer, 1974)

Fig. 3

235

Table 1 shows that the media to which sulpiride was added contained significantly higher concentrations than the control media. The addition of rat hypothalamic extracts inhibited the release of prolactin. On the other hand, the media where hypothalamic extracts plus sulpiride were added contained higher concentrations of prolactin than those where only hypothalamic extracts were added. Paradoxically, the lower dose used seemed to be more effective than the higher one in stimulating prolactin release. Thus it appears that sulpiride acts, at least in part, at the pituitary level.

It is well established that many types of neuroleptic drugs, including phenothiazines, butyrophenones and benzamides increase prolactin secretion *in vivo*. Several of these drugs have been shown to block the inhibitory action of dopamine itself and dopamine agonists on prolactin secretion by pituitary cells *in vitro* (Yeo et al., 1979).

Table 1 — *Effect of sulpiride and hypothalamic extracts on prolactin release by rat pituitaries in vitro*
(From Debeljuk et al., 1974).

Group and treatment [a]	Dose	Prolactin concentration [b]
1 Saline	—	217.6 ± 25.2 [c]
2 Sulpiride	1 mg	272.2 ± 31.0
3 Sulpiride	0.05 mg	352.0 ± 59.4 [d]
4 Rat hypothalamic extract	1.5 hypothalami	120.0 ± 4.4
5 Rat hypothalamic extract plus sulpiride	1.5 hypothalami + 1 mg	221.0 ± 41.2
6 Rat hypothalamic extract plus sulpiride	1.5 hypothalami + 0.05 mg	209.6 ± 36.0

[a] Three beakers containing 5 pituitary halves per each treatment were used. [b] Expressed as ng of NIAMDD-rat prolactin-RP, 1 mg of pituitary weight/ml of medium. [c] The variance analysis showed statistical significance of the differences among groups ($p < 0.05$). [d] Group 3 vs Group 1 : $p < 0.05$ (Duncan's new multiple range test).

Besser et al. (1980) recently investigated the *in vitro* dose response curves for four drugs which are known to increase prolactin release in vivo : Chlorpromazine, haloperidol, metoclopramide and domperidone. They studied the effects of these drugs on the release of prolactin from perfused columns of dispersed rat anterior pituitary cells. All four antagonized the dopamine (5 μM) mediated inhibition of prolactin release at low concentrations (Fig. 4). Haloperidol was effective at 100 pM, metoclopramide and domperidone at 10 nM, and chlorpromazine at 100 nM. Each dopamine antagonist displaced the dose response curve for dopamine induced suppression of prolactin release symmetrically to the right (Fig. 5). At higher concentrations the four drugs became less effective as dopamine antagonists and in the absence of dopamine, the four drugs paradoxically suppressed prolactin secretion by an unknowm mechanism. Recent findings indicate that haloperidol *in vivo* may initially increase prolactin secretion, but that there may be a fall in the serum prolactin after chronic administration. These authors speculate that this fall may be due, at least in part, to the intrinsic prolactin-suppressing effect of high concentrations of haloperidol (Fig. 6).

In summary, the above data have clearly shown that changes of prolactin release in rat anterior pituitary cells in primary culture provide a sensitive, precise, specific and reliable measurement of the agonistic and/or antagonistic action of dopaminergic drugs (Labrie et al., 1978).

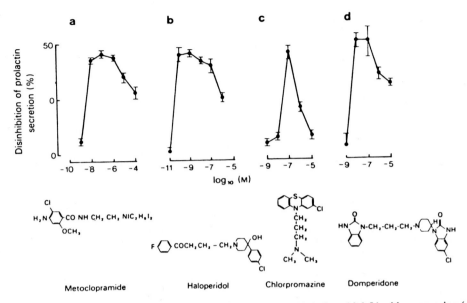

Fig. 4 - Log dose-response curves of the ability of metoclopramide (a), haloperidol (b), chlorpromazine (c) and domperidone (d) to reverse the suppression of prolactin secretion induced by 5 μmol/l dopamine. Each point represents a separate experiment, similar to that illustrated in Figure 1. The prolactin concentrations in each of the last 6 fractions during perfusion with dopamine plus antagonist are expressed as a percentage of the mean concentration when unsuppressed. The values given are the mean ; vertical lines show S.D. A value of 100 % would indicate that the dopamine-induced suppression of prolactin had been completely overcome. (From Besser et al., 1980).

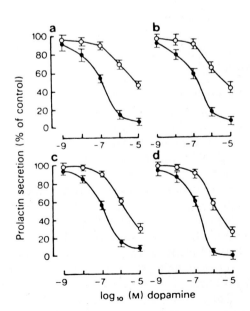

Fig. 5 - Effect of haloperidol (100 pM) (a), chlorpromazine (100 nM) (b), metoclopramide (10 nM) (c) and domperidone (10 nM) (d) on the log dose-response curve for dopamine suppression of prolactin secretion *in vitro* : (●) effect of dopamine alone ; (○) effect of dopamine plus antagonist. Each point represents the mean of 3 separate experiments ; vertical lines indicate S.D. (From Besser et al., 1980)

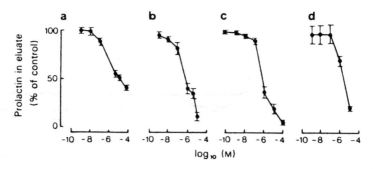

Fig. 6 - Log dose-response curves for the suppression of prolactin secretion from dispersed rat pituitary cell columns by metoclopramide (a), haloperidol (b), chlorpromazine (c) and domperidone (d) in the absence of dopamine. The prolactin concentrations in the last 6 fractions during drug administration are expressed as a percentage of the mean secretion during perfusion with medium to which saline alone was added. Each point represents the mean ; vertical lines indicate S.D. (From Besser et al., 1980)

This system is apparently free of the limitations associated with the use of dopamine receptors and dopamine sensitive adenyl-cyclase assays as screening tests for anti-Parkinsonian, antihyperprolactinemic and antipsychotic drugs.

Indeed, the absence of nerve terminals in the anterior pituitary gland offers the possibility of studying a pure population of post-synaptic receptors and of correlating binding to the dopamine receptor with an easily accessible and highly precise parameter under dopaminergic control.

Thus, Caron et al. (1978) pointed out that the anterior pituitary gland should represent a useful model for detailed study on the mechanisms of dopaminergic action.

Drug affinities for pituitary dopamine receptors

As we have seen, it is now accepted that dopamine has a direct and major physiological role in controlling prolactin secretion (van Mannen and Smelik, 1968, Shar and Clemens, 1976).

Binding studies have suggested that many neuroleptic drugs may act as antagonists at dopamine receptors on pituitary cells.

Calabro and McLeod (1978) initiated a study to identify the receptor through which dopamine interacts with pituitary membranes in order to define the sequence of events at the molecular level resulting in dopamine inhibition of prolactin release. Thus, ^{3}H-dopamine binding to bovine anterior pituitary membranes was measured using sensitive *in vitro* ultrafiltration and centrifugation techniques.

Their results showed that blockade of labelled dopamine binding was produced most effectively by ergocryptine and amphetamine (Table 2).

They showed that very small amounts of perphenazine, haloperidol, pimozide, tiapride and (D)-butaclamol acted as biological dopamine antagonists and thereby

Table 2 — *Blockade of ^{3}H-DA specific binding to bovine adenohypophyseal membranes*
(From Calabro et al., 1978).

Compound	IC_{50} (nM)	Relative Effective Concentration
Ergocryptine	6.9	1
Apomorphine	25	3.6
DA	107	15.5
Norepinephrine	750	109
Perphenazine	750	109
Haloperidol	880	128
Methysergide	1,000	145
Pimozide	>10,000	>1,450
Catechol	>100,000	>14,500
Pyrogallol	>100,000	>14,500

^{3}H-DA binding to membranes was determined as described in Figure 3. Values shown for IC_{50} is the concentration of each compound required to inhibit specific binding of 12.5 nM ^{3}H-DA by 50 %. Selected values were checked using the centrifugation method. Relative IC_{50} values for several compounds are computed in the last column.

maintained prolactin secretion. So, one might infer that these drugs would be extremely efficient competitors for the dopamine receptor site.

Neuroleptics such as haloperidol, metoclopramide and sulpiride were only moderately effective blockers of ^{3}H-dopamine binding to pituitary membranes, and the amounts of drug required were much greater than those needed to inhibit the biological action of dopamine on prolactin secretion (Seeman, 1981). It would appear that the anterior pituitary contains dopamine receptors that meet the criteria of the D_2 receptor, as summarized in Tables 3 and 4 which show that the pattern of binding of ^{3}H-DHEC (dihydroergocryptine) is similar to that for the binding of ^{3}H-butyrophenones. The binding of ^{3}H-dopamine to anterior pituitary tissue is very different from the D_2 site.

Although they readily detected specific binding of ^{3}H-dopamine to rat striata (D_3-sites), Titeler and Seeman (1980) were not able to detect any specific binding of ^{3}H-dopamine in either rat or calf anterior pituitary tissue ; this negative observation is compatible with the idea that high affinity binding of ^{3}H-dopamine may be restricted to nerve terminals (which are not found in the pituitary) suggesting that such sites might be detected in the median eminence (Hökfelt et al., 1977).

In summary, we think that this *in vitro* biochemical model of displacement of labelled ligands from dopamine receptors is certainly of great importance in theoretical research, however, less useful as a screening tool of neuroendocrine effects.

In vivo methods

Monitoring of female rat oestrus cycles during chronic treatment

In order to gain insight into the relationships between hyperprolactinemia and secondary amenorrhea, Lotz and Krause (1978) elaborated an animal test based on the work by Sulman (1970), in which they compared the prolactin releasing activity

239

Table 3 — *Inhibition of ³H-neuroleptic binding to anterior pituitary (from Seeman, 1981)*

	¹H-Spiperone IC₅₀ (nM)		¹H-Haloperidol IC₅₀ (nM)	
	Sheep (r : rat)	Bovine	Rat	Monkey
Neuroleptics				
Spiperone	2.1 (255)	0.6 (243)		
(+)-Butaclamol	3.8 (256)	2.1 (243)		
(−)-Butaclamol	41,000 (256)	20,000 (243)		
Fluphenazine		4.5 (243)		
Pimozide	9.6 (256)			
Haloperidol	29 (255)	7 (243)	6 (102)	0.7 (106)
		9.7 (746)		
Chlorpromazine	41 (255)	39 (243)		
Metoclopramide		158 (746)		10 (106)
(−)-Sulpiride	5,300 (256)		12 (102)	
	r: 700 (788a)			
(+)-Sulpiride	>100,000 (256)			
	r:80,000 (788a)			
Agonists				
Bromocriptine	47 (255)	5.4 (243)		
Apomorphine	560 (255)	525 (243)		
Dopamine	3,400 (255)	16,000 (243)		
Adrenaline	56,000 (255)	140,000 (243)	1,000 (102)	
Noradrenaline	46,000 (255)	450,000 (243)		
Phentolamine	66,000 (255)			
Serotonin	>100,000 (255)	120,000 (243)		

Table 4 — *Inhibition of ³H-agonist binding to anterior pituitary (from Seeman, 1981)*

	¹H-DHEC* IC₅₀ (nM)		¹H-Dopamine IC₅₀ (nM)
	Sheep	Bovine	Bovine
Neuroleptics			
Fluphenazine		15.6 (164)	
Haloperidol	154 (254)	55 (164)	880 (131)
Chlorpromazine		200 (164)	
Agonists			
Bromocriptine	160 (254)	110 (164)	~10 (131)
Apomorphine	190 (254)	360 (164)	25 (131)
Dopamine	1,500 (254)	2,260 (164)	107 (131)
Adrenaline	>10,000 (254)	7,800 (164)	
Noradrenaline	10,000 (254)	14,700 (164)	750 (131)
Phentolamine	10,000 (254)	14,700 (164)	
Serotonin	>100,000 (254)	106,000 (164)	

* DHEC, dihydroergocryptine.

and the influence on the vaginal cycle with the mammotrophic effect of various neuroleptics in rats.

The vaginal cycles of female rats were checked by daily lavage and subsequent cytological analysis (Jadot et al., 1980 ; Jadot, 1981). Indices for evaluation of the mammotrophic effect were defined as follows : 0, resting phase (no lobular stimulation) ; 1, early lobular growth ; 2, more advanced lobular growth with vacuolisation ; 3, marked lobular hyperplasia with ductal fluid ; 4, full lactation.

With this experimental model, treatment with neuroleptics produces dose dependent disruption of the vaginal cycle and stimulation of the mammary tissue. Figure 7 shows the representative example of sulpiride, where chronic oral (13 days) administration of 0.1 mg/kg did not interfere with the vaginal cycle, which was slightly disturbed by a dose of 0.3 mg/kg and markedly disturbed by 1 mg/kg,

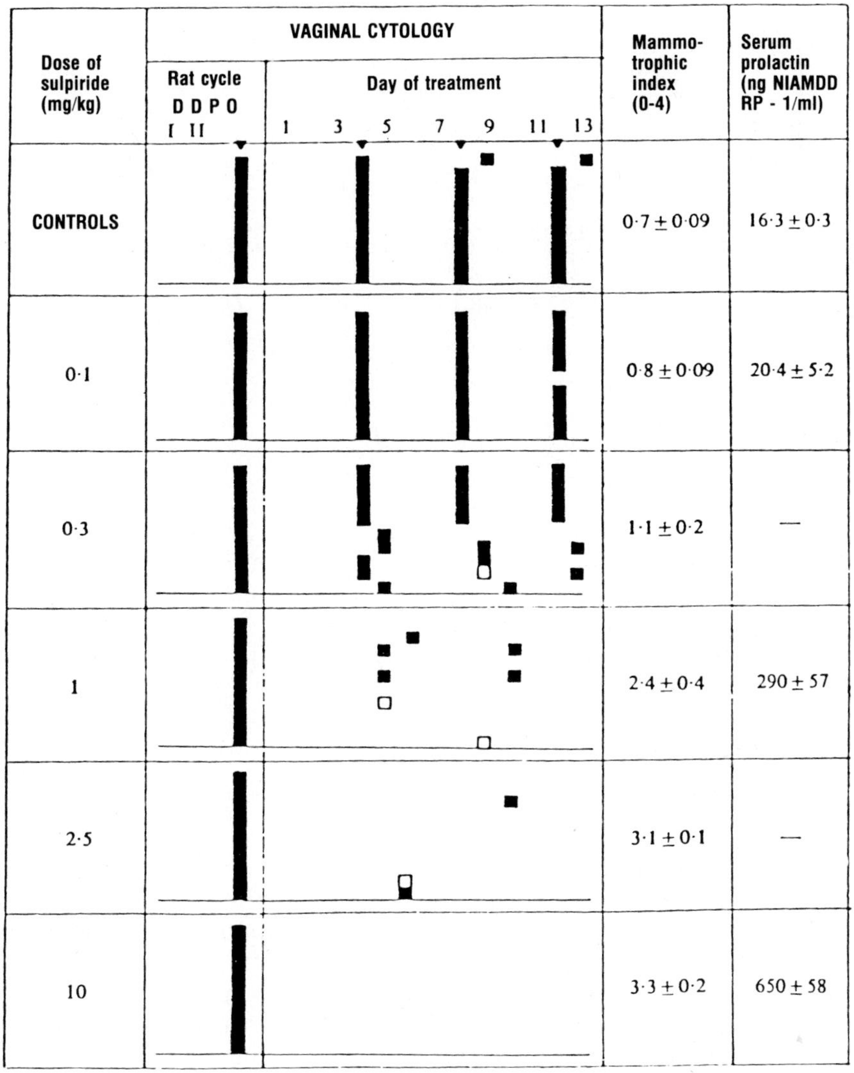

Fig. 7 - Vaginal cytology during treatment and the mammotrophic index and concentration of prolactin in the serum of female rats 30 min after the last of 13 oral applications of graded doses of sulpiride. D, diœstrus ; P, pro-œstrus ; O, œstrus. Results are means ± SEM of nine determinations. Solid squares represent a single œstrous event in a single animal ; open squares represent a single pro-œstrous event not followed by œustrus in a single animal. (From Lotz et al., 1978)

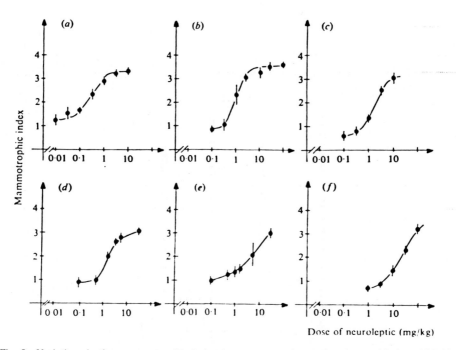

Fig. 8 - Variations in the mammotrophic index in response to increasing doses of haloperidol (*a*), sulpiride (*b*), metoclopramide (*c*), thioridazine (*d*), chlorpromazine (*e*) or clozapine (*f*). Results are means ± SEM of ten determinations. (From Lotz et al., 1978)

when the concentration of prolactin was raised about 17-fold, 30 min after the last of the 13 applications. With doses of 2.5 and 10 mg/kg, the vaginal cycle ceased, all animals showed constant dioestrous and pronounced mammary gland stimulation focally resembling lactation, while the prolactin level was increased about 40-fold.

Figure 8 illustrates the dose dependance of the stimulatory effects of these neuroleptics on the mammary gland. The dose-response curves have a similar shape with different slopes and the neuroleptics can be arranged in the following sequence of potencies based on their ED_{50}: Haloperidol $\geqslant$ sulpiride $\geqslant$ metoclopramide = thioridazine > chlorpromazine > clozapine.

In a similar manner, we presented (Bruguerolle et al., 1981a) a comparative study of four benzamides (metoclopramide, sulpiride, sultopride and tiapride) effects on the same animal model. These compounds were given daily during a 21 day period at the following doses (0.001, 0.01, 0.1 and 1 mg/kg s.c.) on female rats exhibiting three consecutive 4 day cycles.

Our data showed that sulpiride and sultopride supress the oestrous cycle, substituted by a permanent dioestrous blockade, while metoclopramide only extends the duration of the cycle and tiapride has no significant influence (Fig. 9-12).

242

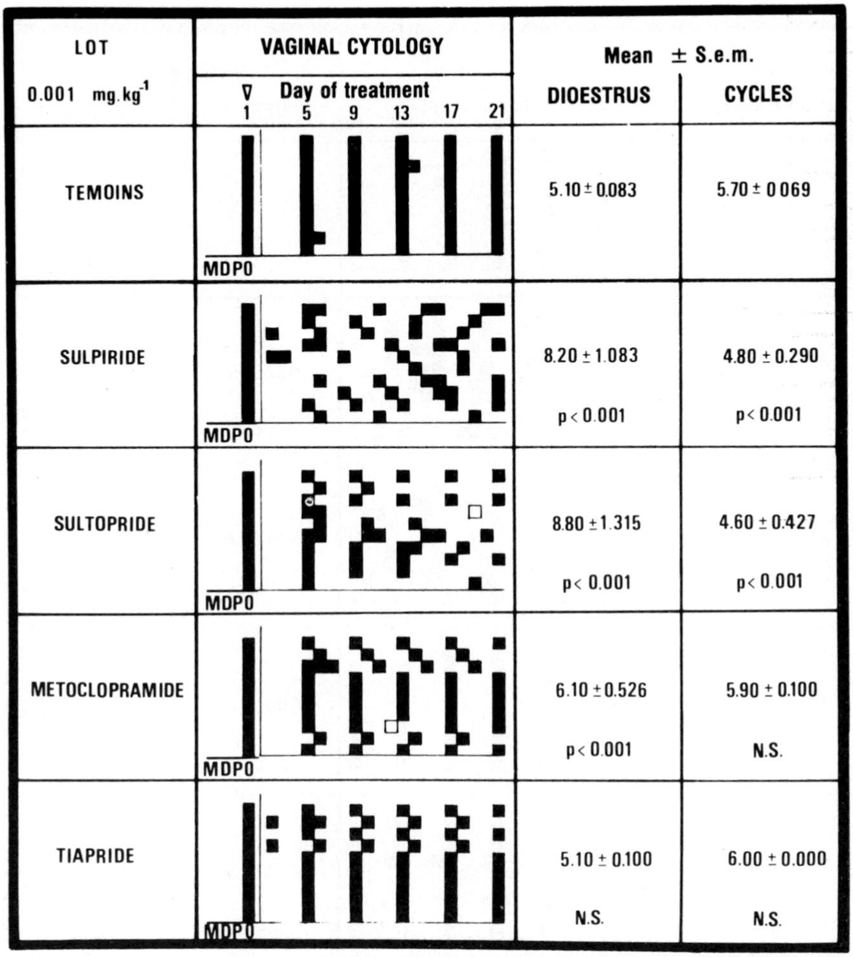

Fig. 9 - Vaginal cytology during treatment of female rats by the four benzamides at the dose of 0.001 mg/kg. Means ±SEM of diœstrus and cycles for each animal compared to controls, during 21 days. For a single animal, a solid square represents a single œstrus, and an open square represents a single prœstrus event not followed by œstrus. (From Bruguerolle et al., 1981).

243

LOT 0.01 mg.kg[-1]	VAGINAL CYTOLOGY ∇ Day of treatment 1 5 9 13 17 21	Mean ± S.e.m. DIOESTRUS	CYCLES
TEMOINS	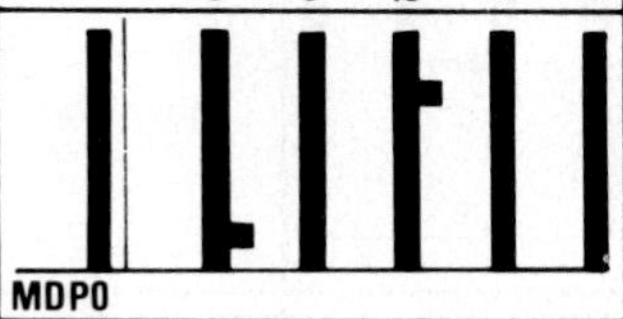 MDPO	5.10 ± 0.083	5.70 ± 0 069
SULPIRIDE	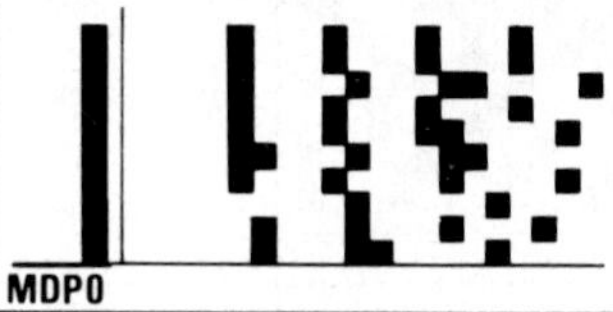 MDPO	9.00 ± 0.715 p < 0.001	5.00 ± 0.258 p < 0.001
SULTOPRIDE	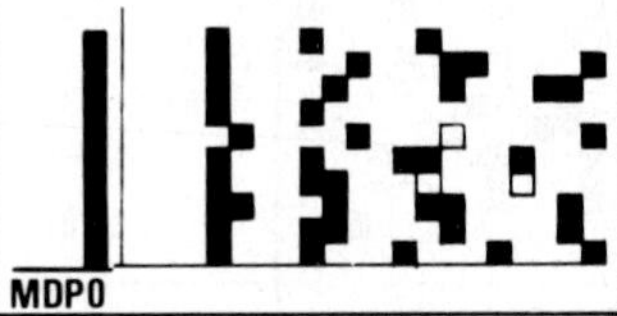 MDPO	8.10 ± 0.795 p < 0.001	5.00 ± 0.210 p < 0.001
METOCLOPRAMIDE	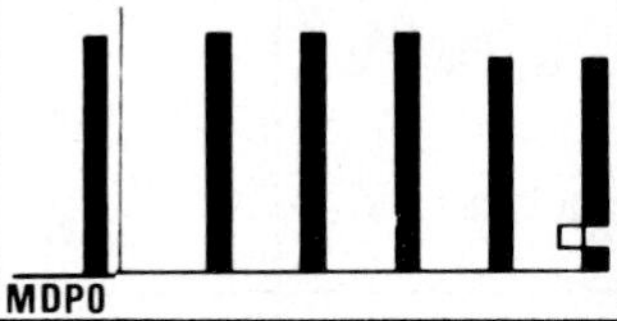 MDPO	6.00 ± 0.471 p < 0.001	5.80 ± 0.200 N.S.
TIAPRIDE	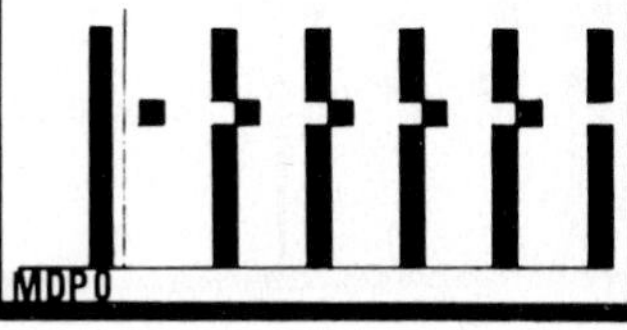 MDPO	5.00 ± 0.000 N.S.	6.00 ± 0.000 N.S.

Fig. 10 - Vaginal cytology during treatment of female rats by the four benzamides at the dose of 0.01 mg/kg. (For details, see Fig. 9)

LOT	VAGINAL CYTOLOGY		Mean ± S.e.m.	
0.1 mg.kg⁻¹	▽ Day of treatment 1 5 9 13 17 21		DIOESTRUS	CYCLES
TEMOINS	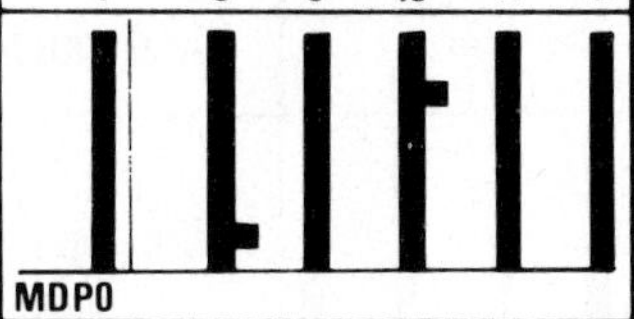 MDPO		5.10 ± 0.083	5.70 ± 0.069
SULPIRIDE	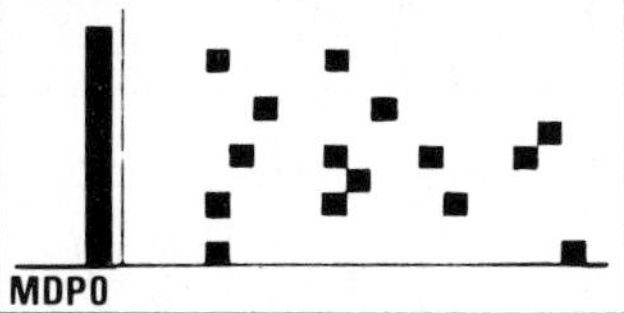 MDPO		15.20 ± 1.298 p < 0.001	2.60 ± 0.499 p < 0.001
SULTOPRIDE	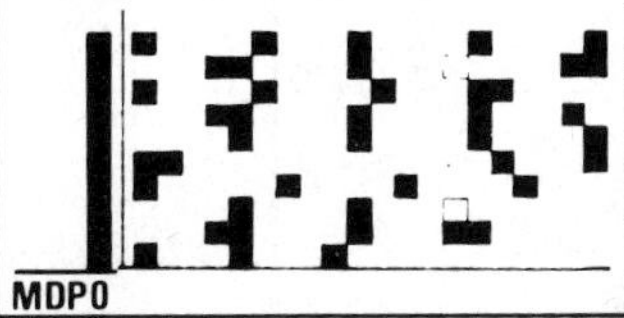 MDPO		10.20 ± 0.680 p < 0.001	4.20 ± 0.249 p < 0.001
METOCLOPRAMIDE	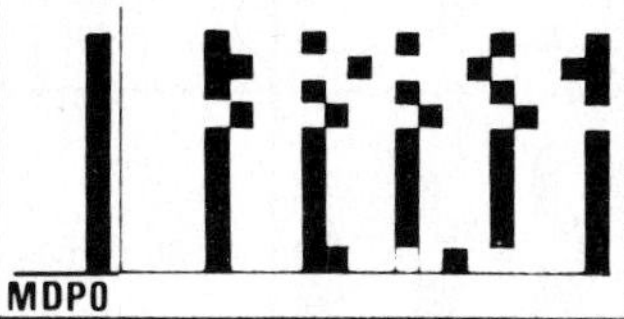 MDPO		6.10 ± 0.348 p < 0.001	5.90 ± 0.100 N.S.
TIAPRIDE	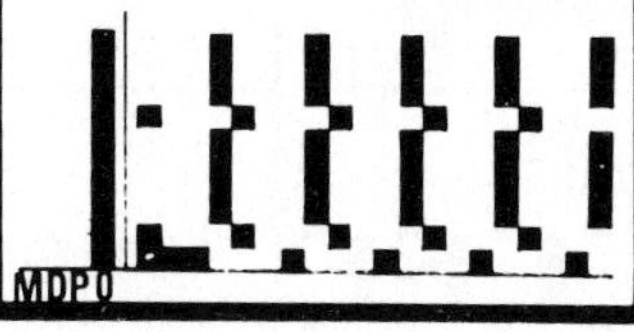 MDPO		5.00 ± 0.000 N.S.	5.90 ± 0.100 N.S.

Fig. 11 - Vaginal cytology during treatment of female rats by the four benzamides at the dose of 0.1 mg/kg. (For details, see Fig. 9)

245

LOT	VAGINAL CYTOLOGY		Mean ± S.e.m.	
1 mg.kg⁻¹	∇ Day of treatment 1 5 9 13 17 21		DIOESTRUS	CYCLES
TEMOINS			5.10 ± 0.083	5.70 ± 0 069
SULPIRIDE			18.20 ± 0.573 p < 0.001	1.80 ± 0.249 p < 0.001
SULTOPRIDE			13.20 ± 0.840 p < 0.001	3.50 ± 0.307 p < 0.001
METOCLOPRAMIDE			7.60 ± 1.046 p < 0.001	4.70 ± 0.335 p < 0.001
TIAPRIDE			5.30 ± 0.213 N.S.	5.60 ± 0.163 N.S.

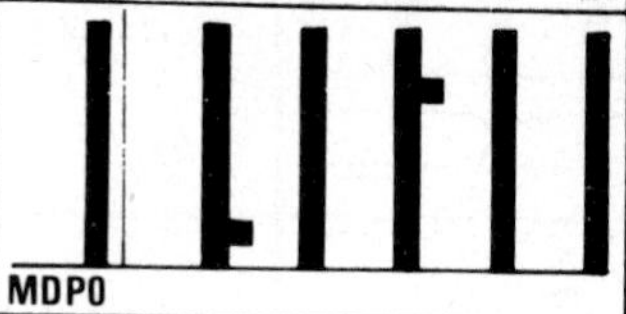

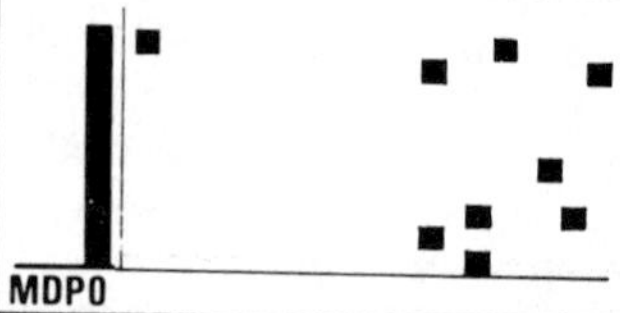

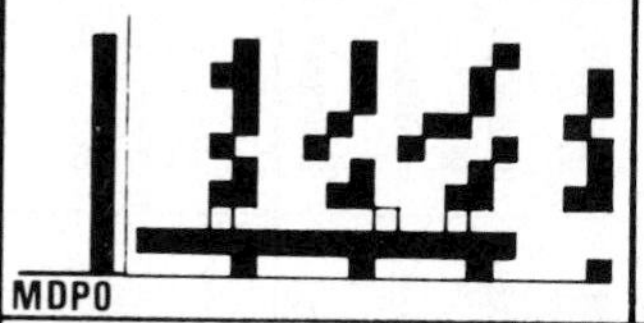

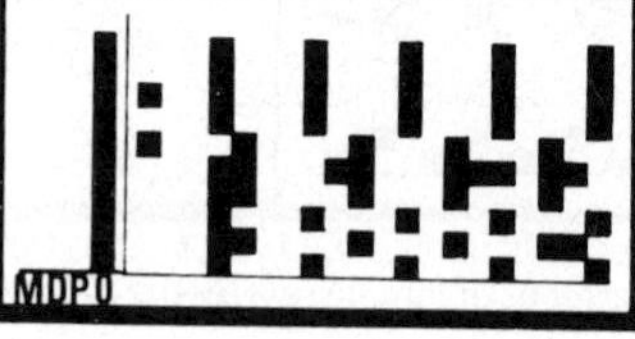

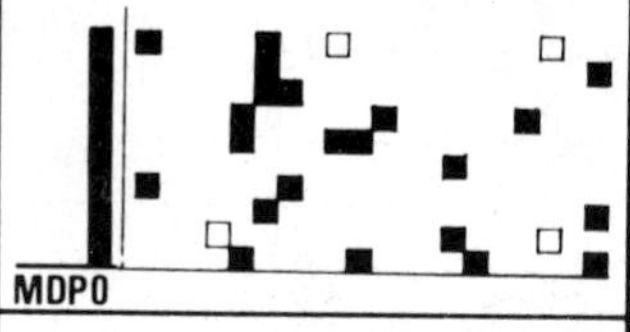

Fig. 12 - Vaginal cytology during treatment of female rats by the four benzamides at the dose of 1 mg/kg. (For details, see Fig. 9)

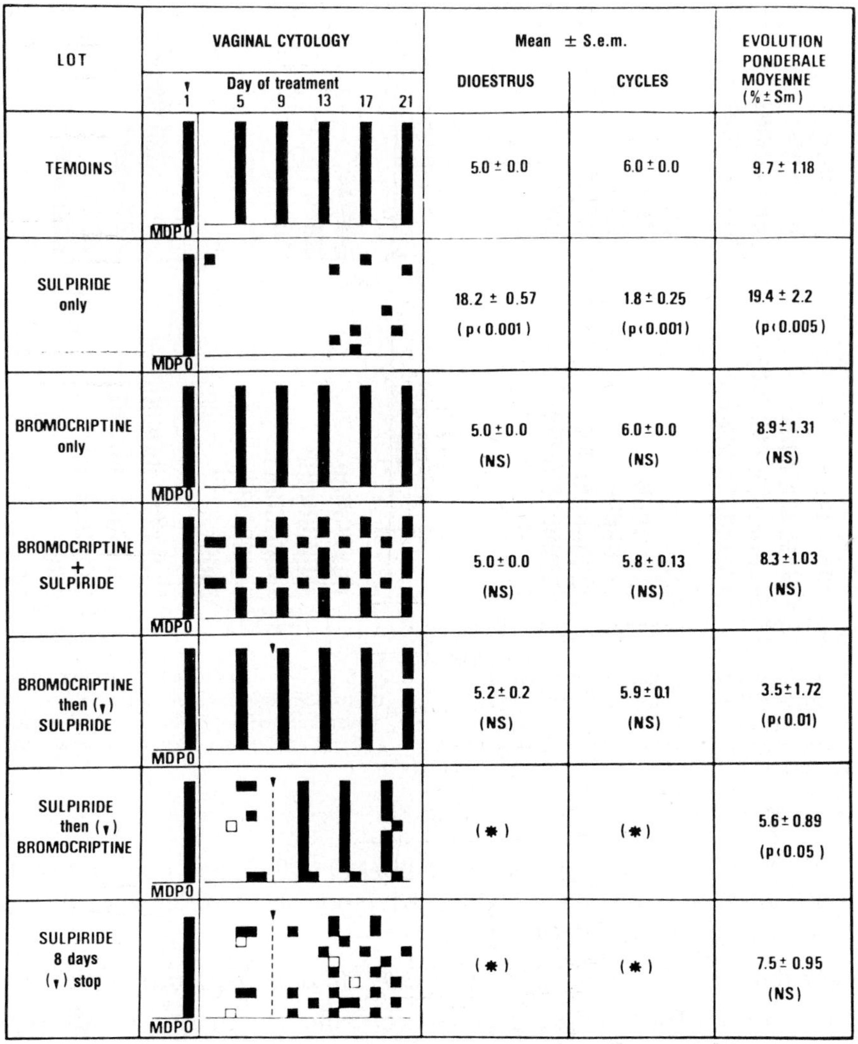

LOT	VAGINAL CYTOLOGY	Mean ± S.e.m.		EVOLUTION PONDERALE MOYENNE (% ± Sm)
	Day of treatment	DIOESTRUS	CYCLES	
TEMOINS	MDP 0	5.0 ± 0.0	6.0 ± 0.0	9.7 ± 1.18
SULPIRIDE only	MDP 0	18.2 ± 0.57 (p < 0.001)	1.8 ± 0.25 (p < 0.001)	19.4 ± 2.2 (p < 0.005)
BROMOCRIPTINE only	MDP 0	5.0 ± 0.0 (NS)	6.0 ± 0.0 (NS)	8.9 ± 1.31 (NS)
BROMOCRIPTINE + SULPIRIDE	MDP 0	5.0 ± 0.0 (NS)	5.8 ± 0.13 (NS)	8.3 ± 1.03 (NS)
BROMOCRIPTINE then (▾) SULPIRIDE	MDP 0	5.2 ± 0.2 (NS)	5.9 ± 0.1 (NS)	3.5 ± 1.72 (p < 0.01)
SULPIRIDE then (▾) BROMOCRIPTINE	MDP 0	(✳)	(✳)	5.6 ± 0.89 (p < 0.05)
SULPIRIDE 8 days (▾) stop	MDP 0	(✳)	(✳)	7.5 ± 0.95 (NS)

Fig. 13 - Vaginal cytoloty, means ± SEM of diœstrus and cycles, and of weight gain for each animal compared to controls, during sulpiride-bromocriptine treatment. (From Valli et al., 1981 ; For details, see Fig. 9).

We also studied (Valli et al., 1981) the effects of a joint treatment by sulpiride and the dopamine agonist bromocriptine on the same model. The results we obtained show that : *(i)* bromocriptine (3 mg/kg) alone does not disturb the oestrous cycle, *(ii)* when given both with sulpiride (1 mg/kg), it prevents this neuroleptic cycle blockade, *(iii)* finally, it leads to the regression of a blockade induced by an 8 day pretreatment with sulpiride (Fig. 13).

In addition, we have previously reported that the repeated administration (3 weeks) of molecules such as cimetidine (Bruguerolle et al., 1979), propranolol

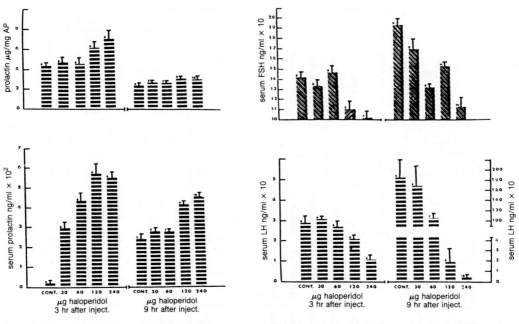

Fig. 14 - Effects of a single s.c. injection of different doses of haloperidol on pituitary and serum prolactin concentration. Haloperidol markedly elevated serum prolactin values (From Dickerman et al., 1974)

Fig. 15 - Effects of a single s.c. injection of different doses of haloperidol on serum FSH and LH concentrations. Haloperidol reduced both serum LH and FSH (From Dickerman et al., 1974)

(Bruguerolle et al., 1981b) or clonidine (Valli et al., 1982) had no significant effects either on the oestrous cycle (lack of blockade), nor on the release of prolactin and gonadotropins from the pituitary.

Serum and pituitary levels of the main anterior pituitary hormones

In order to illustrate these particular screening methods, we will report the following selected data :

Thus, Dickerman et al. (1974) have shown that a single s.c. injection of haloperidol into rats on the morning of proestrus produced up to 22-fold increase in serum prolactin concentration and a significant decrease in serum LH and FSH levels, with a complete blockade of spontaneous ovulation.

Figure 14 shows that 3 hours after injection serum prolactin levels had increased from 24.6 ± 2.7 to 291.9 ± 26.1 ng/ml ($p < 0.01$) by a single injection of 30 μg of haloperidol, to 436.6 ± 48.1 ($p < 0.01$) after 60 μg ; to 588.8 ± 37.9 ($p.< 0.01$) after 120 μg and to 557.6 ± 33.1 ($p < 0.01$) after 240 μg of haloperidol, i.e. a 22-fold increase in prolactin over the control level.

The pituitary prolactin concentration 3 hours after injection of haloperidol remained unchanged when a dose of 30 or 60 μg had been given, but a significant elevation was produced by 120 and 240 μg.

Figure 15 shows that a single s.c. injection of 30 or 60 μg haloperidol did not alter serum LH levels 3 hours later as compared to the control group (29.6 ± 2.6 ng/ml). However there was a decrease in serum LH levels when 120 μg (20.3 ± 2.9 ng/ml ; p < 0.05) or 240 μg haloperidol (11.9 ± 1.9 ng/ml ; p < 0.01) were given.

The same figure also shows the effects on serum FSH values of a single injection of haloperidol at 9.30 a.m. on the day of proestrus. Serum FSH in controls 3 hours after injection was 141.3 ± 3.8 ng/ml. Administration of 30 or 60 μg haloperidol did not significantly alter these values. However, a dose of 120 μg decreased serum FSH to 111.8 ± 7.9 ng/ml, and a dose of 240 μg decreased it to 101.9 ± 8.3 ng/ml.

None of the doses of haloperidol significantly altered pituitary FSH values, regardless of whether or not the rats were killed 3 or 9 hours after injection of haloperidol.

In the same study, the animals were injected on the morning of proestrus and killed on the morning of oestrus and their oviducts were removed and examined for ova. The effects of haloperidol on ovulation can be seen in Table 5. A single injection of 30 or 240 μg of haloperidol produced an 83 % reduction in the number of ovulating rats as compared to controls (100 % ovulation).

Table 5 — *Effects of HAL and exogenous LH injected at a.m. of proestrus on ovulation on day of estrus*

Treatment	Time of injection, proestrus	Laparotomy time, estrus	Number of rats ovulating	Average number of ova per ovulating rat
Corn oil	9.30–10 a.m.	9.30–10 a.m.	7/7	12.8 ± 1
30 μg HAL	9.30–10 a.m.	9.30–10 a.m.	1/6	13.0
240 μg HAL	9.30–10 a.m.	9.30–10 a.m.	1/6	12.0
30 μg HAL + 80 μg LH	9.30–10 a.m. 6.30 p.m.	9.30–10 a.m. –	7/7	10.7 ± 2.4
240 μg HAL 80 μg LH	9.30–10 a.m. 6.30 p.m.	9.30–10 a.m. –	5/7	12.0 ± 1
Corn oil + saline	9.30–10 a.m. 6.30 p.m.	9.30–10 a.m. –	5/5	12.6 ± 1.14

These observations suggest that the drug not only increased both the synthesis and the release of prolactin, but also prevented the release of LH and FSH from the pituitary. The increase in pituitary LH concentrations by the highest dose of haloperidol is believed to reflect the accumulation of LH and the failure of release.

Horowski and Graf (1976) tested the effects of the neuroleptics haloperidol (10 mg/kg i.p.) and sulpiride (25 mg/kg i.p.) 2 hours after injection in male rats. Whereas these two compounds increased the serum prolactin as expected, d-amphetamine, which is thought to act by releasing endogenous dopamine as well

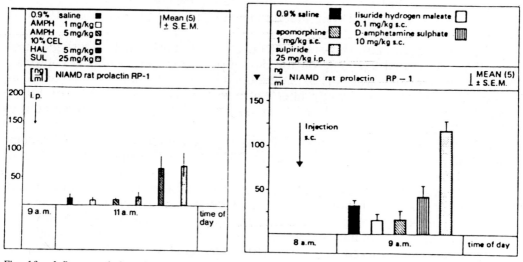

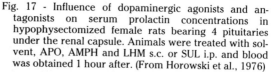

Fig. 16 - Influence of d-amphetamine (AMPH), haloperidol (HAL) and sulpiride (SUL) on serum prolactin concentrations in intact male rats. Animals were treated with AMPH, HAL and SUL, i.p. and blood was obtained 2 hours later. (From Horowski et al., 1976)

Fig. 17 - Influence of dopaminergic agonists and antagonists on serum prolactin concentrations in hypophysectomized female rats bearing 4 pituitaries under the renal capsule. Animals were treated with solvent, APO, AMPH and LHM s.c. or SUL i.p. and blood was obtained 1 hour after. (From Horowski et al., 1976)

as norepinephrine, was without effect in the same animals at 1 and 5 mg/kg i.p. (Fig. 16).

Using hypophysectomized female rats bearing four pituitaries transplanted under the renal capsule, they tested the effect of lisuride, apomorphine, amphetamine and sulpiride. As it can be seen in Figure 17, these animals showed elevated serum prolactin concentrations, which could be lowered by s.c. injection of 0.1 mg/kg lisuride, as well as by 1 mg/kg apomorphine, while 10 mg/kg amphetamine was whithout effect. In contrast, sulpiride (25 mg/kg i.p.) greatly increased serum prolactin in these animals. These results may be explained most easily by the assumption of dopaminergic receptors located within the pituitary itself.

In the case of sulpiride, this work was the first *in vivo* evidence for a direct action of this drug at the pituitary level.

These data support the hypothesis that dopamine has a dominant role as an inhibitor of prolactin secretion by acting itself as the prolactin inhibiting factor (PIF) on dopaminergic receptors located within the pituitary.

Concerning metoclopramide, Carlson et al. (1977) described its dopamine antagonistic action which promotes prolactin secretion. Indeed, 100 μg metoclopramide i.p. resulted in a significant (p < 0.02) increase in serum prolactin levels 60 min later. In contrast, serum growth hormone (GH) was not significantly affected, the mean serum GH level following metoclopramide administration

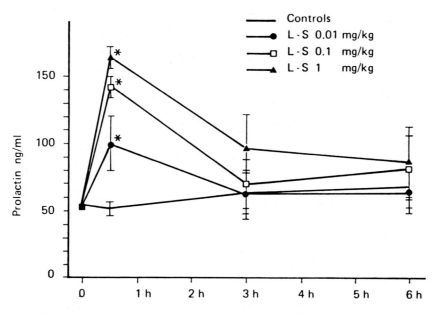

Fig. 18 - Effect of varying doses (1, 0.1, 0.01 mg/kg) of l(—) sulpiride on rat plasma PRL levels. All values are expressed as means ± SEM statistical significance vs basal level : *p < 0,01. (From Scapanigni et al., 1979)

(39 ± 22 ng/ml) was similar to the value of 35 ± 16 ng/ml observed in saline treated controls.

In another way, Scapanigni et al. (1979) have clearly demonstrated that there may exist a different potency between the two isomeric forms of the racemic (±) compound sulpiride in their ability to elevate plasma prolactin in different animal species and in man.

Indeed, the i.p. injection of l (—) sulpiride is much more potent in stimulating prolactin release in male rats in comparison with the d (±) isomer and the racemic (±) compound (Fig. 18, 19).

The effect of l(—) sulpiride has been studied on the hypothalamo-hypophyseal-gonadal axis of the male rat, at the dose of 10 µg/kg i.p. The rats were killed 30 minutes later and the mediobasal hypothalami were dissected out for LH-RH determination, showing that l-sulpiride was able to deplete LH-RH hypothalamic stores of 82,25 % of control values (Fig. 20).

In summary, the *in vivo* rat hormone secretory response seems to be an excellent screening test as a predictor of neuroendocrine potency for dopamine agonists or antagonists ; it has even been proposed as a neuroleptic predictor test of antipsychotic activity (Rubin and Hays, 1980).

In addition, we must also report that the determination of dopamine in the portal blood appears to be a reliable indicator of dopamine secretion from the tuberoinfundibular dopaminergic system (for details, see C. Oliver, this volume), but it re-

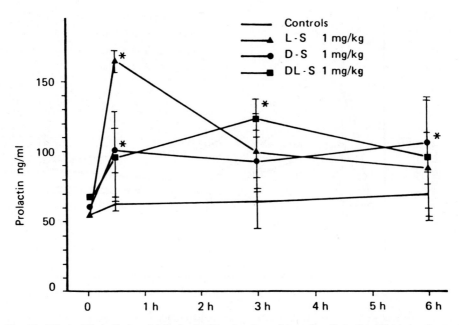

Fig. 19 - Effect of l(—), d(+) and d-l(±) sulpiride at a dose of 1 mg/kg. Note the different pattern of PRL response after the racemic compound (ld) sulpiride, with respect to both enantiomers. (From Scapanigni et al., 1979)

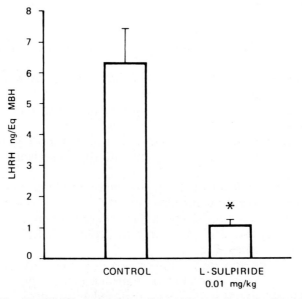

Fig. 20 - LH RH content in mediobasal hypothalami of saline in-jected and l(—) sulpiride (0.01 mg/kg) treated animals 30 min following the i.p. administration. Columns represent the means ± SEM of 10 values.
*Statistical significance p < 0.01
(From Scapanigni et al., 1979)

252

quires unusual manual skilfulness and cannot be applied routinely. For these reasons, Apud et al. (1980) have proposed the measurement of dopamine in the anterior pituitary as a suitable alternative to the previous method. Nevertheless, this remains a cumbersome method of screening for neuroactive drugs able to affect dopaminergic function.

Conclusion

In conclusion, it would appear that in order to evaluate the ability of new psychotropic drugs to induce neuroendocrine effects such as hyperprolactinemia, or the galactorrhea-amenorrhea syndrome in women, the monitoring of oestrous cycles during chronic treatment and the study of serum pituitary hormones — which are simple and accurate methods — are largely sufficient as preclinical screening tools, whereas the other methods we reported which are more sophisticated, may be used to clarify the molecular sites and mechanisms of action of the new molecules at the hypothalamic or pituitary level.

REFERENCES

Apud J., Cocchi D., Iuliano E., Casanueva F., Muller E.E. *1980* — Determination of dopamine in the anterior pituitary as an index of tuberoinfundibular dopaminergic function. *Brain Res., 186 :* 226-231.

Besser G.M., Delitala G., Grossman A., Stubbs W.A., Yeo T. *1980* — Chlorpromazine, haloperidol, metoclopramide and domperidone release prolactin through dopamine antagonism at low concentrations but paradoxically inhibit prolactin secretion at high concentrations. *Br. J. Pharmac., 71 :* 569-573.

Bruguerolle B., Jadot G., Valli M., Bouyard P. *1979* — Recherche des effets de la cimétidine sur le cycle œstral de la ratte. *C.R. Soc. Biol., 173 :* 1095-1098.

Bruguerolle B., Jadot G., Valli M., Bouyard L., Fabregou-Bergier P., Perrot J., Bouyard P. *1981a* — A propos des effets de quatre benzamides (métoclopramide, sulpiride, sultopride, tiapride) sur le cycle oestral de la ratte. *J. Pharmacol. 12 :* 27-36.

Bruguerolle B., Valli M., Jadot G., Baret A., Bouyard P. *1981b* — Recherche des effets éventuels du propranolol sur le cycle oestral de la ratte. *C.R. Soc. Biol., 175 :* 87-90.

Calabro M.A., McLeod R.M. *1978* — Binding of dopamine to bovine anterior pituitary gland membranes. *Neuroendocrinology, 25 :* 32-46.

Carlson H.E., Briggs J.E., McCallum R.W. *1977* — Stimulation of prolactin secretion by metoclopramide in the rat. *Proc. Soc. Exp. Med., 154 :* 476-478.

Caron M.G., Beaulieu M., Raymond V., Gagne B., Drouin J., Lefkowitz R.J., Labrie F. *1978* — Dopaminergic receptors in the anterior pituitary gland : correlation of [3H]-dihydroergocryptine binding with the dopaminergic control of prolactin release. *J. Biol. Chem., 253 :* 2244-2253.

Debeljuk I., Daskal H., Rozados R., Guitelman A. *1974* — Effect of sulpiride on prolactin release by rat pituitaries in vitro. *Experientia, 30 :* 1355-1356.

Dickerman S., Kledzik G., Gelato M., Chen H.J., Meites J. *1974* — Effects of haloperidol on serum pituitary prolactin, LH and FSH and hypothalamic PIF and LRF. *Neuroendocrinology, 15 :* 10-20.

Hökfelt T., Johansson O., Fuxe K., Elde R., Goldstein M., Park D., Efendic S., Luft R., Fraser H., Jeffcoate S. *1977* — Hypothalamic dopamine neurons and hypothalamic peptides. *Advanc. Biochem. Psychopharmacol., 16 :* 99-108.

Horowski R., Gräf K.J. *1976* — Influence of dopaminergic agonists and antagonists on serum prolactin concentrations in the rat. *Neuroendocrinology, 22 :* 273-286.

Jadot G. *1981* — *Le rat de laboratoire. I.-Réactif biologique,* pp. 34-36. Paris, Masson.

Jadot G., Bruguerolle B., Bouyard, L., Fabregou P., Bouyard P. *1980* — Etude statistique comparative de l'action de deux antiémétiques, le métoclopramide et la métopimazine, sur le cycle oestral de la ratte. *Pathol. Biol.,* 68-72.

Kordon C., Enjalbert A., Hery, M., Joseph-Bravo P.I., Rotsztejn W., Ruberg M. *1980* — Role of the neurotransmitters in the control of adenohypophyseal secretion. *In : Handbook of the hypothalamus.* Morgane P.J., Panksepp J. (eds), pp. 235-306. New York-Basel, M. Dekker.

Labrie F., Beaulieu M., Caron M.G., Raymond V. *1978* — Adenohypophyseal receptor : specificity and modulation of its activity by estradiol. *In : Progress in prolactin physiology and pathology.* Robyn C., Harter M. (eds) pp. 121-136 Amsterdam Elsevier-North Holland Biomedical Press.

Lotz W., Krause R. *1978* — Correlation between the effects of neuroleptics on prolactin release, mammary stimulation and the vaginal cycle in rats. *J. Endocrinol., 76 :* 507-515.

McLeod R.M., Lehmeyer J.E., *1974* — Studies on the mechanism of dopamine mediated inhibition of prolactin secretion. *Endocrinology, 94 : 1077-1085.*

Meites J., Sonntag W.E. *1981* — Hypothalamic hypophysiotropic hormones and neurotransmitter regulation : current views. *Ann. Rev. Pharmacol. Toxicol., 21 :* 295-322.

Rubin R.T., Hays S.E. *1980* — The prolactin secretory response to neuroleptic drugs : mechanisms, applications and limitations. *Psychoneuroendocrinology, 5 :* 121-137.

Scapagnini U., Clementi G., Fiore L., Marchetti B., Prato A., Fonzo D., Nistico G., Germana G., Bronzetti B. *1979* — Action of sulpiride's isomers on hypothalamic-hypophyseal-prolactin and hypothalamic-hypophyseal-gonadal axis. In : *Sulpiride and other Benzamides.* Spano P.F., Trabucchi M., Corsini G.U., Gessa G.L. (eds) pp. 193-205. Milan Italian, Brain Research Foundation Press.

Seeman P. *1981* — Brain dopamine receptors. *Pharmacol. Rev., 32 :* 229-313.

Shar C.J., Clemens J.A. *1976* — A catecholamine as a prolactin inhibiting factor (PIF). *Fed. Proc. Am. Soc. Exp. Biol. 35 :* 305.

Simpson G.M., Pi E.H., Sramek J.J. *1981* — Adverse effects of antipsychotic agents. *Drugs, 21 :* 138-151.

Titeler M., Seeman P. *1980* — Radioreceptor labeling of presynaptic and postsynaptic dopamine receptors. *Advan. Biochem. Psychopharmacol., 24 :* 159-165.

Valli M., Bruguerolle B., Jadot G., Bouyard P. *1981* — Étude expérimentale de l'association sulpiride-bromocriptine sur le cycle œstral de la ratte. *Ann. Endocrinol. 42 :* 49-55.

Valli M., Bruguerolle B., Jadot G., Bouyard P., Courtiere A., Baret A. *1982* — Études des effets neuroendocriniens de l'administration chronique de clonidine chez la ratte. *C.R. Soc. Biol.,* (in press).

Van Mannen J.H., Smelik P.G. *1968* — Induction of pseudopregnancy in rats following local depletion of monoamines in the median eminence of the hypothalamus. *Neuroendocrinology, 3 :* 177-186.

Yeo T., Thorner M.O., Jones A., Lowry P.J., Besser G.M. *1979* — The effects of dopamine, bromocriptine, lergotrile, and metoclopramide on prolactin release from continuously perfused columns of rat isolated pituitary cells. *Clin. Endocrinol., 10 :* 123-130.

DISCUSSION

C. Hagen
Have you looked for the binding of spiroperidol to isolated pituitary cells ?

M. Valli
No, we did not try that.

K. Fuxe
I would like to add that I think it is good that you measured dopamine in the portal vessels and in the anterior pituitary gland. However, I think that some investigators seem to forget that there are very important axo-axonic interactions going on in the median eminence and that it is only a portion of the tuberoinfundibular dopamine neurons that act by releasing dopamine as a PIF into this system. Thus, you are missing all the other interactions and therefore, it would be better for a more penetrative analysis to add also an analysis of the dopamine levels and the dopamine turnovers in the median eminence in order to understand possible interactions with the LHRH and TRH systems for instance.

M. Valli
Yes, I totally agree with you.

J. Mendlewicz
There are several investigators in this group, who work also very systematically with healthy volunteers, looking at hormonal levels as well as neuroendocrine responses. I wonder whether you feel there would be any value in that kind of approach for assessing the neuroendocrine effect of psychoactive drugs ?

M. Valli
I think it would be very interesting.

J. Mendlewicz
I meant in particular the work of Profs. Ackenheil and Matussek.

M. Valli
Yes, but you know this report was only focused on animal models, so it is difficult for me to tell you about the use of this practice in humans.

J. Mendlewicz
Yes, I think you concentrated mainly on animal work and gonadotrophines and prolactin.

M. Valli
Yes.

G. Sedvall
I was very interested to see the prolactin release you obtained. When you gave sulpiride did you study the dose-response curves for the prolactin elevation ? Did you study the binding of the ligands to these glands ? As I was astonished to see that you could find this effect, even if you do not have an inhibitory effect of the dopamine in this condition. Could there be some other factor besides dopamine, that would be inhibited by the neuroleptic treatment ?

M. Valli
Of course, it would be of very great interest, but it was not done in this study.

G. Sedvall
And the prolactin you measured, was that of the same order after transplantation as before transplantation ?

M. Valli
Yes, it was exactly the same.

G. Sedvall
And that was after one dose of the neuroleptic ?

M. Valli
Yes, it was only an acute administration.

J. Mendlewicz
Do you expect to have a supersensitivity of dopamine receptors in these after the transplantation ? It would be interesting to study the time course for this effect after transplantation, as you may have a development of supersensitivity.

M. Valli
Yes, that may be so.

K Fuxe
I think perhaps the circulating dopamine levels in the blood may be sufficient to activate the dopamine receptors of this transplant.

M. Ackenheil
You relate all your effects or at least most of the effects to the influence on dopaminergic neurons, but it is known that one can block the secretion of prolactin with anti-serotonergic drugs, such as methysergide. In your system, did you try to see if there are receptors for serotonin or if there are different receptors for the regulation of prolactin secretion ?

M. Valli
No.

Dopaminergic system and hypophyseal function

C. Oliver[1,2], B. Conte-Devolx[1,3], P. Giraud[2], E. Castanas[1,4], F. Boudouresque[1,3], G. Gunz[2]

1) Department of Endocrinology and Metabolic Disorders, Hospital of the Conception, Marseille, France.
2) Experimental Medicine Laboratory, Northern University, Marseille, France.
3) Physiology and 4) Biochemistry Laboratories, Timone University, Marseille, France.

Summary : the secretion of pituitary hormones is regulated by the production of several hypothalamic peptides such as thyrotropin releasing hormone, luteinizing releasing hormone, somatostatin and corticotrophin releasing hormone. In addition to these peptides, dopamine and other monoamines participate in the regulation of anterior pituitary function.

The dopaminergic tuberoinfundibular pathway consists of short neurons with cell bodies in the arcuate nuclei and terminals both in the external layer of the median eminence at the level of the hypophyseal portal vessels and in the neurointermediate lobe. Dopamine, but not norepinephrine or epinephrine, has been found in hypophyseal portal blood collected in anaesthetized rats at concentrations higher than in the systemic circulation. Dopamine can change adenohypophyseal secretion by acting directly on the pituitary gland or indirectly at the level of stroma, dendrites or axons of neurons secreting hypothalamic hormones. Receptors for dopamine agonists and antagonists have been demonstrated in the anterior pituitary gland and median eminence. They have the same characteristics as receptors already known in the nigro-striatal system. However, no pre-synaptic receptors for dopamine have been found and re-uptake of dopamine is very low.

There is now good evidence that dopamine is the physiological prolactin inhibiting factor (PIF). Indeed, no peptide with PIF activity has been found in the hypothalamus. The administration of L-dopa and dopamine is followed by a fall in plasma prolactin levels, through a direct effect on pituitary mammotrophs. In humans, a large increase in plasma prolactin is observed after acute or chronic administration of dopamine-receptor blocking agents (such as chlorpormazine, sulpiride and metoclopramide). Much attention has been devoted recently to the effect of ergot compounds which are dopamine agonists on prolactin secretion. Among them, bromocriptine was selected because of its strong inhibitory action on prolactin secretion. It is now currently used in the inhibition of post-partum lactation as well as in the treatment of hyperprolactinemia due to pituitary tumors.

There are still contradictory data on the dopaminergic control of growth hormone (GH) release. In the rat, dopamine stimulates somatostatin release by the hypothalamus and lowers GH secretion. In opposition, in man, dopamine agonists have a stimulatory effect on the secretion of GH. However, in acromegalic patients, a paradoxical decrease in GH plasma levels is observed and bromocriptine is used as a therapeutic tool in these patients. Dopamine has been postulated to have both an excitatory and an inhibitory action in the regulation of gonadotrophin secretion. However, recent histochemical evidence supports the hypothesis that hypothalamic dopaminergic neurons cause inhibition of LH release while hypothalamic noradrenergic neurons induce stimulation of gonadotrophin secretion from the pituitary. Dopamine does not act directly on the anterior pituitary to affect LH release, so any observed effects must be indirect through the hypothalamus.

Dopamine does not appear to have a major role in the control of ACTH secretory mechanisms. The administration of L-dopa is reported to have no effect or only a slight stimulative effect on ACTH secretion.

Neither L-dopa administration, nor the infusion of dopamine cause any definite change in TSH secretion in unthyroid subjects. However, in primary hypothyroidism, L-dopa administration lowers TSH secretion.

Introduction

The secretion of the pituitary gland is largely dependent upon hypothalamic hypophysiotropic hormones that reach the anterior portion of the gland via the hypophyseal-portal vessels.

Four hypophysiotropic hormones or factors have already been discovered: Thyrotropin-releasing hormone (TRH) which stimulates the secretion of TSH and prolactin; luteinizing hormone-releasing hormone (LH-RH) which increases the secretion of ACTH and β-endorphin; somatostatin which inhibits the secretion of GH and TSH. Prolactin-releasing hormone (PRH) and growth hormone-releasing hormone (GH-RH) which are postulated to stimulate the secretion of prolactin and GH respectively have not yet been discovered. As discussed below, it seems likely that dopamine serves as the physiological prolactin-inhibiting hormone (PIH) and melanocyte-stimulating hormone-inhibiting hormone (MIH) (Bowers et al. 1979). Unlike gonadotropins, TSH, GH, prolactin and ACTH which are secreted by the anterior lobe, α-melanocyte-stimulating hormone (α-MSH) is mainly produced by the intermediate lobe.

Using immunocytochemical techniques, TRH-containing neurons have been identified with cell bodies in the dorsomedical nucleus and the perifornical area, and nerve terminals in the medial part of the external layer of the median eminence and in many hypothalamic areas. The cell bodies containing LHRH are located in the preoptic, anterior hypothalamus and arcuate nucleus and they send axons that converge on the median eminence. Somatostatin is secreted in the median eminence from the endings of neurons with cell bodies in the preoptic and anterior hypothalamic area (Hökfelt et al., 1977). The secretion of these hypothalamic hormones is modulated by neurotransmitters released by noradrenergic, dopaminergic and serotoninergic neurons from various nuclei of the brain. It now appears that dopamine is an important factor in the regulation of pituitary hormones secretion.

Organization of dopaminergic neurons

In the mammalian hypothalamus, the dopaminergic pathways can be divided into two major systems: The tuberohypophyseal dopamine system and the incerto-hypothalamic dopamine system.

The cell bodies of the tubero-hypophyseal system in the rat are located in the arcuate nucleus of the hypothalamus and the immediately adjacent periventricular nucleus. The neurons represent approximately 7 % of the cell bodies of this nucleus. One group of axons projects ventrally through the arcuate nucleus and then turns medially into the zona externa of the median eminence. The terminals are abundant in the external layer where they are packed in a palisade-like manner, close to the capillaries of the portal vessels. The anterior portion of the arcuate nucleus projects upon the pars intermedia of the pituitary. The region just caudal to that portion projects to the pars nervosa. It has not been well established if the arcuate-periventricular dopaminergic neurons are the only source of dopaminergic innervation in the median eminence. According to some authors, part of the hypothalamic dopamine is contributed by the incerto-hypothalamic system. However, other investigators found no change in median eminence dopaminergic innervation after hypothalamic de-afferentation. The incerto-hypothalamic fiber system, so far identified only in the rat, originates from dorsal and caudal hypothalamic cell groups (A11-A13) and periventricular cells of the A14 cell group. The system projects for short distance into the medial preoptic, suprachiasmatic, dorsomedial and anterior hypothalamic nuclei. (Björklund, 1978).

258

Approaches to the analysis of the action of dopamine on the pituitary gland :

There are several possible sites at which brain dopamine can act to affect pituitary secretion (Weiner and Ganong, 1978).

There is now evidence that dopamine is secreted into the portal hypophyseal vessels at the level of the median eminence. The dopamine released in portal blood appears to act directly on the lactotrophs to inhibit their secretion.

Another possibility is that dopamine produces local vasomotor changes in the portal vascular bed.

Dopamine may also act via release at synaptic endings in or near the neurons that secrete the hypophysiotropic hormones. Indeed the dopaminergic axons terminate in proximity with TRH, LH-RH, and somatostatin-secreting neurons. Synaptic endings may be located on dendrites and cell bodies of these neurons or on their axonal terminations in the median eminence.

The role of brain dopamine in the regulation of pituitary function has been studied using the following methods.

1. *Correlation between dopamine concentration,* turnover in the hypothalamus or secretion in hypophysial portal blood and pituitary hormones secretion.

2. *Pharmacological methods :* Measurement of plasma prolactin after :
— administration of drugs interfering with the biosynthesis of dopamine or antagonizing its action on its receptors. However, the drugs available are never entirely specific, — or direct intraventricular or systemic administration of dopamine.

3. *In vivo methods :* Measurement of plasma prolactin after electrical lesion or stimulation of the arcuate nucleus.

4. *In vitro methods :* Measurement of prolactin released by pituitary glands or determination of hypothalamic hormones released by hypothalamic fragments or synaptosomes during *in vitro* incubations.

Dopamine and prolactin secretion

It has been known since 1961 that acid extracts from hypothalamic tissue inhibit the *in vitro* secretion of prolactin. Since these extracts contain dopamine which can inhibit prolactin secretion by a direct action on the pituitary, the question has been raised : Is dopamine itself PIH. ? There is now evidence that dopamine is indeed PIH. Hypothalamic extracts lose their ability to inhibit prolactin secretion after enzymatic digestion with monoamine oxidase which destroys dopamine. There is a good correlation between PIH. activity and dopamine content of the hypothalamic extracts. Using pituitaries incubated *in vitro*, it has been shown that the secretion and synthesis of prolactin is inhibited by 10^{-7} to 10^{-9} dopamine. *In vivo* studies using rats with pituitary grafts under the renal capsule with high prolactin have shown that L-dopa inhibits prolactin release probably via a direct effect on the pituitary transplant. In intact rats, the infusion of dopamine into hypophysial portal vessels is followed by a significant decrease of prolactin secretion (Neill, 1980).

Dopaminergic receptors have been identified in anterior pituitaries. *In vitro* experiments with bovine anterior pituitary membranes show that dopamine antagonists compete stereospecifically for dopamine receptors. Their competition for ^{3}H-dihydroergocryptine, a dopamine agonist, parallel their capacity to inhibit the *in vitro* release of prolactin from cultured rat pituitary cells in the following rank order : Apomorphine > dopamine > epinephrine > norepinephrine > clonidine = isoproterenol (Labrie et al., 1980).

Dopamine, but not norepinephrine or epinephrine is present in rat hypophysial stalk blood in higher concentrations than found in the peripheral circulation, establishing dopamine as a secretory product of the median eminence (Ben-Jonathan et al. 1977). The physiological significance of dopamine in hypophyse portal blood has been established showing that they are sufficient to inhibit prolactin secretion *in vivo* and *in vitro*. Rats in which the median eminence has been destroyed in order to inhibit dopamine synthesis, show a decrease in prolactin secretion when dopamine is infused into the peripheral circulation at a rate sufficient to achieve plasma concentrations (6 to 9 ng/ml) similar to those found in hypophysial stalk plasma (Gibbs and Neill, 1978). It appears likely that changes in dopamine secretion account for changes in prolactin release during the estrous cycle after cervical stimulation or suckling. Ben-Jonathan et al. (1977) have reported that dopamine levels in stalk blood are moderately, but significantly lower at proestrus than at estrus, suggesting that dopamine plays a physiological role in prolactin secretion. Plotsky and Neill (1982) have recently shown that a 62,5 % decrease in dopamine secretion in portal blood occurs within 1-4 minutes after initiation of mammary nerve stimulation. This momentary but profound decrease in hypothalamic dopamine secretion precedes or accompanies the rise in prolactin secretion evoked by the same stimulus. Similary, cervical stimulation is followed by a decrease of dopamine levels in portal blood (Neill, 1980).

However, factors other than dopamine may be of importance in the regulation of prolactin secretion. Among these factors, one can enumerate oestrogens, peptides such as TRH, vasoactive intestinal peptide and monoamines such as serotonin which are known to stimulate prolactin release directly at the level of the pituitary gland.

The secretion of dopamine into portal blood can be modulated by hormonal changes. For example, short-term treatment with 17 β-estradiol lowers dopamine release into hypophysial portal blood. This oestrogen-induced suppression of the release of hypothalamic dopamine may facilitate the proestrus surge of prolactin secretion.

In contrast, long-term treatment of rats with 17 β-estradiol results in a marked increase in the secretion of dopamine. In the rat, gestation is also associated with a high dopamine secretion in hypophysial portal blood. During gestation as well as after estrogen-treatment, plasma prolactin levels are high. Increased dopamine secretion in both conditions can be explained by the so-called short-loop feed-back of pituitary hormones on the hypothalamus. Since prolactin has been shown to increase dopamine levels in portal blood, the stimulatory effect of long-term estrogen treatment or gestation on hypothalamic dopamine secretion may be a consequence of hyperprolactinemia (Porter et al., 1980). The recent demonstration of a

260

retrograde blood flow in the pituitary stalk supports the hypothesis that pituitary hormones which circulate at high levels in the hypothalamus can influence hypothalamic dopamine secretion (Oliver et al., 1977).

A number of pharmacologic agents, mainly tricyclic neuroleptics elevate plasma prolactin by blocking specific dopamine receptors. Sulpiride and metoclopramide are used in the clinical evaluation of prolactin reserve.

The effect of ergot compounds on the dopaminergic system controlling prolactin secretion has been extensively studied (Del Pozo and Lancranjan, 1978). Among them, bromocriptine (CB 154, Parlodel[R]) inhibits basal plasma prolactin in normal women and has been subsequently used in postpartum women for inhibiting milk secretion. The effect of bromocriptine in prolactinomas has been well documented. Treatment with bromocriptine is followed by normal ovulatory cycles and disappearance of galactorrhea. A regression of pituitary tumors has even been observed in some observations (Wass et al., 1979).

Dopamine and the control of gonadotropin secretion

While most neuroendocrinologists agree that norepinephrine stimulates the gonadotropin release, the role of dopamine remains controversial.

The finding that the dopamine content of the median eminence undergoes changes during the estrous cycle and is modified by endocrine manipulations inducing changes in the secretion of FSH and LH led to the hypothesis that dopamine is involved in the control of gonadotropins. Increased hypothalamic dopamine turnover is observed when LH and FSH levels are low (estrus, after therapy with estradiol). By contrast, dopamine turnover is low when LH and FSH are high (proestrus, castration). These results suggest that dopamine has an inhibitory effect on gonadotropin secretion (Fuxe et al., 1978). Measurements of dopamine in hypophysial portal blood are in good agreement with these histophysiological experiments in which fluorescence methods are used to measure dopamine turnover. However, no definite conclusion can be drawn from these experiments since prolactin and estrogens, which are known to vary during the estrous cycle, can modify the release of dopamine. Thus, the changes in dopamine secretion may be only the consequence of prolactin and estrogen variations rather than the cause of changes in gonadotropin secretion (Fuxe et al., 1978).

Data from pharmacological experiments do not allow a definite conclusion (Barraclough and Wise, 1982). In several laboratories, it has been reported that the administration of dopamine or dopamine agonists (intraventricularly or intraperitoneally) stimulates LH release. This effect has been substantiated both in intact rats and in ovariectomized, estradiol- or progesterone-primed rats. In some experiments, it has been dramatically related to the dose of dopamine. For example, Vijayan and McCann (1978) recently observed an increase of LH following injection of 4 and 20 μg dopamine into the third ventricle of estradiol- and progesterone-primed rats whereas no effect was observed with 2 and 10 μg.

In contrast to these studies which advocate a stimulatory role for dopamine there are reports from many other laboratories suggesting that norepinephrine, rather than dopamine activates the release of gonadotropins (Sawyer, 1975).

In other experiments, dopamine has also been shown to inhibit gonadotropin secretion in the rat as well as in other species. In the rabbit, dopamine has also been shown to inhibit LH secretion directly at the pituitary level, this effect being observed only within a restricted dose-range (Dailey et al., 1978). In humans, several studies suggest that dopamine and its agonists are inhibitory to gonadotropin secretion. Dopamine-induced inhibition of LH secretion in men is associated with a reduction in both pulse frequency and amplitude of LH secretion. Furthermore, the observation that partial inhibition of LH secretion occurs even in the presence of a continuous LH-RH and dopamine infusion, suggests that dopamine may also modulate the gonadotrope response to LH-RH (Huseman et al., 1980).

Although the action of dopamine on gonadotropin secretion remains to be clarified there have been speculations on its mechanism of action. Dopamine has no effect on gonadotropin secretion when tested on *in vitro* pituitary incubations. An indirect effect through the hypothalamus is more likely. Axo-axonal contacts between dopamine and LH-RH containing terminals have not been conclusively demonstrated, but the close anatomical proximity of the dopamine system terminals to LH-RH terminals in the median eminence makes possible an action of dopamine on the release of LH-RH into the hypophysial portal system. The large concentrations and turnover rates of dopamine in the median eminence can easily flood the extracellular space between the LH-RH and dopamine terminals without the need for specialized axo-axonal endings (McNeill and Sladek, 1978). No measurements of immunoreactive LH-RH in portal blood after dopamine administration are available. When tested *in vitro* on synaptosomes or fragments from the mediobasal hypothalamus, dopamine stimulates LH-RH release. The effect of dopamine is dose-dependent and can be inhibited by dopamine antagonists (Rotsztejn et al., 1977). The significance of this finding still needs to be clarified.

Dopamine and growth hormone secretion

Most authors agree that norepinephrine, dopamine and serotonin stimulate GH secretion in humans. The results are more controversial in other animal species in which large variations have been observed in the regulation of GH secretion (Martin, 1976). For example, it appears that the regulation of GH secretion is opposite in primates and rodents. Indeed, GH release after stress increases in primates and decreases in rodents. In humans, L-dopa the precursor of both dopamine and norepinephrine has been shown to increase GH secretion, an effect that is suppressed by phentolamine, an α-adrenoceptor blocking agent. These findings suggest that norepinephrine and not dopamine, is involved in the stimulation of GH release. The role of α-adrenergic receptors in GH control is supported further by the report that clonidine, a central α-agonist, causes GH release. However, it appears than in humans, dopamine can also exert a stimulatory influence on GH secretion. Apomorphine significantly increases GH secretion and a single dose of bromocriptine is able to release GH in normal men. Further indirect proof for the dopaminergic control of GH secretion is provided by the report that pimozide, a dopamine-receptor blocker, significantly reduces GH release following exercice and arginine. By contrast, L-dopa and apomorphine both cause inhibition of GH release in the rat, an effect mediated by the stimulation of somatostatin secretion (Chihara et al., 1979).

During the last few years, dopaminergic drugs have been used for their unexpected therapeutic effect on acromegaly. Indeed the paradoxical decrease in GH release recorded by apomorphine and bromocriptine in acromegaly led to the possibility that dopaminergic drugs might be used as therapeutic tools in this disease. An interesting study was reported by Besser et al. (1980) who demonstrated clinical and biochemical improvement in 94 % and 77 % respectively of 101 patients treated with bromocriptine. The mechanism of paradoxical effect of dopamine in acromegalic patients has recently been investigated by Marcovitz et al. (1982). These authors have shown that when tested *in vitro* on normal pituitary tissue as well as on somatotrophic adenoma, dopamine lowers GH release.

The increased GH release observed *in vivo* in normal subjects is the consequence of a strong stimulatory extra-pituitary action of dopamine which overwhelms its inhibitory effect on the pituitary gland. In some acromegalic patients, the extra-pituitary effect of dopamine has disappeared and only the action on the pituitary gland is recorded.

Dopamine and the regulation of ACTH secretion

Most experiments suggest that dopamine does not play a very important role in the control of ACTH. For most authors, norepinephrine, and not dopamine, has an inhibitory effect on ACTH release. This conclusion is consistent with the inability of dopamine to affect CRH release *in vitro* (Weiner and Ganong, 1978). Bromocriptine has recently been used as a therapeutic agent in a few cases of Cushing's disease without conclusive results (Del Pozo and Lancranjan, 1978).

Dopamine and the control of TSH secretion

A moderate inhibitory role of dopamine in TSH release has been shown in humans using dopamine receptor-blocking drugs. This effect is seen most clearly in hypothyroid patients in whom the dominant negative feedback of thyroid hormones is reduced. In euthyroid subjects, the inhibitory role of dopamine on TSH secretion is also demonstrated using a sensitive radioimmunoassay for human TSH, this effect being greatest at night. The finding that dopamine infusion produces an acute suppression of the TSH response to TRH in normal subjects suggests that dopamine lowers TSH release by a direct effect on the pituitary gland (Scanlon et al., 1980).

Dopamine and α-MSH secretion

α-MSH is a peptide with melanotropic activity and is found in high concentrations in the pars intermedia. This part of the pituitary gland contains an enzymatic system which acts on the proopiomelanocorticotropin precursor to produce α-MSH. Since the development of the pars intermedia varies according to the species, the α-MSH level in the pituitary is variable : Very low in adult human, high in human fetus and other species such as the rat. The secretion of α-MSH in mammals is under predominantly inhibitory control by the central nervous system. The pars intermedia is poorly vascularized, but receives a dense dopaminergic system originating in the arcuate nucleus. The hypothesis that a tripeptide Pro-Leu-Gly-NH$_2$ named M.I.H. represents the physiologically relevant MSH release-inhibiting factor, has not been confirmed. However, there is now evidence that dopamine is in fact the physiological M.I.H. In the rat, apomorphine and bromocriptine lower plasma α-MSH levels. In the same animal, the injection of dopamine-receptor blocking agents (haloperidol and pimozide) is followed by a rapid increase in circulating α-MSH levels. Dopamine acts directly at the level of the pars intermedia cells (Tilders and Smelik, 1977).

Conclusion

Dopamine has a direct action on the pituitary gland inhibiting prolactin and α-MSH secretion. The intra-hypothalamic dopaminergic neurons send axons close to the hypophysial portal vessels which carry dopamine until its binding to specific receptors on the pituitary cells. Experimental studies suggest that dopamine is indeed both a physiological P.I.H. and M.I.H. The data concerning the influence of dopamine on the secretion of other pituitary hormones are controversial.

The effect of dopamine may be either indirect passing through the hypothalamus (for GH and gonadotropins) or only slight (for TSH).

Both possibilities may account for difficulties encountered in the experimental studies and controversies in the interpretations of the data.

Acknowledgements :
The authors thank Mrs R. Garozzo for her excellent secretarial assistance.

REFERENCES

Barraclough C.A., Wise P.M., *1982* — The role of catecholamines in the regulation of pituitary luteinizing hormone and Follicle-Stimulating Hormone. *Endocrine Reviews, 3 :* 91-119.

Ben-Jonathan N., Oliver C., Weiner H.J., Mical R.S., Porter J.C., *1977* — Dopamine in hypophysial portal plasma of the rat during the estrous cycle and throughout pregnancy. *Endocrinology, 100 :* 452-458.

Besser G.M., Wass J.A.H., Thorner M.O., *1980* — Bromocriptine in the medical management of acromegaly. *In : Ergot Compounds and Brain Function : Neuroendocrine and neuropsychiatric aspects.* Goldstein, D.B. Calne, A. Lieberman, M.O. Thorner (eds) pp. 191-198 New York, Raven Press.

Björklund A. *1978* — Organization of catecholamine neurons involved in endocrine functions. *In : Biologie cellulaire des processus neurosécrétoires hypothalamiques.* J.D. Vincent and C. Kordon (eds) pp. 280, 81-100, Paris, Ed. du C.N.R.S.

Bowers C.Y., Folkers K., Knudsen R., Lam Y.K., Wan Y.P., Humphries J., Chang D. *1979* — Hypothalamic peptide hormones ; chemistry and physiology. *In : Endocrinology. 1* L.J. DeGroot (ed), pp. 65-93. New York, Grune and Statton.

Chihara K., Arimura A., Schally A.V., *1979* — Effect of intraventricular injection of dopamine, norepinephrine, acetylcholine and 5-hydroxytryptamine on immunoreactive somatostatin release into rat hypophyseal portal blood. *Endocrinology, 104 :* 1656-1662.

Dailey R.A., Tsou R.C., Tindall G.T., Neill J.D. *1978* — Direct hypophysial inhibition of Luteinizing Hormone release by dopamine in rabbit. *Life Sc., 22 :* 1491-1498.

Del Pozo E., Lancranjan I., *1978.* — Clinical use of drugs modifying the release of anterior pituitary hormones. *In : Frontiers in Neuroendocrinology. 5* W.F. Ganong and L. Martini (eds), pp. 207-247 New York, Raven Press.

Fuxe K., Löfström A., Hökfelt T., Ferland L., Andersson K., Agnati L., Eneroth P., Gustafsson J.A., Skett P., *1978* — Influence of central catecholamines on LHRH-containing pathways. *Clin. Obstet. and Gynecol. 5 :* 251-269.

Gibbs D.M., Neill J.D., *1978.* — Dopamine levels in hypophysial stalk blood in rat are sufficient to inhibit Prolactin secretion in vivo. *Endocrinology, 102 :* 1895-1900.

Hökfelt T., Johansson O., Fuxe K., Elde R., Goldstein M., Park D., Efendic S., Luft R., Fraser H., Jeffcoate S., *1977.* — Hypothalamic dopamine neurons and hypothalamic peptides. *In : Advances in Biochemical Psychopharmacology. 16* E. Costa and G.L. Gessa (eds), pp. 99-108. New York, Raven Press.

Huseman C.A., Kugler J.A., Schneider I.G. *1980* — Mechanism of dopaminergic suppression of gonadotropin secretion in men. *J. clin. Endocrinol. Metab., 51 :* 209-213.

Labrie F., Di Paolo T., Raymond V., Ferland L., Beaulieu M., *1980* — The pituitary dopamine receptor. *In : Ergot Compounds and Brain Function : Neuroendocrine and neuropsychiatric aspects.* M. Goldstein, D.B. Calne, A. Lieberman, M.O. Thorner, (eds) pp. 217-227. New York, Raven Press.

Marcovitz S., Goodyer C.G., Guyda H., Gardiner R.J., Hardy J. *1982* — Comparative study of human fetal, normal adult, and somatotropic adenoma pituitary function in tissue culture. *J. clin. Endocrinol. Metab., 54 :* 6-16.

McNeill T.H., Sladek J.R. Jr *1978* — Fluorescence-immunocytochemistry : simultaneous localization of catecholamines and gonadotropin-releasing hormone. *Science, 200 :* 72-74.

Martin J.B., *1976* — Brain regulation of Growth Hormone secretion. In : *Frontiers in Neuroendocrinology, 4.* L. Martini and W.F. Ganong (eds) pp. 129-168. New York, Raven Press.

Neill J.D. *1980* — Neuroendocrine regulation of Prolactin secretion. *In : Frontiers in Neuroendocrinology,* L. Martini and W.F. Ganong (eds) *6,* 129-155. New York, Raven Press.

Oliver C., Mical R.S., Porter J.C. *1977* — Hypothalamic-Pituitary vasculature : evidence for retrograde blood flow in the pituitary stalk. *Endocrinology, 101 :* 598-604.

Plotsky P.M., Neill J.D., *1982* — The decrease in hypothalamic dopamine secretion induced by suckling : comparison of voltametric and radioisotopic methods of measurement. *Endocrinology, 110 :* 691-696.

Porter J.C., Gudelsky G.A., Nansel D.D., Foreman M.M., Reymond M.J., Tilders F.J.H. *1980.* — Regulation of hypothalamic secretion of dopamine into hypophysial portal blood : role of pituitary hormones. *In : Progress in psychoneuroendocrinology.* F. Brambilla, G. Eacagni, D. de Wied (eds), pp. 349-358. Amsterdam, Elsevier.

Rotsztejn W.H., Charli J.L., Pattou E., Kordon C., *1977* — Stimulation by dopamine of luteinizing hormone-releasing hormone (LHRH) release from mediobasal hypothalamus in male rats. *Endocrinology, 101 :* 1475-1483.

Sawyer C.H., *1975* — Some recent developments in brain-pituitary-ovarian physiology. *Neuroendocrinol. 17 :* 97-124.

Scanlon M.F., Lewis M., Weightman D.R., Chan V., Hall R., *1980* — The neuroregulation of human thyrotropin secretion. *In : Frontiers in Neuroendocrinology 6.* L. Martini and W.F. Ganong (eds), pp. 333-380. New York, Raven Press.

Tilders F.J.H., Smelik P.G., *1977* — Direct neural control of MSH secretion in mammals : the involvement of dopaminergic tubero-hypophysial neurons. *In : Frontiers in Hormone Research, 4.* F.J.H. Tilders, D.F. Swaab, Tj. B. Van Wimersma Greidanus (eds) pp. 80-93, Basel, Karger.

Vijayan E., McCann S.M., *1978* — Re-evaluation of the role of catecholamines in control of gonadotropin and prolactin release. *Neuroendocrinol., 25 :* 150-165.

Wass J.A.H., Moult P.J.A., Thorner M.O., Dacie J.E., Charlesworth M., Jones A.E., Besser G.M., *1979* — Reduction of pituitary tumor size in patients with prolactinomas and acromegaly treated with bromocriptine with or without radiotherapy. *Lancet, 2 :* 66-69.

Weiner R.I., Ganong W.F., *1978* — Role of brain monoamines and histamine in regulation of anterior pituitary secretion. *Physiological Rev., 58 :* 905-976.

DISCUSSION

C. Hagen

First of all, just a comment : We have recently published the first double blind study on the treatment of acromegaly with bromocryptine and found no effect in the treatment of 18 patients. The study has not excluded that a sub-population of patients will respond, but an overall response could not be demonstrated. On your slide you showed that apomorphine and bromocryptine induced GH release of about 10 ng/ml and we and others have recently found that metoclopramide is also able to stimulate GH secretion and this does not seem to be related with nausea or any discomfort of the patients. Do you have a comment on that ?

Ch. Oliver

Regarding your comment on the treatment of acromegaly by bromocryptine, I believe that Besser et al. got almost 100 % good results using this drug. On the other hand, you find almost zero percent good results. In Marseille we find an improvement of the symptoms in about 40 to 60 % of the patients.

P. Grof

I wonder could you mention the dosage you used, just to give some understanding to this controversy ?

Ch. Oliver

We used between 15 — 20 mg/die per patient. Dr. Hagen, I cannot give a satisfactory explanation about the stimulatory effect of both metoclopramide and apomorphine on GH secretion

K. Fuxe

I think that part of this problem with dopamine agonists and antagonists producing the same final action on the anterior pituitary secretion, e.g. GH secretion could in part be related to the fact that the dopamine nerve terminals do not only regulate the somatostatin secretion, but also the GRF secretion. In fact, there may be a possibility that a drug can produce increases or decreases of GH secretion depending upon whether the dominating effect is on the somatostatin or GRF neurons. No doubt the results show the importance, not only of the pharmacological approach, but also as introduced in the sixties' by us, of a more physiological approach, which involves a correlative effect between the neurochemical changes in the hypothalamus and the changes of hormone secretion, in order to better define which type of neuron systems are involved in the regulation of that hormone. I think this was a fine review and as you are probably aware, I have opposed the view of MaCann and Kordon for over 10 years, claiming that dopamine releases LHRH. More and more evidence supports our hypothesis that some dopamine tuberoinfundibular neurons are inhibitory systems inhibiting the release of LHRH. Then I would like to mention a few additional studies that you did not mention in your lecture. In recent years, we have also really done quite careful intraindividual correlations by which we can relate in an animal the levels of the hormone, e.g. LH to the dopamine levels or the dopamine turnover in the median eminence. In this type of analysis we have always found intraindividual correlations showing that whenever there is an enhancement of dopamine turnover in the lateral palisade zone, there is also a lowering of LH secretion. Indeed, the dopamine turnover increase was secondary and related to changes in prolactin or gonadal steroid hormone secretion, leading to an increase of dopamine turnover producing LH release, then we would have had the opposite type of correlation, which we have never been able to observe. This type of intraindividual correlation is quite an important aspect to this type of discussion on various hypotheses on the role of dopamine in LHRH release. Another problem in this field has been that the median eminence dopamine receptors must, in my mind, be very humorally regulated. There is a substantial regulation by the hormones of the properties of the dopamine receptors in the median eminence. Thus, differences in the humoral environment with regard to e.g. steroid hormones and prolactin can change the coupling of the dopamine receptors and the number. Such modulations can explain why you get such different types of results with various dopamine receptor agonists and antagonists in the different humoral conditions. This gonadotropin-induced ovulation in the pre-pubertal rat can be impressively inhibited by dopamine receptor agonist actions, which you could counteract with dopamine receptor antagonists. Instead, in the adult female rat the inhibitors' effect of dopamine agonists are much less pronounced. It may well be that you need a sensitization of the median eminence dopamine receptor in some endocrine estates to really demonstrate the powerful inhibitory action in LHRH release by dopamine agonists. The mechanism involved in our mind would be one of the pre-synaptic inhibition. This means that the dopamine terminals would be more inhibitory when you have a large number of action potentials coming down the LHRH to a partly depolarized nerve terminal due to the action of dopamine. Under these conditions, the action potentials coming down cannot release as much LHRH as normal. On the other hand, if you have a silent LHRH sytem, then you might even obtain some LHRH release by dopamine receptor activation, because of the small depolarization produced by dopamine itself. Well, those are some of the thoughts we have on the complexity of dopamine synapses in the median eminence. The neurochemical approaches have really made it possible to penetrate the problems in neuroendocrinology in a much better fashion. Of course, previously we just had the pharmacological approach. Now, we can perform for example elegant measurement of dopamine in the portal blood, as very beautifully illustrated in this lecture. The results illustrate the importance of bringing neurochemistry into the field of neuroendocrinology.

N. Matussek
You mentioned that you get an increase of dopamine after giving prolactin to animals. In your opinion, is the dopamine and HVA increase after neuroleptics due to prolactin or to post-synaptic receptor blockade ?

Ch. Oliver
In Dr. Porter's group (Dallas, Texas) it has been shown that haloperidol injections in rats are followed by a large increase in dopamine secretion in portal blood. If, under the same experimental conditions, a prolactin-antiserum is injected into the rat, there is a decrease in dopamine release in portal blood. That leads to the conclusion that the increase in dopamine secretion observed after haloperidol is due to the increase in prolactin release.

267

Effects of tiapride and sulpiride infusions on plasma levels of beta-endorphin, prolactin and dopamine in patients with neoplastic pain

C. Gennari, R. Nami, G. Francini, S. Gonnelli and C. Bianchini.

Institute of Medical Semeiotics, University of Siena, Italy.

Summary : Tiapride, a substituted benzamide, exerts an analgesic effect in man. To examine the possibility that tiapride analgesia might be related to a mechanism involving a release of endogenous opioids, the acute effects of an intravenous injection of the drug on plasma radioimmunoassayable beta-endorphin were studied in patients with pain from cancer (placebo-tiapride double-blind randomized trial). Another group of patients with pain from cancer was studied in the same way, using a different substituted benzamide, sulpiride (placebo-sulpiride double blind randomized trial).

As substituted benzamides affect prolactin secretion, the plasma levels of prolactin and dopamine, a known inhibitor of prolactin release, were studied as well. The tiapride infusion produced a slight but significant increase in plasma beta-endorphin, an early and significant increase in plasma prolactin, and a sudden and highly significant decrease in plasma dopamine. These results are compatible with the hypothesis that tiapride influences the neuroendocrine system.

The sulpiride infusion produced the same modification of prolactin and dopamine circulating levels as observed after tiapride infusion, but did not affect the plasma beta-endorphin level. These results demonstrate that the effects of the two drugs on the neuroendocrine system are not completely superimposable.

Introduction

Tiapride is a substituted benzamide drug employed in the fields of psychiatry and gastroenterology for its ability to cause dopamine blockade. In the therapeutic application of tiapride an analgesic effect in headache and facial pain (Brion and Guerin, 1977 ; Sambin, 1977) and in patients with cancer pain (Lepille and Bastit, 1979 ; Clavel and Pommatau, 1980) has been observed. In addition the drug is employed for the relief of pain following the withdrawal of cerebrospinal fluid or the injection of radio opaque contrast for myelography or cerebral arteriography.

Recent studies suggest that endogenous opiates may play a central part in modulating the perception of pain (Belluzzi et al., 1976 ; Akil et al., 1978 ; Krieger and Liotta, 1979). Beta-endorphin (B-END) seems to be the main pituitary peptide with opiate activity. In man B-END given intravenously is 3 to 4 times more potent than morphine and has an even more powerful effect when given intracerebrally (Tseng et al., 1976 ; Catliin et al., 1977 ; Hosobuchi and Li, 1978).

Adrenocorticotropin (ACTH), betalipotropin (B-LPH) and B-END are derived from a common precursor, propiocortin (Mains and Eipper 1977, 1979). B-END is the 61-91 C-terminal portion of the B-LPH segment, which is considered the immediate precursor of B-END (Bradbury et al., 1976). ACTH, B-END and B-LPH are released simultaneously from the pituitary into the blood in response to many types of stress stimuli (Nakao et al., 1979 ; Guillemin et al., 1977 ; Carr et al., 1981 ; Gambert et al., 1981). Recently it has been demonstrated that B-END is present along with ACTH in the corticotrophs of the human adenohypophysis (Mendelsohn et al., 1979 ; Weber et al., 1979 ; Allen et al., 1980).

Although it still remains to be shown that the changes in plasma B-END levels could be related to analgesia, evidence is, however, accumulating that some drugs exhibiting an analgesic effect stimulate the release of B-END (Gennari, 1981).

The mechanism of tiapride's analgesic effect is still unknown. In order to examine the possibility that tiapride induced analgesia may be related to a mechanism of B-END release from the pituitary gland, we studied the acute effects of intravenous injection of tiapride on plasma B-END levels in 10 patients with pain from cancer. Another group of 10 patients with cancer pain were studied using a different substituted benzamide, sulpiride. In both cases, the studies were conducted in a double-blind randomized trial with placebo. At the same time, because substituted benzamides affect prolactin secretion, we have studied the plasma levels of prolactin (PRL) and dopamine (DA) a known factor inhibiting PRL release.

Materials and methods

Ten patients, 7 males and 3 females, aged 66 -76 years, with different kinds of neoplasia-related pain, were submitted to a double-blind randomized study to estimate the acute effects of tiapride when compared to placebo. All patients were in an advance stage of neoplasia with multiple metastases (origin of cancer : gut 3, breast 2, lung 2, uterus 1, pancreas 1, prostate 1). The fasting patients were infused at 8:00 a.m. with tiapride (200 mg in 100 ml of saline, infusion time 15 minutes) or placebo (100 ml of saline). The intravenous infusion (tiapride or placebo) was repeated in the same patient 2 days later, so that randomized sequence of infusions was tiapride-placebo in 5 cases, and placebo-tiapride in the other 5 cases.

Ten patients, 4 males and 6 females, aged 53 -79 years, with different kinds of neoplasia-related pain (origin of cancer : gut 5, breast 1, lung 3, Hodgkin's disease 1) were submitted to a double-blind, randomized study to evaluate the acute effects of sulpiride when compared to placebo. The fasting patients were infused at 8:00 a.m. with sulpiride (200 mg in 100 ml of saline, infusion time 15 minutes) or placebo (100 ml of saline). The intravenous infusion (sulpiride or placebo) was repeated in the same patients 2 days later, so that the randomized sequence of infusions was sulpiride-placebo in 5 cases, and placebo-sulpiride in the other 5 cases.

Blood samples were taken at —15, 0, 15, 30, 60, 90, 120 and 240 minutes from the start of the infusion. All blood samples were withdrawn into chilled plastic syringes and transferred to chilled, siliconized disposable glass tubes which contained trasylol (300 kallikrein inactivator units/ml) and EDTA (1 mg/ml) ; plasma was separated by centrifugation in a refrigerated centrifuge. Aliquots of plasma were immediately frozen at —20° C for radioimmunoassay of PRL, B-END and for radioenzymatic assay of DA.

The measurement of circulating PRL was performed by the Prolactin RIA Kit (Diagnostic Products Corp., Los Angeles, USA). In our laboratory the normal range was 10-25 ng/ml ; in women, values were slightly higher than in men.

The measurement of circulating DA was performed by the Catecholamine Radioenzymatic Assay Kit (Upjohn Diagnostic, Kalamazoo, USA) according to the procedure described in detail elsewhere (Gennari et al., 1981). In our laboratory the DA plasma values in normal fasting subjects at 8:00 a.m. ranged from 180 to 500 pg/ml. Before and during the study the administration of substances interfering with DA metabolism was avoided.

The plasma values of B-END were determined with the B-END RIA Kit (New England Nuclear, Boston USA) according to the procedure reported in detail elsewhere (Gennari et al., 1981). In our laboratory, the values of plasma B-END in normal fasting subjects at 8:00 a.m. ranged from 10-25 pg/ml.

For the chromatographic study of plasma pools, used to profile the B-END and B-LPH immunoreactivity, 1 ml plasma aliquots from different subjects were pooled from blood samples taken before (—15, 0 min) and after (15, 30 min) the infusion of tiapride or sulpiride. The peptides were extracted with salycic acid, eluted with acetic acid in acetone, and lyophilized. Lyophilates were reconstituted and chromatographed over G-50 Sephadex columns in 0.1 % bovine serum albumin : 0.1 M acetic acid. Fractions were assayed in duplicate using the same assay employed for the measurement of circulating B-END level, but with a separate plasma-free standard curve. The antibody had equimolar cross-reactivity to B-END and B-LPH (50 %).

The significance of changes in blood levels of PRL, B-END and DA was estimated by a paired t-test.

The analgesic effect of tiapride, sulpiride and placebo was evaluated according to the visual analogue scale method of Huskisson (1974) ; pain relief was measured by subtracting the pain score, 4 hours after the infusion, from the initial pain score.

Results

Of the 10 patients infused with tiapride, 8 demonstrated an improvement in pain lasting 4 to 8 hours after the i.v. infusion of the drug. A moderate improvement in pain after placebo was observed in two cases. When pain relief was measured by substracting the pain score after infusions from the initial pain score, a relationship was found between pain relief and initial pain score after tiapride but not after placebo (Fig. 1). Of the 10 patients infused with sulpiride, only three demonstrated a moderate improvement in pain and a slight improvement in pain was observed after placebo in two cases. In the sulpiride treated group, no relationship was found between pain relief and initial pain score after both sulpiride and placebo (Fig. 2).

The behavior of B-END plasma levels is shown in Figure 3. The mean B-END plasma level in the ten patients treated with tiapride was 15.9 ± 0.6 pg/ml (M $\pm$ SE) before the drug infusion and 15.0 ± 0.5 before the placebo infusion. Tiapride infusion caused a significant increase in B-END levels at 15, 30, 60, 90 minutes ; no significant changes were observed after placebo infusion. The mean B-END plasma level in the ten patients treated with sulpiride was 28.7 ± 2.7 pg/ml before the sulpiride infusion and 21.6 ± 1.5 before placebo infusion. Sulpiride and placebo infusions did not significantly modify the circulating levels of B-END (Fig. 3).

Gel chromatography of plasma extracts obtained from two sample pools, before (—15, 0 min) and after (15, 30 min) initiation of drug infusion, indicated an increase in B-END, but no change in B-LPH after tiapride and no change in either hormone after sulpiride (Fig. 4).

In comparison to pre-infusion values, PRL plasma levels after tiapride showed

271

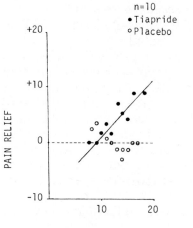

Fig. 1 - Pain relief as measured by a visual analogue scale in 10 patients with pain from cancer after placebo or tiapride intravenous infusion.

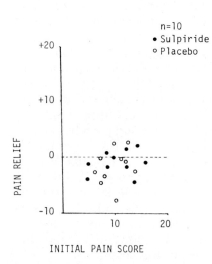

Fig. 2 - Pain relief as measured by a visual analogue scale in 10 patients with pain from cancer after placebo or sulpiride intravenous infusion.

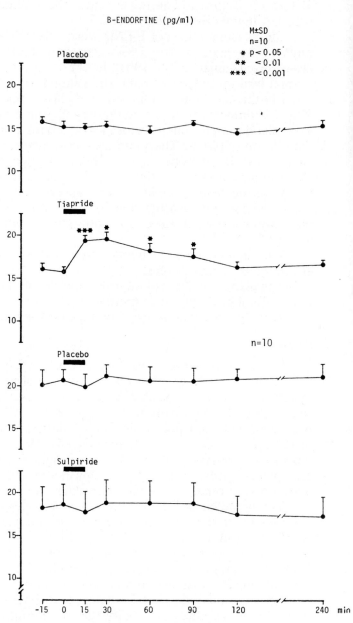

Fig. 3 - Effect of placebo, tiapride or sulpiride intravenous infusion on B-END circulating levels.

272

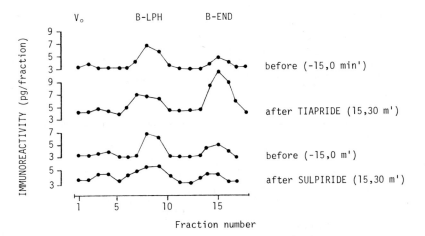

Fig. 4 - Gel chromatography of plasma pools before and after tiapride or sulpiride infusions. The positions of void volume (Vo), B-LPH and B-END are indicated in the uppermost part of the graph.

an early and highly significant increase, reaching peak values within 30 min. PRL levels subsequently decreased slowly, so that after 4 hours, levels were still elevated (Fig. 5). The same behavior of circulating PRL levels was observed with sulpiride infusion (Fig. 5). In both patient groups placebo infusion did not cause any significant change in PRL levels.

The tiapride infusion caused a sudden and highly significant decrease in plasma DA levels ; after which DA levels rose again reaching basal levels after 2 hours from initiation of infusion (Fig. 6). The sulpiride infusion also produced an immediate decrease in circulating DA levels, but in this case low levels of DA persisted until 4 hours after the beginning of infusion (Fig. 6). DA levels in plasma were not significantly affected by the placebo infusion.

Examining the plots of PRL and DA response to infusions, a reciprocal behavior in the two parameters causes one to consider a relationship between the two effects. In fact a statistically significant correlation between PR and DA levels was shown to exist (Fig. 7 and 8).

Discussion

In recent years the class of compounds known as the substituted benzamides, including drugs such as metoclopramide, sulpiride, sultopiride and tiapride, has been introduced into clinical use : Most are potent antiemetics, while some exhibit antipsychotic activity. There are also important differences in their clinical properties, particularly concerning tiapride, which produces an antidyskinetic effect and mild analgesia. Neither the peripheral nor central mechanism of action of these drugs is clearly understood.

273

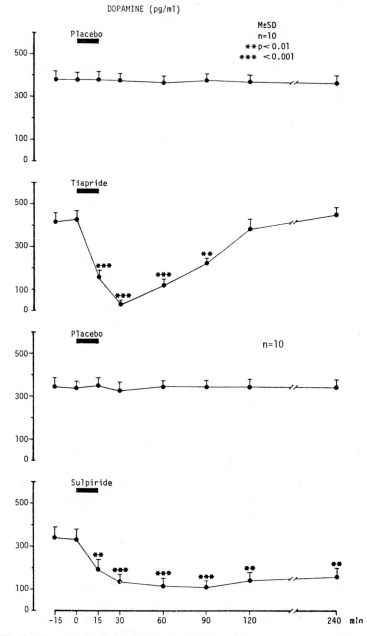

Fig. 5 - Effect of placebo, tiapride or sulpiride intravenous infusion on dopamine circulating levels.

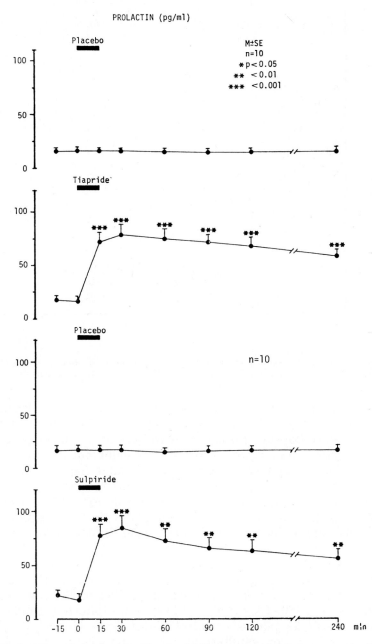

Fig. 6 - Effect of placebo, tiapride or sulpiride intravenous infusion on prolactin circulating levels.

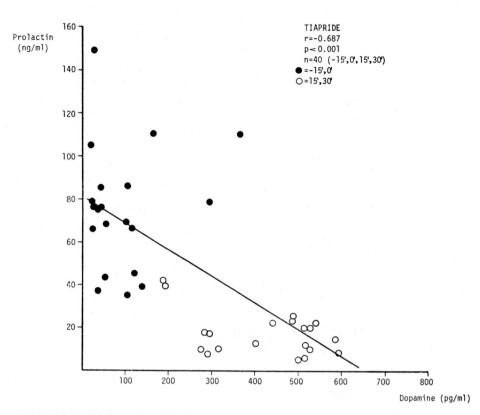

Fig. 7 - Relationship between prolactin and dopamine plasma levels before (closed cycles) and after (open cycles) an intravenous infusion of tiapride in 10 patients with cancer pain.

In this study the analgesic effect of tiapride was studied despite a limited number of patients and difficulties in evaluating pain modifications. The intravenous infusion of tiapride in patients with pain from cancer produced significant analgesia after 4 hours, which followed a slight but significant increase in plasma B-END. Plasma concentrations of B-END after tiapride were well below those needed to produce analgesia with systemic B-END administration (Rossier et al., 1977). However, our data suggest a possible role for B-END in mediating the analgesic effect of tiapride. On the other hand, sulpiride infusion demonstrated neither pain relief nor an increase in circulating B-END levels in patients with pain from cancer.

The sources of B-END have not yet been defined. B-END has been isolated from brain and pituitary gland (Donald, 1980) and measured in human cerebrospinal fluid and plasma (Nakai et al., 1978 ; McLoughlin et al., 1980 ; Clement-Jones et al., 1980 ; Carr et al., 1981). It seems that circulating peptides with opioid activity are under pituitary control (Goldstein et al., 1977). Concerning B-END, a retrograde flow from pituitary to hypothalmus via the hypophyseal portal system has been described (Bergland and Page, 1978). Conversely, a moderate cerebrovascular permeability, sufficient to produce significant brain uptake of B-END within a few minutes after a steep rise in plasma concentrations of B-END, has

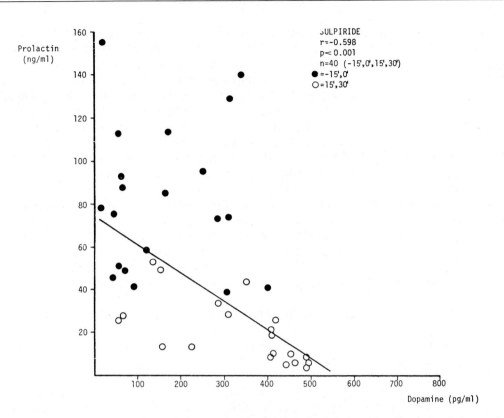

Fig. 8 - Relationship between prolactin and dopamine plasma levels before (closed cycles) and after (open cycles) an intravenous infusion of sulpiride in 10 patients with cancer pain.

been demonstrated (Rapoport et al., 1980). Thus, it may be that brain areas mediating pain inhibition are reached by opioids in concentrations sufficient to cause analgesia.

The fact that only one of the two substituted benzamides tested, tiapride, produced a release of B-END in the blood, indicates that the sites of action of the two drugs could be different, at least in part.

B-END and B-LPH are synthesized and stored together within anterior pituitary cells. Gel filtration chromatographic studies in animals and in man indicate that the pars distalis (PD) of the pituitary gland contains two major forms of opioid-like immunoreactivity corresponding to B-END and B-LPH (Liotta et al., 1978; Lissitsky et al., 1978; Eipper and Mains, 1978; Smyth and Zakarian 1980), while virtually all of the opioid-like immunoreactivity secreted by the cells of the pars intermedia (PI) of the pituitary corresponds to B-END (Eipper and Mains, 1978; Mains and Eipper 1979; Vermes et al., 1980; Pettibone and Mueller, 1982). Our chromatographic studies indicating that the increase in opioid-like immunoreactivity elicited by tiapride is due to B-END could suggest that tiapride acts, directly or indirectly, on the PI of the pituitary, which is directly innervated by tubero-hypophyseal neurons (Bjorklund et al., 1973).

277

It is known that substituted benzamide drugs increase plasma PRL levels (Mc-Callum et al., 1976 ; Mancini et al., 1976). This effect, recently studied for tiapride (Gennari et al., 1981), is thought to be associated with interference with dopaminergic mechanisms. Substituted benzamides increase DA turnover on acute administration, as shown by the elevation of the central DA metabolites, probably by acting on post-synaptic DA receptors (Jenner and Marsden, 1979). In our patients the intravenous infusion of both tiapride and sulpiride caused an early increase in plasma PRL, combined with a sudden decrease in plasma DA. These data support the concept that tiapride and sulpiride act on the brain-neuroendocrine system which stimulates the secretion of PRL, and that the resulting hyperprolactinaemia is correlated with the turnover of DA.

The decrease in DA circulating levels observed in our studies may reflect abnormally low release or augmented uptake by specific dopaminergic receptors. However, the face of released DA appears to be quite complicated (Van Loon and Sole, 1980), since a portion of DA could be taken up by the neuron for storage in new cytoplasmic granules. Finally, we must consider that a part of the circulating DA may be metabolically inactivated. In fact, it has been demonstrated that metoclopramide induces an acceleration in DA turnover in mice and rat, evidenced by an elevation of the homovanillic acid levels (Peringer et al., 1976 ; Mangoni et al., 1976). Unfortunately, we did not measure the plasma concentration of homovanillic acid, the major metabolite of DA, so that from our data it is not possible to deduce the mechanism through which tiapride and sulpiride reduce circulating DA levels.

Strong evidence has been obtained which suggests that DA acts as an inhibitor of PRL secretion : Under physiological conditions of low PRL release, hypothalamic DA secretion is elevated, and when PRL release is elevated DA secretion is reduced (Ben-Jonathan et al., 1980). Hypothalamic DA is considered the predominant factor regulating pituitary secretion of PRL. It has been demonstrated that DA is secreted into hypophyseal portal vessels (McLeod, 1976), and that DA and DA-agonists bind with high affinity to anterior pituitary receptors, which mediate the inhibition of PRL release (Cronin et al., 1980). Tiapride and sulpiride are probably competitive antagonists of DA thereby blocking neurotransmission at dopaminergic receptors. Conceivably, substituted benzamides, in addition to their postulated central action on the hypothalamus (Jenner and Marsden, 1979), might have direct effects on anterior pituitary cells, thereby blocking the effect of DA and permitting PRL release. This direct action on the pituitary has been demonstrated with sulpiride (McLeod and Robyn, 1977).

Probably, the mechanism through which substituted benzamides modify the PRL secretion is more complex than previously thought. Recently, it has been suggested that the theory of substituted benzamides inhibiting only hypothalamic DA and thus stimulating PRL release appears to be incomplete (Fang and Shian, 1981). Pretreatment of rats with mianserin, a specific serotonin receptor blocker, reduced the PRL response to metoclopramide (Fang and Shian, 1981). This effect is also consistent with the hypothesis that metoclopramide acts on serotoninergic receptors.

On the other hand, it has been demonstrated that the release of B-END from the pituitary of mammals appears to be under inhibitory control by DA (Loh and Jenks, 1981 ; Farah et al., 1982). But, in recent studies with rats, evidence was presented that a serotoninergic mechanism also stimulates the secretion of pituitary B-END (Sapun et al., 1981). In fact, stimuli which increase serotonin neurotransmission produce analgesia in man (Messing and Lytle, 1977 ; Johansson and Von Knorring, 1979 ; Hosobuchi and Li., 1981). So both mechanisms, that of PRL secretion and that of B-END secretion, depend in part on dopamine and serotonin.

Finally, recent evidence has been presented demonstrating that B-END stimulates PRL secretion in man (Von Graffenried et al., 1978) and that B-END enhances PRL release through an interaction with the hypothalamic dopaminergic system in rats (Van Vugt et al., 1979).

From our studies it is difficult to draw conclusions regarding the mechanisms by which two different substituted benzamides act on the pituitary ; the first, in which tiapride stimulates PRL and B-END release, the second, in which sulpiride stimulates PRL but not B-END release. Both drugs decrease the circulation levels of DA. In this regard, it is possible to conclude that the two drugs act on neuroendocrine systems with mechanisms that are not superimposable and which are still partially unclear.

REFERENCES

Akil, H., Richardson, D.E., Barchas, J.D., Li, C.H. *1978.* — Appearance of beta-endorphin-like immunoreactivity in human ventricular cerebrospinal fluid upon analgesic electrical stimulation. *Proc. Nat. Acad. Sci., 75 :* 5170.

Allen, R.G., Orwoll, E., Kendall, J.W., Herbert, E., Paxton, H. *1980.* — The distribution of forms of adrenocorticotropin and beta-endorphin in normal, tumorous, and autopsy human anterior pituitary tissue : virtual absence of 13 K adrenocorticotropin. *J. Clin. Endocrinol. Metab., 51 :* 376.

Belluzzi, J.D., Grant, N., Garsky, V., Sarantakis, D., Wise, C.D., Stein, L. *1976.* — Analgesia reduced *in vivo* by central administration of enkephalin in rat. *Nature, 260 :* 625.

Ben-Jonathan, N., Neill, M.A., Arbogast, L.A., Peters, L.L., Hoefer M.T. *1980.* — Dopamine in hypophysial portal blood : relationship to circulating prolactin in pregnant and lactating rats. *Endocrinology, 106 :* 690.

Bergland, R.M., Page, R.B. *1978.* — Can the pituitary secrete directly to the brain ? (Affirmative anatomical evidence). *Endocrinology, 102 :* 1325.

Bjorklund, A., Moore, R.Y., Nobin, A., Stenevi, U. *1973.* — The organization of tuberohypophyseal and reticuloinfundibular catecholamine neuron systems in the rat brain. *Brain Res., 51 :* 171.

Bradbury, A.F., Smyth, D.G., Snell, C.R. *1976.* — Lipotropin : precursor to two biologically active peptides. *Biochem. Biophys. Res. Commun, 69 :* 950.

Brion, S., Guerin R. *1977.* — Action d'une molécule neurotrope originale dans certains syndromes neurologiques (mouvements anormaux et algies diverses). *Sem. Hôp. Paris, 53 :* 40.

Carr D.B., Bullen B.A., Skrinar G.S., Arnold M.A., Rosenblatt M., Beitins I.Z., Martin J.B., McArthur J.W. *1981.* — Physical conditioning facilitates the exercise-induced secretion of beta-endorphin and beta-lipotropin in women. *Engl. J. Med., 305 :* 560.

Catliin, D.H., Hui, K.K., Loh, H.H., Li, C.H. *1977.* — Pharmacologic activity of beta-endorphin in man. *Psychopharmacology, 1 :* 493.

Clavel M., Pommatau E. *1980.* — Etude de l'effect antalgique du tiapride chez l'homme. *Sem. Hôp. Paris, 56 :* 430.

Clement-Jones, V., McLoughlin, L., Tomlin, S., Besser, G.M., Rees, L.H., Wen, H.L. *1980.* — Increased beta-endorphin but not met-enkephalin levels in human cerebrospinal fluid after acupuncture for recurrent pain. *Lancet, ii :* 946.

Cronin, M.J., Faure, N., Martial, J.A., Weiner, R.I. *1980.* — Absence of high affinity dopamine receptors in GH_3 cells : a prolactin-secreting clone resistant to the inhibitory action of dopamine. *Endocrinology, 106 :* 718.

Donald, R.A. *1980.* — ACTH and related peptides. *Clin Endocrinol., 12 :* 491.

Eipper, B.A. Mains, R.E. *1978.* — Existence of a common precursor to ACTH and endorphin in the anterior and intermediate lobes of the rat pituitary. *J. Supramol. Struct., 8 :* 25.

Fang, U.S., Shian, L. *1981.* — A serotonergic mechanism of the prolactin-stimulating action of metoclopramide. *Endocrinology, 108 :* 1622.

Farah, J.M., Malcom, D.S., Mueller, G.P. *1982.* — Dopaminergic inhibition of pituitary beta-endorphin-like immunoreactivity secretion in the rat. *Endocrinology, 110 :* 657.

Gambert S.R., Hagen T.C., Garthwaite T.L., Duthie E.H., McCarty D.J. *1981.* — Exercise and the endogenous opioids. *N. Engl. J. Med., 305 :* 1590.

Gennari C., *1981.* — Calcitonin and bone metastases of cancer. *In : Calcitonin 1980.* A. Pecile (ed.) p. 277. *Amsterdam, Excerpta Medica.*

Gennari, C., Nami, R., Pizzuti, M., D'Ascenzo, G., Bianchini, C. *1981.* — Effects of tiapride infusion on plasma levels of beta-endorphin, prolactin and dopamine in patients with pain from cancer. *Pathol. Biol. 29 :* 105.

Goldstein, A., Cox, B.M., Gentleman, S., Lowney, L.I., Cheung, A.L. *1977.* — Pituitary and brain opioid peptides (endorphins). *Ann. New York Acad. Sci., 297 :* 108.

Guillemin, R., Vargo, T., Rossier, J., Minick, S., Ling, N., Rivier, C., Vale, W., Bloom, F. *1977.* — Beta-endorphin and adrenocorticotropin are secreted concomitantly by the pituitary gland. *Science, 197 :* 1367.

Hosobuchi, Y., Li, C.H. *1978.* — The analgesic activity of human beta-endorphin in man. *Commun. in Psychopharmacol., 2 :* 33.

Hosobuchi, Y., Lamb, S., Bascom, D. *1981.* — Tryptophan loating may reverse tolerance to opiate analgesics in humans : a preliminary report. *Pain, 9 :* 161.

Huskisson, E.C. *1974.* — Measurement of pain. *Lancet, 2 :* 1127.

Jenner, P., Marsden, C.D. *1979.* — The substituted benzamides. A novel class of dopamine antagonists. *Life Sci., 25 :* 479.

Johansson, F., Von Knorring, L. *1979.* — A double-blind controlled study of serotonin uptake inhibitor (zimelidine) versus placebo in chronic pain patients. *Pain, 7 :* 69.

Krieger, D.T., Liotta, A.S., *1979.* — Pituitary hormones in brain : where, how, and why ? *Science, 205 :* 366.

Lepille, D., Bastit, Ph. *1979.* — Essai thérapeutique dans les algies néoplastiques. *Sem. Hôp. Paris, 55 :* 1.

Liotta, A.S., Suda, T., Krieger, D.T. *1978.* — Beta-lipotropin is the major opioid-like peptide of human pituitary and rat pars distalis : lack of significant beta-endorphin. *Proc. Nat. Acad. Sci, 75 :* 2950.

Lissitsky, J.D., Morin, O., Dupont, A., Labrie, F., Seidah, N.G., Cretien, M., Lis, M., Coy, D.H. *1978.* — Content of beta-LPH and its fragments (including endorphins) in anterior and intermediate lobes of the bovine pituitary gland. *Life Sci., 22 :* 1715.

Loh, Y.P., Jenks, B.G. *1981.* — Evidence for two different turnover pools of adrenocorticotropin, alfa-melanocyte-stimulating hormone, and endorphin-related peptides released by the frog pituitary neurointermediate lobe. *Endocrinology, 109 :* 54.

McCallum, R.W., Sowers, J.R., Hershman, J.M., Sturdevant, R.A.L. *1976.* — Metoclopramide stimulates prolactin secretion in man. *J. Clin. Endocrinol. Metab., 42 :* 1148.

McLeod, R.M. *1976.* — Regulation of prolactin secretion, *In : Frontiers in Neuroendocrinology, Vol. 1,* Martini L. and W.F. Ganong (eds), p. 169. New York, Raren Press.

McLeod, R.M., Robyn, C. *1977.* — Mechanism of increased prolactin secretion by sulpiride. *J. Endocrinol., 72 :* 273.

McLoughlin, L., Lowry, P.J., Ratter, S., Besser, G.M., Rees L.H. *1980.* — Beta-endorphin and beta-MSH in human plasma. *Clin. Endocrinol., 12 :* 287.

Mains, R.E., Eipper, B.A., Ling N. *1977.* — Common precursor to corticotropins and endorphins. *Proc. Nat. Acad. Sci., 74 :* 3014.

Mains R.E., Eipper B.A. *1979.* — Synthesis and secretion of corticotropins, melanotropins and endorphins by rat intermediate pituitary cells. *J. Biol. Chem. 254 :* 7885.

Mancini, A.M., Guitelman, A., Vargas, C.A., Debeljuk, L., Aparico, N.J. *1976.* — Effect of sulpiride on serum prolactin levels in humans. *J. Clin. Endocrinol. Metab. 42 :* 181.

Mangoni, A., Corsini, G.U., Piccardi, M.P., Gessa, G.L. *1976.* — Increase of brain homovanillic acid level induced by metoclopramide. *Neuropharmacology, 14 :* 333.

Mendelsohn, G., D'Agostino, R., Eggleston, J.C., Baylin, S.B. *1979.* — Distribution of beta-endorphin immunoreactivity in normal human pituitary. *J. Clin. Invest. 63 :* 1297.

Messing, R.B., Lytle, L.D. *1977.* — Serotonin-containing neurons : their possible role in pain and analgesia. *Pain, 4 :* 1.

Nakai, Y., Nakao, K., Oki, S., Imura, H., Li, C.H. *1978.* — Presence of immunoreactive beta-endorphin in plasma of patients with Nelson's syndrome and Addison's disease. *Life Sci., 23 :* 2293.

Nakao, K., Nakai, Y., Jingami, H., Oki, S., Fukata, J., Imura, H. *1979.* — Substantial rise of plasma beta-endorphin levels after insulin-induced hypoglycemia in human subjects. *J. Clin. Endocrinol. Metab. 49 :* 838.

Peringer, E., Jenner, P., Donaldson, I.M., Marsden, C.D., Miller, R. *1976.* — Metoclopramide and dopamine receptor blockade. *Neuropharmacology, 15 :* 463.

Pettibone, D.J., Mueller, G.P. *1982.* — Evidence for independent secretion of beta-endorphin immunoreactivity from rat pars distalis in vivo. *Endocrinology, 110 :* 469.

Rapoport, S.I., Klee, W.A., Pettigrew, K.D., Ohno, K. *1980.* — Entry of opioid peptides into the central nervous system. *Science, 207 :* 84.

Rossier, J., French, E.D., Rivier, C., Ling, N., Guillemin, R., Bloom, F.E. *1977.* — Footshock induced stress increases beta-endorphin levels in blood but not brain. *Nature, 270 :* 618.

Sambin P. *1977.* — Le tiapride dans les céphalalgies. *Sem. Hôp. Paris, 53 :* 45.

Sapun, D.I., Farah, J.M., Mueller, G.P. *1981.* — Evidence that a serotonergic mechanism stimulates the secretion of pituitary beta-endorphin-like immunoreactivity in the rat. *Endocrinology, 109 :* 421.

Smyth, D.G., Zakarian, S. *1980.* — Selective processing of beta-endorphin in regions of porcine pituitary. *Nature, 288 :* 613.

Tseng, L.F., Loh, H.H., Li, C.H. *1976.* — Beta-endorphin as a potent analgesic by intravenous injection. *Nature, 263 :* 239.

Van Loon, G.R., Sole, M.J. *1980.* — Plasma dopamine : source, regulation, and significance. *Metabolism, 29 :* 1119.

Van Vugt, D.A., Bruni, J.F., Sylvester, P.W., Chen, H.T., Ieiri, T., Meites J. *1979.* — Interaction between opiates and hypothalamic dopamine on prolactin release. *Life Sci., 24 :* 2361.

Vermes, I., Mulder, P.G., Smelik, P.G., Tilders, F.J.H. *1980.* — Differential control of beta-endorphin/beta-lipotropin secretion from anterior and intermediate lobes of the rat pituitary gland in vitro. *Life Sci., 27 :* 1761.

Von Graffenried, B., Del Pozo, E., Roubicek, J., Krebs, E., Poldinger, W., Burmeister, P., Kerp L. *1978.* — Effects of the synthetic enkephalin analogue FK 33-824 in man. *Nature, 272 :* 729.

Weber, E., Martin, R., Voigt, K.G. *1979.* — Corticotropin/beta-endorphin precursor : concomitant storage of its fragments in the secretory granules of anterior pituitary corticotropin/endorphin cells. *Life Sci., 25 :* 1111.

DISCUSSION

S.Z. Langer
In your opinion, what is the origin of dopamine in circulation ?

C. Gennari
A good question. In a recent paper the probable sources of circulating dopamine were described : Many tissues have been suggested, but I think that the main sites generating dopamine peripherally are the adrenal glands and sympathetic nerves, so I cannot tell you the precise origin of the dopamine which appears in blood.

S.Z. Langer
I think there is a recent publication showing that very low doses of apomorphine in man reduce the levels of HVA in plasma and this is somewhat paradoxical with your findings that the acute infusion of sulpiride or tiapride decreases the levels of dopamine plasma.

C. Gennari
I do not know, as I have not used apomorphine.

W.H. Vogel
I think there is another source of circulating dopamine and that source is the intestinal bacteria. It has been shown that rats given neomycine, which cleans out the bacterial flora, show a decrease in circulating dopamine levels. If the antibiotic is stopped, the dopamine levels rise again. So, there are two sources ; one comes from the body and another one comes from the bacteria. Do you think that the drugs could perhaps effect the intestinal flora ?

C. Gennari
I have no data to support this hypothesis. I can only say that this type of patient was treated by chemotherapeutic agents, which could influence the intestinal flora.

Ch. Oliver
I am surprised by the dopamine levels you reported in plasma. I am surprised you find such high levels using a radio-enzymatic assay, we find usually between 10 and 40 pg/ml. I would like to ask you if you add a dopa-decarboxylase inhibitor to your preparation of catechol-o-methyl-transferase? If not, I wonder if you are perhaps measuring dopa instead of dopamine?

C. Gennari
We have used the radio-enzymatic assay kit and it is true that there are great discrepancies in the values from different laboratories. In my laboratory, samples were collected using special tubes containing anti-coagulant EDTA and anti-oxydants. The preparation of catechol-o-methyl-transferase is employed to catalyse the transfer of a tritiated methyl group from s-adenosyl-l-methionine to dopamine. The resulting product, which is the tritiated 3-methoxy-tyramine, was isolated with thin layer chromatography. With this method I am sure that the values circulating are over 40 pg/ml, but in our case the effect observed was not an increase, but a decrease in circulating dopamine

U. Corsini
Just a comment on this point. HVA and DOPAC in plasma come from the brain, at least 40 % according to a paper by Roth and others, but dopamine is probably only from the periphery. We have no data indicating that dopamine comes from the brain. In other words, these data found with tiapride may be interpreted absolutely in another way, like the data interpreted with apomorphine.

P. Grof
I was thinking that you could decipher for us some of the relationships that you have by looking at more time points in your observations. It sounded as though you looked at the analgesic effect only after 4 hours, whereas the changes in β-endorphin were already over in 90 minutes.

C. Gennari
I agree with you. We should look into this.

Abnormal circadian pattern of melatonin cortisol and growth hormone secretion in cluster headache : Biological criteria for drug design

G. Chazot[1], B. Claustrat[2], J. Brun[2], G. Sassolas[3] and B. Schott[1]

1) Neurometabolism Department, 2) Nuclear Medicine Center, and 3) Radioanalysis Unit Neurologic Hospital, Lyons, France

Summary : Cluster headache represents a primary headache disorder. The attacks occur in series interrupted by extended periods of remission. The major characteristics of cluster headache are the seasonal frequency (spring, autumn) and the occurence of symtoms during night-time. Melatonin (5-methoxy-N-acetyl-serotonin) is mainly secreted during the night by the pineal gland, which is claimed to be an internal clock with seasonal variations in its activity. In a group of 12 cluster headache patients, the 24-hour patterns of hormones were determined by radio-immunoassay in plasma. We observed a significant decrease in nocturnal melatonin levels associated with a shift in cortisol and growth hormone acrophase. These abnormalities could be explained on the basis of aminergic neuroendocrine mechanisms and of peripheral action of melatonin on platelets. In addition the effectiveness of lithium in cluster headache could also be explained by a direct action of this drug on N-acetyl-transferase, a pineal enzyme which controls melatonin synthesis.

Introduction

Episodic cluster headache is a primary headache disorder. Paroxysms or attacks occur in series, interrupted by extented periods of remission. The attacks often occur regularly, at times frequently, throughout the cluster period.

A major characteristic of these attacks is the frequency of occurence at night-time. Cluster periods also seem associated with the seasons, particularly spring and autumn, or more likely with temperature fluctuations. In addition cluster headache can occur after shift work, jet-lag or summer/winter time change or vice versa.

The pineal gland, an endogenous clock plays a central role in the circadian organisation of biological rhythms in several species including man. Melatonin, an indolic compound which is mainly secreted by this gland, can be considered as a good marker of pineal cyclic activity : Blood concentrations of this hormone rise markedly during the night and show seasonal variations (Arendt et al., 1979).

Therefore we studied, in cases of cluster headache, the 24-hour profiles of plasma melatonin, cortisol, growth hormone, and prolactin. To our knowledge, no data are available about the possible role of a disruption of the temporal organisation of hormonal secretions to help understand the pathogenesis of this affection. However, such an approach is of interest in explaining the activity of drugs (such as lithium, benzamides) and to determine more effective chronotherapy in cluster headache.

Materials and methods

Eleven patients (10 men, 1 woman, mean age of 39 years, range 23-67 years) suffering from episodic cluster headache were selected according to the international classification *. They were studied during a « cluster » severe enough to warrant hospitalisation. They did not take any drug for at least one week except an analgesic (glafenine) in the acute phase. The patients were confined to bed throughout the investigation and had normal breakfast, lunch and dinner at 7 a.m, midday and 7 p.m respectively. Lights were out from 10 p.m to 7 a.m. At 2 p.m an indwelling catheter was introduced and a very slow infusion of heparinised saline was constantly pumped through the system to keep the vein open. Saline was removed before sampling. Blood samples were taken every 2 hours during the day and every hour between 10 p.m and 4 a.m ; they were kept at 4 oC until the experiment ended, then decanted before storing the plasma at —20 oC until radioimmunoassay.

The control subjects in this study were eight consenting healthy males, with a mean age of 27 years (range, 25-34 years). They were normal metabolically, neuropsychiatrically and in their sleep patterns and free from drug intake. They were rigorously submitted to the same protocol as the sick in April and May, a period during which plasma melatonin levels are claimed to be the lowest (Arendt et al., 1979). Hormonal values were determined by radioimmunological methods using specific antibodies prepared in our laboratory.

Results

Compared to the controls, most of the patients had a lower nocturnal melatonin secretion, particularly in the early part of the night (Fig. 1 and 2). In one patient the rhythm was completely abolished. The magnitude of this rhythm was significantly decreased and the acrophase was often displaced from its physiological location (Fig. 3).

For cortisol secretion, there was a shift in the acrophase which occurred, on average, at about 6 a.m. The mean cortisol level over the 24-hour cycle was normal (Fig. 4).

An abnormal pattern of GH secretion was observed during the night : In some patients a bimodal pattern was obtained, a supplementary peak being observed in the late evening or in the early morning (Fig. 5). In the absence of polygraphic sleep recording, no conclusion was drawn.

No significant alteration in prolactin secretion was observed and plasma levels were within a physiological range (Fig. 6).

* Ad hoc Committee on classification of headache. *1962 — JAMA, 179* : 717.
World Federation of Neurology's Research Group on Migraine and Headache. *1969 — J. Neurol. Sci., 9* : 202.

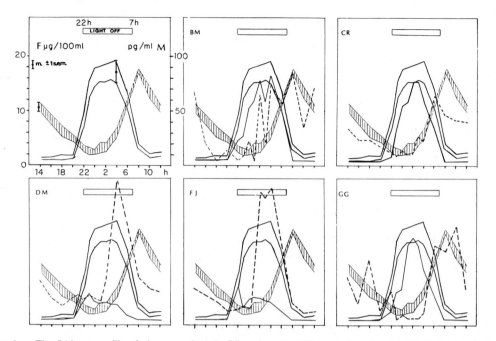

Fig. 1 — The 24-hour profile of plasma melatonin (M) and cortisol (F) levels in patients with cluster headache. Dotted lines represent cortisol and continuous lines melatonin. Shaded area represents normal range for cortisol and white area normal range for melatonin.

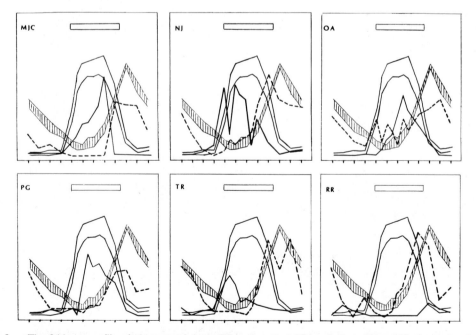

Fig. 2 — The 24-hour profile of plasma melatonin (M) and cortisol (F) levels in patients with cluster headache. Dotted lines represent cortisol and continuous lines melatonin. Shaded area represents normal range for cortisol and white area normal range for melatonin.

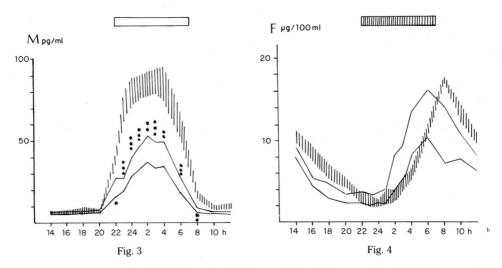

Fig. 3

Fig. 4

Fig. 3 — Transverse mean ± SEM of the sets of 24-hour profiles of plasma melatonin in cluster headache.
Fig. 4 — Transverse mean ± SEM of the sets of 24-hour profiles of plasma cortisol in cluster headache.

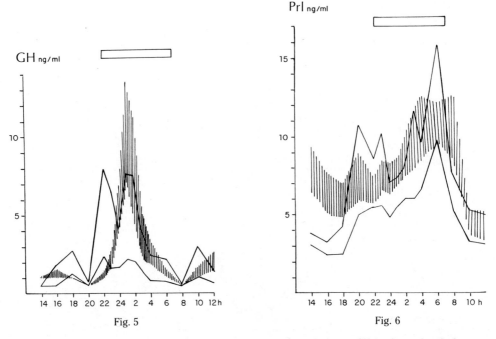

Fig. 5

Fig. 6

Fig. 5 — Transverse mean ± SEM of the sets of 24-hour profiles of plasma GH in cluster headache.
Fig. 6 — Transverse mean ± SEM of the sets of 24-hour profiles of plasma prolactin in cluster headache.

Discussion

Our data clearly show abnormal circadian patterns of melatonin, cortisol and GH secretions. These findings are of interest as regards the clinical characteristics of cluster headache.

This multi-abnormality is likely to be related to an alteration of the suprachiasmatic nucleus — which can control at the same time, cortisol, melatonin and GH secretions (Willoughby and Martin, 1978) — and a noradrenergic defect. This hypothesis could be clarified by studying the 24-hour profile of plasma catecholamines.

The decreased levels of plasma melatonin, mainly during the early part of the night, reflect a disturbance in the sympathetic control of the pineal gland via the superior cervical ganglion (Cardinal et al., 1981). Because of the antagonism of melatonin for prostaglandin E secretion by platelets (Gimeno et al., 1980), our data could suggest a relation with abnormalities of PGE.

In pharmacological screening, one must choose, as the most effective and the most physiological drugs, those having a synchronising effect on the endogenous rhythms. Lithium can be considered as the leader in this pharmacological group (Friedman and Yocca, 1981 ; Eachrom et al., 1982). Other drugs, such as benzamides, proposed in the acute phase of the disease, must be tested in the human model.

REFERENCES

Arendt, J., Wirz-Justice, A., Bradtke, J., Kornemar,, M. *1979* — Long-term studies on immunoreactive human melatonin. *Ann. Clin. Biochemist., 16* : 307-312.

Cardinal, D.P., Vacas, M.I., Gejman, P.V. *1981* — The sympathetic superior cervical ganglia as peripheral neuroendocrine centers. *J. Neural. Transmis., 52* : 1-21.

Friedman, E., Yocca, F.D. *1981* — The effect of chronic lithium treatment of rat pineal N-acetyltransferase rhythm. *Pharmacol. Experiment. Therapeut., 219* : 121-124.

Gimeno, M.F., Ritta, M.N., Bonacossa, A., Lazzari, M., Gimeno, A.L. Cardinali D.P. *1980* — Inhibition by melatonin of prostaglandin synthesis in hypothalamus, uterus and platelets. *In : Melatonin : Current Status and Perspectives*, Birau N., Schloot W. (eds), pp. 147-150. (Advances in the Biosciences, 29), Oxford and New York, Pergamon Press.

McEachron, D.L., Kripke, D.F., Hawkins R., Haus, E., Pavlinac D., Deftos L. *1982* — Lithium delays biochemical circadian rhythms in rats. *Neuropsychobiology, 8* : 12-29.

Willoughby, J.O., Martin, J.B. *1978* — The suprachiasmatic nucleus synchronizes growth hormone secretory rhythms with the light-dark cycle. *Brain Res., 151* : 413-417.

DISCUSSION

J. Mendlewicz
I would first like to congratulate you on this very nice study and I think the observations that there seems to be a disturbance in melatonin circadian secretion is very interesting. Since you mentioned that in cluster headache the attacks sometimes occur during the night and that these patients may have very severe sleep disturbances, would that not be a reason why you would expect the nocturnal melatonin secretion to be altered and that you may see suppression of night melatonin secretion as a result of sleep disturbances?

G. Chazot
In Weissman's study it seems that cluster pain appeared linked with the REM sleep stage and the mechanism is probably before pain, but we have no data on this.

N. Matussek
In what affective state are your patients? Do they also have some depressive symptoms?

G. Chazot
No, they are not depressive, but in the 24-hour profile of cortisol or melatonin in depression, there is a rise in cortisol.

N. Matussek
Did you also find a phase advance shift of the cortisol rhythm, as Sachar did, in depressed patients for instance?

G. Chazot
It should decrease at 8 o'clock, but there was a rise at 8 o'clock. Yes, cortisol secretion is phase advanced.

N. Matussek
Did you use a self-rating scale for depression in these patients?

G. Chazot
No, but it is possible that some migranous patients or cluster headache patients are linked genetically with depression. There is probably a sub-group of patients with depressive and migranous background.

P. Grof
I have a number of questions in mind. The similarity between what you have been presenting and what one sees in primary affective disorders is tremendously striking. First of all, all the clinical phenomena that you mentioned, the seasonal frequency, relationship to jet lag, relationship to shift work that can precipitate attacks of cluster headaches, are present in affective disorders. Secondly, the resemblance with the neuroendocrine findings in depression is particularly striking in the change in melatonin. And finally, the tremendous parallel with treatment results, where one finds lithium efficatious in both the affective disorders and cluster headache. This illustrates one very interesting general point, which I think has recently emerged as interesting, that lithium probably works on some kind of episodic dysregulations of the CNS. These dysregulations can manifest with psychiatric symptoms and in that case abnormal mood is the disturbance. Or, they can manifest as a neurological episodic dysregulation, as you are pointing out here with cluster headaches. Or otherwise, they can manifest as dysregulations that internists see, as duodenal ulcers for instance, which again have certain clinical and therapeutic resemblances.
The data on the melatonin supression of the rhythm is very interesting. It would be interesting to test also the β-endorphin-like immuno-reactivity, because this is linked to the same family. Concerning the rhythm, recently Dent and collaborators published a paper regarding the diurnal rhythm of plasma immuno-reactive β-endorphin and this relationship to sleep stages and plasma rhythms of cortisol and prolactin. In volunteers these results have shown a close relationship between prolactin and the β-endorphin and also with cortisol.

288

J. Mendlewicz
When we observe your cortisol profiles, it looks as though there is a shift, like some kind of a phase advanced phenomena. It looks like there is a hypercortisol secretion in some of your patients, so I think it may be interesting to do the dexamethasone suppression test in these patients.

P. Grof
I have the same impression from the slide, that if one calculated the area under the curve, one would find hypersecretion of cortisol.

G. Chazot
Corticosteroids have been proposed for the treatment of cluster headaches at night.

P. Grof
I was wondering : When you treat cluster headache with lithium, do you have to treat patients chronically or can you concentrate on the spring and autumn periods ?

G. Chazot
Only in the spring.

P. Grof
That way you get around the side effects related to chronic treatment ?

G. Chazot
We treat with lithium only after 4 weeks of treatment and we have no controls.

Cl. Hagen
Were any of the patients alcoholics, because these patients often have abnormal secretion of pituitary hormones including ACTH and thus cortisol secretion ?

G. Chazot
Alcoholism often provokes the attack of cluster headaches, but in our patients we have no alcoholics

Effect of estrogens on the dopamine turnover increase induced by sulpiride

G.U. Corsini, F. Bernardi, M.P. Piccardi, A. Bocchetta.

Clinical Pharmacology, University of Cagliari, Cagliari, Italy.

Abstract*

Recent evidence indicates that female hormones modulate dopamine (DA) receptor sensitivity. More recently, electrophysiological, behavioral and biochemical data have suggested that estrogen treatment is able to induce a down-regulation of DA autoreceptors in rats and this effect may account for some clinical observations. DA agonists such as apomorphine, 2-α-bromocriptine, 3-PPP and n-propylnorapomorphine failed to induce hypomotility and DA turnover decrease when administered to estrogen-pretreated animals. In the present study we observed the effect of estrogen pretreatment (17 β estradiol benzoate 10 μg/kg s.c. for 3 days) on the behavioral and biochemical responses induced by substituted benzamides, such as sulpiride (5-25 mg/kg) in rats. Estrogens markedly potentiated the motility response and the increase in DA turnover elicited by sulpiride, suggesting that female hormones increase DA autoreceptor sensitivity to DA receptor blockers.

* *We regret that Prof. Corsini's results were not available for publication.*

DISCUSSION

G. Groß
In which phase of the estrous cycle were the rats and have you tested male and female rats ?

G.U. Corsini
All these experiments shown were done in male rats, but we also did this experiment in female and in ovariectomized rats, and we found in ovariectomized rats that estrogen pre-treatment completely abolished the apomorphine response, but in female animals this effect was less evident but we did not check the animals for the cycle phase. This is probably one of the reasons for the lower response to estrogens in this respect.

N. Matussek
Are there also studies with females during menstruation, since in such cases you would expect the same effects of neuroleptics or maybe of dopamine agonists ? Are there results on such influences in females ?

G.U. Corsini
It is true, it seems that females during menstruation respond differently to neuroleptics for instance and also to the neuroleptic-induced Parkinsonian syndrome as well as with regard to tardive

dyskinesia. This occurs more often in females than in males, so these differences and others shown by various authors with other drugs may be due to a really different sensitivity of dopamine autoreceptors rather than of post-synaptic dopamine receptors. Another point, which could be interesting for your study on depression : It has been shown that estrogens have some antidepressant activity, either when exogenously administered or during the menstrual cycle. The female seems to be depressed at the end of the cycle when estrogens are down and not depressed in the middle of the cycle, when estrogens are up. Several authors have correlated estrogen levels with antidepressant activity. However, I cannot switch from the extrapyramidal to the limbic system, in order to say that these mechanisms we presented may be also involved in antidepressant activity of estrogen, but it seems there is a possibility.

P. Grof

I think the issue of estrogens and depression is still rather confusing. In the forties' a large number of studies were carried out trying to use estrogens in the treatment of depression and to measure plasma levels. It was impossible to find any significant correlation with the improvement of depression. Recently, some of the studies looking at the inter-play between estrogens and catecholamines seem to be more promising, but it is still an unresolved, blurred issue.

W.H. Vogel

How do your results fit with the observation that female patients treated with antipsychotic medication seem to show a higher incidence of tardive dyskinesia than male patients ?

U. Corsini

It is difficult to answer that question, but one possibility may result from the fact that estrogens induced a hyposensitivity of dopamine autoreceptors, thus increasing dopaminergic activity, so perhaps long-term treatment with neuroleptics induces a more pronounced response to the neurons pre-synaptically. This could be one possibility, or a hypersensitivity of the post-synaptic dopamine receptors as shown by other authors.

D. Lefaucheur

This increase of dopaminergic activity could be due to the fact that the estrogens are competitive for the enzymes implied in the catabolism of catecholamines and can be transformed into catechol-estrogen. This decrease in the catabolism of catecholamines can induce an accumulation of catecholamines.

G.U. Corsini

Which is the mechanism through which these estrogens act on the receptors ? One possibility suggested by different authors is through the pituitary or through an active metabolite of estrogens. It has been shown that catechol-estrogens, in other words the true hydroxylated estradiol, is the real hormone estrogen for the brain estrogen is specifically hydroxylated at position two in the brain and is a specific example of this activity. Catechol-estrogens may mediate all the effects of estrogens in the brain. Catechol-estrogens may interfere as shown very clearly with the COMT activity for instance as well as with other enzymatic activities. This may modify and alter the picture I gave before, but all the same I still do not think that it is a good possibility, because the amount of catechol-estrogens formed in the brain after such a low dose of estrogens is very low and thus, does not block the COMT activity for instance, but since catechol-estrogens are also important for the dopamine receptors, these hormones may affect the dopamine receptors, so maybe this is one mechanism, but it has to be shown completely.

B.E. Leonard

If I remember rightly, about 10 years ago it was shown that women taking the high estrogen pill tended to show quite a high instance of depression and when this was studied by a group of investigators of the Hammersmith hospital, it was found that tryptophane-pyrolase activity in the liver was enhanced ; this could ultimately lead to a decrease in serotonin concentration in the brain. So there did seem to be some sort of connection then between the increase in circulating estrogen levels and decrease in brain tryptophane and serotonin, which could underline depression. Indeed in those patients treated with vitamin B-6, it was found that the depression was attenuated. I was therefore wondering, and this is the question, have you tried other doses of estrogen in your studies ? It could be that you are getting a sort of dose/response effect and the changes are dependent upon whether the estrogen is inducing hepatic enzyme activity and/or affecting amine uptake mechanisms in the brain.

G.U. Corsini

We only used doses of 10 μg/kg for 3 days, a very standard treatment and we have not used other dosages. I do agree with you that probably if we increase the dosage or if we alter the hormonal treatment, we may obtain some different results. The group of Hruska inject only one dose and a high one of estradiol valerate for instance, so they are different hormonal treatments that could lead to different results. I know that estrogens modify the liver metabolism, in other words, they alter different liver enzymes and this complicates the picture of the effect of these hormones on all catecholamines, because one very strong effect of these hormones is to decrease the metabolizing enzymes. The P-450 system shows that many of the effects observed after drug treatment are due to these effects, rather than a direct effect in the brain. Due to a decrease in P-450 systems, estrogens increase the effect of neuroleptics, but in our study with apomorphine we can exclude that this effect is on the P-450 system, just because we observe an antagonistic rather than a potentiating effect.

Ph. Protais

You have shown results indicating that estrogen modifies hypokinesia and that such treatment modifies also the effect of sulpiride. Have you tried to observe the effect of apomorphine in rats simultaneously treated with neuroleptics and estrogen ? In other terms, are you sure that the results you show depend on an interaction on dopamine autoreceptors ?

G.U. Corsini

As far as we know now, the low dose effect of apomorphine seems to be due to a dopamine autoreceptor stimulation. This is one hypothesis and the most well-known one at the moment. I agree that this is an indirect study, but these two phenomena seem to be mediated through a dopamine autoreceptor stimulation, so, in other words, since we saw these effects of estrogens on these two behaviors, we believe them to be mediated by the dopamine autoreceptors.

The role of dopamine in the modulation of pituitary gonadotrophin secretion. Evidence for increased dopaminergic activity in hyperprolactinaemic patients and in women with hypothalamic functional amenorrhoea

C. Hagen, H. Djursing, K. Petersen and A. Nyboe Andersen.

Departments of Endocrinology and Gynaecology, University Hospital, Hvidovre, Denmark.

Summary : The pituitary gonadotrophins LH and FSH are regulated by a stimulatory effect of gonadotrophin releasing hormone (GnRH) and an inhibition by sex steroids and inhibin, as well as a stimulatory effect of estrogens in the female. To explain the changes in gonadotrophins during the menstrual cycle one has to invoke other regulatory mechanisms.

Dopamine is the physiological inhibitor of prolactin secretion, but has a variable effect on gonadotrophin secretion. In normal women in the early follicular phase dopamine infusion lowers basal LH levels without changing FSH and this effect seems to be increased around the midcycle. Similar changes in gonadotrophins have been found in hyperprolactinaemic women, women with primary ovarian failure and in the polycystic ovarian syndrome. By contrast, numerous investigators have been unable to demonstrate a change in LH secretion caused by L-dopa, bromocriptine, lergotrile or apomorphine drugs which stimulate the dopamine receptor, although, an inhibitory effect of bromocriptine on GnRH stimulated LH levels in hyperprolactinaemic patients has been reported. Furthermore, sulpiride, metoclopramide and haloperidol (dopamine receptor blockers) have been ineffective in altering either basal LH release or the midcycle surge in normal women and men. In normoprolactinaemic women with hypothalamic amenorrhea, a stimulatory effect of short as well as long term administration of metoclopramide on gonadotrophins has been found. It is concluded that hypothalamic dopamine neurons probably inhibit the secretion of GnRH and LH release, and we suggest that in hyperprolactinaemic women as well as in a proportion of normoprolactinaemic women with hypothalamic amenorrhoea an increased dopamine activity is responsible for the low gonadotrophins. In addition, in a proportion of normoprolactinaemic amenorrhoic women it may be possible to stimulate the gonadotrophins by the administration of dopamine receptor blockers and subsequently restore normal pituitary-ovarian function.

Introduction

In the last decade a rich peptidergic network in the hypothalamus has been described, and it has become obvious that a delicate balance between a number of these peptide neurotransmitters and the monoamines influence the secretion of gonadotrophin releasing hormone (GnRH). Experiments in the rat (Fuxe et al., 1980 ; McCann and Moss, 1975) and the Rhesus monkey (Knobil, 1980) suggest that the neuronal component of the system is located in the basal hypothalamus. However, in the rat, extrahypothalamic CNS structures including the limbic system also influence gonadotrophin secretion. The perikarya of the GnRH containing neurons which is essential for the synthesis and release of luteinizing hormone (LH)

295

and follicle stimulating hormone (FSH) are mainly located in nuclei of the suprachiasmatic and preoptic region of the medial basal hypothalamus (Fuxe et al., 1980 ; McCann and Moss, 1975 ; Knobil, 1974 ; Okon and Koch, 1976 ; Barraclough and Wise, 1982). The axons from these neurons terminate in the central portion of the basal hypothalamus, the lateral region of the median eminence, which is partly outside the blood brain barrier. Immunohistochemical data (Fuxe et al., 1980 ; McNeil and Sladek, 1978), electrophysiological data (Sawyer, 1975) and *in vivo* experiments (Leblanc et al., 1976 ; Judd et al., 1978 ; Barraclough and Wise, 1982) suggest that the dopaminergic system is an important modulator of GnRH secretion and that an axon-axonic regulation may exist in the median eminence close to the release of GnRH into the portal circulation by which GnRH reach the anterior pituitary gland. This review concentrates on the recent advances in our understanding of the dopaminergic regulation of gonadotrophin secretion and attempts to integrate this knowledge with the recent hypothesis of increased hypothalamic dopamine neurosecretion in patients with hyperprolactinaemia (Quigley et al., 1980 ; Evans et al., 1980 ; Djursing et al., 1981) and in a proportion of patients with hypothalamic normoprolactinaemic functional amenorrhoea (HFA) (Quigley et al., 1980 ; Djursing et al., 1981).

Dopamine neurons and receptors

Dopamine (DA) and norepinephrine (NE) are synthesized from tyrosine. The initial and rate limiting step in DA synthesis is the hydroxylation of tyrosine to dopa which is controlled by end-product inhibition. The hydroxylation rate is also influenced by tyrosine levels in the brain since tyrosine hydroxylase is not fully saturated with substrate at normal tyrosine concentration (Wurtman et al., 1974). It should thus be possible to accelerate tyrosine hydroxylation *in vivo* by adding tyrosine.

Specific DA-pathways have been localized in the rat brain (Fuxe et al., 1980 ; McCann and Moss, 1975 ; Barraclough and Wise, 1982) and it was found that DA containing nerve cells in the arcuate nucleus and the periventricular nucleus of the mediobasal hypothalamus project axons to the median eminence forming the tuberoinfundibular DA system. These DA secreting neurons interact functionally with neuropeptides and thus GnRH neurons, or secrete DA directly into portal blood (Fuxe et al., 1980 ; McCann and Moss, 1975 ; McNeil and Sladek, 1978 ; Gudelsky et al., 1981).

The regulatory mechanisms which determine the activity of DA neurons are not fully understood. There is a large amount of evidence, that the usual neuronal feedback mechanism is not operating (Müller et al., 1981), whereas prolactin (PRL) via its short loop feedback mechanism (Fuxe et al., 1980 ; Gudelsky et al., 1980, 1981 ; Selmanoff, 1981) and oestradiol (Gudelsky et al., 1980, 1981 ; Heritage et al., 1980 ; Labrie et al., 1980 ; Barroclough and Wise, 1982) increase the DA-turnover in the neurons. In addition intra- and extrahypothalamic pathways modulate DA activity. The biological effect of the DA system is dependent on the DA-turnover and the state of the receptors. The concept of multiple rather than a single class of DA receptors has been accepted, whereas the characteristic of the various receptors has not been agreed upon. The dopamine receptors that are associated with cAMP

296

have been designated D_1 receptors, and those that are not dependent on cAMP have been termed D_2 receptors (Kebabian and Calne, 1979 ; Creese et al., 1981). The D_1 receptors have been localized in a number of areas of the brain including substantia nigra, nucleus caudatus, the pituitary gland and by one group but not by others in the median eminence. These receptors bind tritiated dopamine, apomorphin and flupenthixol but not spiroperidol and haloperidol.

The dopamine receptor blockers sulpiride and metoclopramide have no effect on these receptors, whereas bromocriptine has an antagonistic effect (Creese et al., 1981 ; Snyder and Goodman, 1980). The D_2 receptors have been localized in most areas of the brain including the corticostriate pathway, the hypothalamus and the pituitary gland and they bind tritiated dopamine, spiroperidol and haloperidol. Bromocriptine has the known agonistic action on these receptors whereas haloperidol, spiroperidol, sulpiride and metoclopramide have an antagonistic action (Creese et al., 1981 ; Snyder and Goodman, 1980 ; Jenner and Marsden, 1979).

Most DA-receptors of the anterior pituitary gland are coupled to the adenylate cyclase system (D_1 receptors) which theoretically imply that bromocriptine should have a weak antagonistic action on PRL secretion. Furthermore, conflicting results have appeared concerning the effect of DA and bromocriptine on adenylate cyclase activity (Snyder and Goodman, 1980) although DA binding to the receptor seems to inhibit the enzym in the lactotrophs. At the moment it seems likely that the DA-receptors involved in the inhibition of PRL-secretion are closer to the classical type D_2 receptor than to type D_1 receptor (Kebabian and Calne, 1979 ; Creese et al., 1981). Recently it has been suggested that more than one type of receptor is present on the pituitary PRL-secreting cells.

In contrast to dopamine (Oldendorf, 1971), bromocriptine and metoclopramide cross the blood-brain barrier and may act at pituitary DA receptors as well as at the hypothalamic level to influence DA activity.

Secretion pattern of gonadotrophins in normal women

The gonadotrophins circulate in plasma in an unbound form and the half-life of LH and FSH in plasma has been estimated to about 30 minutes and 4 hours respectively (see Hagen, 1978). Plasma clearance of the gonadotrophins occurs by hepatic and kidney uptake and renal excretion, and do not seem to change significantly throughout reproductive age. Therefore, changes in basal plasma levels of gonadotrophins mainly reflect changes in pituitary secretion.

The secretory patterns of the gonadotrophins can be considered as tonic and phasic. The tonic secretion is regulated by the negative feedback of steroids and inhibin. The sites for this negative feedback are in both the hypothalamus and a direct effect on the pituitary gland. Studies in the monkey using surgical isolation of the hypothalamus from the rest of the brain indicate that the neural component of the negative feedback system resides in the basal medial hypothalamus (Plant et al., 1978 ; Ferin et al., 1974 ; Barraclough and Wise, 1982). Oestrogens increase DA turnover in the tuberoinfundibular dopamine system *in vitro* (Fuxe et al., 1980 ; Gudelsky, 1981 ; Ferin et al., 1974) and increase PRL secretion by a direct action on the lactotroph (Kamberi et al., 1971 ; McLeod and Lehmeyer, 1974 ; Shaar and Clemens, 1974 ; Raymond et al., 1978) and may indirectly by way of the short loop feedback action of PRL on the dopaminergic system induce an elevation of DA turnover in the median eminence and consequently a decrease in GnRH secretion (Fuxe et al., 1980 ; Sawyer, 1975 ; Gudelsky et al., 1981 ; Labrie et al., 1980 ; Gudelsky and Porter, 1980). Recently a blunted postcastration gonadotrophin rise was found during bromocriptine administration to normal females (Melis et al., 1981), suggesting that the tonic pattern of secretion is partly under dopaminergic inhibitory control. *In vitro*, oestrogens decrease the stimulatory effect of NE at the receptor sites of the GnRH neurons (Sawyer, 1975 ; Sawyer et al., 1978 ; Inaba and Kamata, 1979). Sex steroids may therefore theoretically inhibit LH secretion via NE as well.

Pulsatile secretion of LH and FSH is probably caused by the periodic increase in the secretion of GnRH (Carmel et al., 1976 ; Sarda et al., 1981 ; Belchetz et al., 1978). There is evidence that the pulsatile GnRH release may be mediated by the stimulatory effect of NE and the inhibitory effect of DA (Sawyer, 1975 ; Drouva and Gallo, 1976 ; Negro-Vilar et al., 1979 ; Barraclough and Wise, 1982). Furthermore it has been suggested that progesterone suppresses LH secretion by a central action to decrease the frequency of GnRH pulses whereas oestradiol decreases the responsiveness of the pituitary gland to stimulation by GnRH (Goodman and Karsch, 1980 ; Chappel et al., 1981 ; Yen et al., 1975 ; Baird, 1978). Thus normal ovulatory women have a pattern of low amplitude and high frequency pulses during the follicular phase when the effect of oestradiol prominents and high amplitude and low frequency pulses during the luteal phase of the cycle when progesterone is high (Yen et al., 1975 ; Santen and Bardin, 1973).

Cyclic gonadotrophin secretion involves a stimulatory feedback of incremental levels of circulating oestrogens and this ovarian signal initiates the syncronous preovulatory release of LH and FSH in normally menstruating females. This effect is dependent on oestrogen levels and duration of the stimulus (Yen and Lein, 1976). The combination of events required for a positive feedback action of oestradiol on gonadotrophin release at the time of the midcycle surge is a pituitary gland sensitive to GnRH, partly mediated by an increase in the number of GnRH receptors on the gonadotrophs (Adams et al., 1981), which have built up large pools of releasable LH and FSH to support the midcycle surge. In the rhesus monkey the site of oestrogen action seems almost exclusively to be the anterior pituitary gland (Knobil et al., 1980) whereas in the rat there is also an increase in NE turnover in the suprachiasmatic nucleus and a reduction in medial basal hypothalamic DA turnover leading to an acute GnRH discharge on the day of the LH surge (Rush et al., 1980 ; Sarkar and Fink, 1981 ; Wise et al., 1981 ; Selmanoff et al., 1976). In humans oestradiol has a positive feedback effect directly on the pituitary gland and prolonged administration of oestradiol to normal women in the early follicular phase is accompanied by an augmented LH response to GnRH administration (Djursing et al., 1981 ; Yen et al., 1975).

Secretion pattern of gonadotrophins in patients with hypothalamic functional amenorrhoea (HFA) and in hyperprolactinaemia

Basal gonadotrophin concentrations are variable in patients with HFA but most patients have either normal or low levels and they usually have a secretory

298

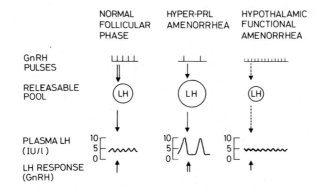

Fig. 1 - The frequency of gonadotrophin releasing hormone (GnRH) pulses and size of pituitary luteinizing hormone (LH) releasable pool in normal women in the early follicular phase, in a proportion of hyperprolactinaemic patients with small pituitary tumors and amenorrhoea and in women with hypothalamic functional amenorrhoea. This hypothesis is based on the known pulsatile secretion of plasma LH and the rise of plasma LH concentration after i.v. injection of GnRH in normal women and in patients.

pattern of low amplitude and high frequency (Santen and Bardin, 1973 ; Buckman et al., 1981) suggesting rapid but minor pulses of GnRH but a normal or a small releasable pool of LH (Fig. 1).

The mean LH and FSH concentrations in hyperprolactinaemic patients with small tumors are usually not different from those of normal women (Moult et al., 1982 ; Buckman et al., 1981 ; Thorner et al., 1974a) and some patients comprise a LH pattern of high amplitude and low frequency (Santen and Bardin, 1973 ; Moult et al., 1982) (Fig. 1). In addition, in these patients, as well as in patients with HFA, the negative feedback of oestrogens is intact, but there is a loss of the normal rise in LH secretion in response to the administration of oestrogens (Djursing et al., 1981 ; Glass et al., 1976 ; Shaw et al., 1975) (Fig. 2).

GnRH stimulation

It is possible to study the pituitary sensitivity to GnRH and the dynamic reserve or readily releasable pool of pituitary gonadotrophins by the use of a bolus injection of GnRH whereas assessment of the synthetic capacity of the gonodotrophin secreting cell is done by the use of intermittent, repetitive low doses of GnRH (Yen et al., 1975). The degree of previous exposure of the gonadotrophin secreting cells to endogenous GnRH appears to affect both the magnitude and quality of LH and FSH responses to an intravenous dose of GnRH (Yen et al., 1975 ; Yen and Lein, 1976 ; Kletzky et al., 1977).

The LH and FSH responses following the administration of GnRH to hyperprolactinaemic women with or without a pituitary tumor has been shown to be decreased (Spellacy et al., 1978), normal or exaggerated (Djursing et al., 1981 ; Glass et al., 1976 ; Thorner et al., 1974a ; Lachelin et al., 1977a). Recently, an increased readily releasable pool and synthetic capacity of the gonadotrophin secreting cells was demonstrated in a group of these patients harbouring a pituitary

299

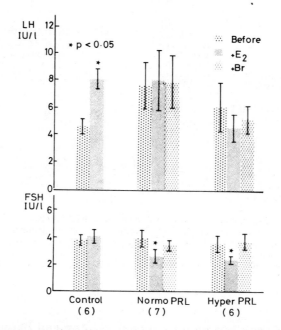

Fig. 2 - Basal plasma concentrations of LH and FSH before and after 4 days of œstradiol (2 mg/day), and after 5 days of bromocriptine (5 mg/day) administration to normal women day 2-5 of the menstrual cycle (control), normoprolactinaemic women with hypothalamic functional amenorrhoea (Normo PRL) and hyperprolactinaemic women with amenorrhoea (Hyper PRL) Mean ± SEM, *significantly (p < 0.05) different from before. Reproduced with permission from Djursing et al. (1981).

tumor (Monroe et al., 1981). The differences recorded may be due to the variable PRL levels and tumor size of the patients studied. In patients with large tumors the tumor itself, and the high PRL levels via its short-loop feedback action, may inhibit gonadotrophin secretion. In contrast most HFA patients have either a normal or increased gonadotrophin response to GnRH (Djursing et al., 1981 ; Rebar et al., 1978) (Fig. 3).

Other neurotransmitters

Apart from DA and NE other neurotransmitters may also participate in the regulation of GnRH secretion and thus gonadotrophin release. There is experimental evidence that acetylcholine and gammaaminobutyric acid (Ondo, 1974) stimulate and that serotonin (Baumgarten et al., 1978 ; Kamberi et al., 1971b) and the opiates (Olson et al., 1981) inhibit the release of LH. Most studies point to an effect of these neurotransmitters via the tuberoinfundibular dopaminergic tract.

Dopamine and gonadotrophin secretion

In animals administration of DA has a stimulatory (Kamberi et al., 1971 ; Schneider and McCann, 1969 ; Vijayan and McCann, 1978), inhibitory (Fuxe et al.,

1977 ; Dailey et al., 1978 ; Gallo, 1980 ; Beck et al., 1978) or absent effect (Sawyer et al., 1978 ; Blake, 1976) on GnRH and gonadotrophin release. At the moment there is no explanation for the variability of results because a stimulatory as well as inhibitory effect have been found during similar experimental conditions. However, it has recently been suggested that the differences may have a physiological explanation (Barraclough and Wise, 1982) because not only the concentration of DA but also the duration of time that DA is presented to the receptor may determine whether DA-stimuli become stimulatory or inhibitory to GnRH release.

In normal men and women most authors report an inhibitory role of DA on LH secretion without any effect on FSH (Leblanc et al., 1976 ; Judd et al., 1978 ; Travaglini et al., 1981 ; Huseman et al., 1980 ; Kaptein et al., 1980 ; Ferrari et al., 1981 ; Martin et al., 1981). On the other hand Leebaw et al. (1978) found that in 6 normal men DA was ineffective in suppressing basal gonadotrophin levels but decreased LH response to GnRH. In one study (Pucci et al., 1981) DA infusion to normal women on day 6 of the mentrual cycle even enhanced the LH response to GnRH.

The inhibitory effect of DA infusion on LH release in normal women was similar during the early and late follicular phases of the cycle but increased on day 14 (Judd et al., 1978). In addition the DA lowering effect on LH levels was much more pronounced in postmenopausal women than in normal women on day 2 of the cycle (Judd et al., 1979). The finding that DA inhibition of LH secretion is increased when basal LH levels are high, probably due to enhanced GnRH secretion, supports the hypothesis that DA acts directly on GnRH secreting neurons. Furthermore, DA seems unable to inhibit gonadotrophin secretion when added to rat pituitary tissue *in vitro* (Chiocchio et al., 1980). The change in sensitivity to DA in the menstrual cycle (Judd et al., 1978) support the theory that the positive oestrogen feedback on GnRH secretion may act at least partly by reducing the hypothalamic DA activity.

In hyperprolactinaemic patients and women with the polycystic ovarian syndrome an inhibitory effect of DA on basal LH levels without changes in FSH levels has been reported (Reschini et al., 1980).

Bromocriptine and gonadotrophin secretion

Bromocriptine (2-bromo-alpha-ergocryptine) is an ergot derivative with dopamine receptor agonistic actions (Müller et al., 1981 ; Thorner et al., 1980). The drug lowers PRL in blood by inhibiting PRL secretion from the pituitary gland by a direct action on the prolactin cell.

In normal women investigations of the acute effect of bromocriptine administration on gonadotrophin secretion have given conflicting results. Two studies (Martin et al., 1981 ; Tolis et al., 1975) were unable to demonstrate any changes in plasma LH concentrations after an oral dose of bromocriptine despite marked suppression of PRL levels. In contrast Pontiroli et al. (1980) were able to demonstrate a fall in plasma LH concentration after bromocriptine. In addition these same authors and others (Lachelin et al., 1977 b) found a decrease in circulating LH levels after L-dopa administration to six normal women, but others (Zarate et al., 1973 ; Polansky et al., 1976 ; Pinter et al., 1975) have not been able to confirm this finding. In agreement with the inhibitory action of bromocriptine on LH secretion, Melis et al. (1981) found that in 12 normal women 7 days of bromocriptine administration induced a blunted increase in basal and GnRH stimulated LH levels at day 14 after castration. However, bromocriptine administration during the normal menstrual cycle decreased plasma PRL and progesterone concentrations but did not change basal LH, FSH and oestradiol levels (Del Pozo et al., 1975).

In hyperprolactinaemic patients the raised plasma PRL concentration may increase the activity of the dopaminergic neurons in the hypothalamus by its short loop feedback action. The raised dopaminergic tone might inhibit the GnRH secretion into the portal vessels and thus explain the low gonadotrophin levels despite low oestrogens in these patients (Quigley et al., 1980 ; Evans et al., 1980 ; Djursing et al., 1981). Therefore, additional dopamine receptor stimulation by bromocriptine might not lead to further inhibition of GnRH and thus to decreased basal LH levels. To explain the elevated PRL levels in these patients a reduced availability of DA at the receptor site of the PRL-secreting cells has been suggested (Fine and Frohman, 1978). In most studies bromocriptine administration to hyperprolactinaemic patients did not induce any changes in basal gonadotrophin levels within the first 4 days of treatment (Evans et al., 1980 ; Djursing et al., 1981 ; Strauch et al., 1977) (Fig. 2). In contrast, Lachelin et al. (1977a) demonstrated a fall in basal LH levels within 3 hours of bromocriptine administration in these patients. In addition, we (Djursing et al., 1981) found decreased pituitary sensitivity of the gonadotrophin secreting cells after 4 days of bromocriptine treatment (Fig. 3) and a normal rate of LH pulsatility can be restored by bromocriptine in hyperprolactinaemic women prior to any alteration in serum oestradiol (Moult et al., 1982).

In normoprolactinaemic, normo- or hypogonadotrophic women with functional amerorrhoea (HFA) bromocriptine appears not to have an effect on gonadotrophin secretion (Djursing et al., 1981) (Fig. 2, 3). This may indicate that these patients have an increased dopaminergic activity at the hypothalamic level. Alternatively, the release of LH is not influenced by DA in these patients. A third possibility is that DA is functional but that the DA-receptor complex does not respond to bromocriptine.

It has been shown, that in hyperprolactinaemic women as well as patients with HFA, the negative feedback of oestrogens is intact but positive feedback is suppressed (Djursing et al., 1981 ; Glass et al., 1976 ; Shaw et al., 1975). It was found that positive feedback is restored in hyperprolactinaemic women when PRL levels are lowered with bromocriptine therapy (Faglia et al., 1977). As the positive feedback depends not only on intact gonadotrophin secretion but also on GnRH release one could speculate that absence of a positive feedback represents an inhibition of GnRH secretion.

Bromocriptine therapy in women with hyperprolactinaemic amenorrhoea is associated with the suppression of raised plasma PRL levels and a return to normal cyclic pattern of gonadotrophin and ovulatory cycles (Thorner et al., 1974a ; del Pozo et al., 1974 ; Bergh et al., 1978). Therefore, the long term effect, if any, of bromocriptine on gonadotrophin secretion seems not to be of pathophysiological significance.

The discrepancy between DA and bromocriptine to induce an effect on plasma LH levels suggest the existence of a number of different DA receptors and the sim-

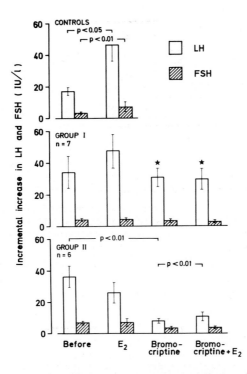

Fig. 3 - Increases in plasma LH and FSH concentrations after i.v. injection of 50 μg of gonadotrophin releasing hormone to normal women in the early follicular phase (controls), women with hypothalamic functional amenorrhoea (group I) and hyperprolactinaemic women with amenorrhoea (group II). The patients were studied before and after 4 days of œstradiol (2 mg/day, E_2) and after 5 days of bromocriptine (5 mg/day) and after 9 days of bromocriptine (5mg/day) plus 4 days of œstradiol (2 mg/day) administration. Mean ± SEM.
*Significant (p < 0.02) difference between group I and II. Reproduced with permission from Djursing et al. (1981).

ple D_1 and D_2 classification of receptors may be an over-simplification (Kebabian and Calne, 1979 ; Creese et al., 1981 ; Snyder and Goodman, 1980) .

On the basis of these results we extend the hypotheses for the relation between gonadotrophin secretion and hypothalamic dopaminergic activity (Fig. 1 and 4). In normoprolactinaemic patients with amenorrhoea increased dopaminergic activity inhibits GnRH secretion which is counteracted by an increased sensitivity of the gonadotrophs which may be due to an alteration in the number and/or affinity of GnRH receptors. This is supported by normal basal gonadotrophin concentrations and enhanced LH and FSH responses to GnRH in some of these patients. With a further increase in inhibition of GnRH an increased sensitivity of the gonadotrophs is no longer sufficient to maintain normal basal levels. Therefore, basal gonadotrophin concentrations as well as responses to GnRH decrease to subnormal and normal levels respectively. This phenomenon is probably seen in a proportion of normoprolactinaemic women with HFA, and perhaps in some cases with

303

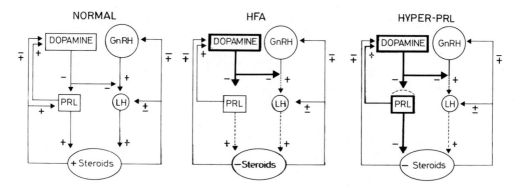

Fig. 4 - Illustration of the possible regulation of pituitary prolactin (PRL) and luteinizing hormone (LH) by œstradiol, dopamine and gonadotrophin releasing hormone (GnRH) in normal women, patients with hyperprolactinaemia and amenorrhoea and in a proportion of patients with hypothalamic functional amenorrhoea. Prolactin increases hypothalamic dopaminergic activity via its short-loop feedback action and presumably decrease GnRH secretion. Patients with hypothalamic functional amenorrhoea (HFA) may have a increased hypothalamic dopaminergic activity not related to changes in PRL levels.

long standing hyperprolactinaemic amenorrhoea and small tumours. If dopaminergic tone is further increased, basal as well as GnRH stimulated gonadotrophin levels will show an additional decrease. These changes in gonadotrophin secretion have been found in diabetic patients with HFA (Djursing et al., 1982 ; Hagen et al., 1982) who had hormonal parameters in accordance with maximal DA activity, although the etiology and mechanism of the increased inhibitory dopaminergic activity on gonadotrophin secretion cannot be determined from the available data.

Benzamides and gonadotrophin secretion.

Metoclopramide (MTC) and sulpiride (SPR) are substituted benzamides with a DA receptor blocking action. These drugs antagonize DA receptors in D_2 receptors containing areas of the cerebrum (Creese et al., 1981 ; Snyder and Goodman, 1980 ; Jenner and Marsden, 1979).

Both MTC and SPR are potent releasers of PRL in normal men and women (Thorner et al., 1974 ; Judd et al., 1976 ; Sowers et al., 1976). It is generally accepted that the PRL response to MTC and SPR is significantly greater than that obtained with maximal thyrotrophin releasing hormone (TRH) stimulation (Hagen et al., 1981 ; Thorner et al., 1974). This may in part be due to an effect of continuous secretion of DA during the TRH test which limits the release of stored PRL and the synthesis of new PRL. The administration of surprisingly small doses of MTC (1 mg i.v. : Healy and Burger, 1977 ; Kitaoka et al., 1980) and of SPR (6.25 mg : Tormey et al., 1981) induces a significant increase in PRL levels. Pretreatment with L-dopa suppresses the PRL responses to MTC and SPR due to a competition for DA receptors in the hypothalamus and the pituitary gland (Judd et al., 1976 ; Sowers et al., 1976 ; Kitaoka et al., 1980 ; L'Hermite et al., 1978b ; Spitz et al., 1979).

In normal women and men, investigations of the acute administration of MTC

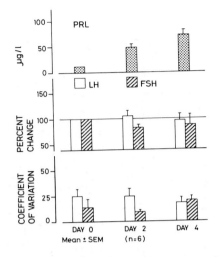

Fig. 5 - Basal plasma concentrations of prolactin (PRL), and percentage changes of basal levels of luteinizing hormone (LH) and follicle stimulating hormone (FSH) before (day 0) and after 2 days of
sulpiride (200 mg/day p.o.) (day 2) and after additional 2 days of sulpiride (400 mg/day p.o.) (day 4) in
6 normal men. In each subject bloodsamples were collected every 15 min for 3 hours before, on day
2 and day 4. On the basis of these repeated LH and FSH determinations the coefficient of variations
were calculated. No significant (p > 0.05) changes in percent changes and coefficient of variations
were found.

and SPR on gonadotrophin secretion point to its lack of effect (Judd et al., 1976;
Healy and Burger, 1977; L'Hermite et al., 1978b; Spitz et al., 1979; Quigley et al.,
1979; Andersen et al., 1979). Only Sowers et al. (1976) demonstrated a small but
significant fall in LH levels after oral administration of MTC (10 mg) to eleven normal males. We (Hagen et al., 1982a) found decreased basal LH levels without any
change in FSH after 4 weeks of MTC administration to normal women in the early
follicular phase of the cycle. In contrast the administration of MTC (10 mg, 3 times
daily) for one week to normal women in the follicular phase caused an increased
response of both LH and FSH to GnRH (Andersen et al., 1982). During the luteal
phase of the cycle the basal and GnRH stimulated plasma FSH concentration increased during three weeks of SPR administration, whereas LH levels did not
change significantly (L'Hermite et al., 1978b). In 5 normal men Falaschi et al. (1978)
found a fall in sperm counts without any changes in basal gonadotrophin levels nor
in their responses to GnRH, during 6 weeks of MTC administration. In addition we
found no changes in either basal levels or secretion pattern of LH and FSH during
5 days of SPR administration to normal men (Fig. 5). Galactorrhoea and menstrual
disorders have been reported to occur frequently during long term MTC and SPR
administration and are typically reversible on drug withdrawal (L'Hermite et al.,
1972; Aono et al., 1978). Furthermore, deteriorated corpus luteum function is
found during treatment with SPR, in doses causing true hyperprolactinaemia
(Robyn et al., 1977), and treatment with either SPR or MTC inhibits the positive
feedback of œstrogens on LH release (L'Hermite et al., 1978b; Schmidt-Gollwitzer

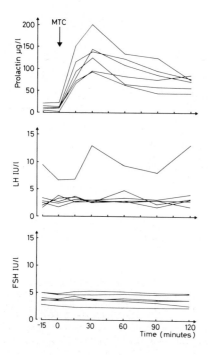

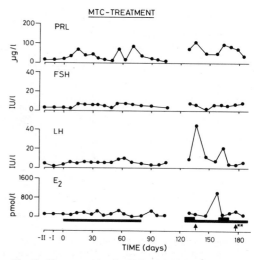

Fig. 6 - Individual plasma prolactin, luteinizing hormone (LH) and follicle stimulating hormone (FSH) responses to i.v. administration of 10 mg of metoclopramide (MTC) in 6 patients with hypothalamic functional amenorrhoea.

Fig. 7 - Plasma prolactin (PRL), follicle stimulating hormone (FSH), luteinizing hormone (LH) and œstradiol-17β (E₂) concentrations before and during continuous (7.5 mg/day) as well as sequential (20 mg/day for 10 days followed by 7.5 mg/day for 20 days) metoclopramide administration to one women with hypothalamic functional amenorrhoea.

↑ indicate detectable levels of progesterone
** indicate bleeding episodes
— dose of MTC.

et al., 1979 ; Nansel et al., 1979) and may augment the negative feedback (Andersen et al., 1982)

If the concept of inhibition of GnRH release by DA is accepted and that an increased DA inhibition of GnRH is found in hyperprolactinaemic patients, MTC and SPR should be able to stimulate gonadotrophin secretion in hyperprolactinaemic patients. A gonadotrophin response to 10 mg of MTC has in fact been demonstrated (Quigley et al., 1979 ; White et al., 1981).

Conflicting data exist regarding the effect of MTC on gonadotrophin levels in patients with HFA. Quigley et al. (1980) studied a group of 8 HFA patients and found that the four women with the lowest ideal body weight and highest plasma LH and œstradiol concentrations responded with a rise in LH and FSH levels during the MTC-test. We were unable to confirm this finding in a similar study of 6 women with HFA (Fig. 6) but were able to demonstrate a rise in basal plasma concentrations of PRL, FSH and œstradiol within 5 weeks of oral MTC treatment (7.5 mg/day) and in LH levels within 10 weeks of treatment of the same 6 patients (Hagen et al., 1982b). Furthermore, in one woman, ovulatory cycles returned during treatment. After an interval of two to three months without treatment, 5 of the women started sequential MTC therapy in a dose of 5 mg four times a day for 10 days followed by a

306

dose of 2.5 mg three times a day for 20 days and then repeated the sequence. This therapeutic scheme was chosen on basis of the known secretion of GnRH. The first 10 days of treatment might lead to an increased secretion of GnRH and thereby a build-up of LH in the pituitary gland and at the same time an enhanced LH secretion, whereas the low dose of MTC should just be able to prevent the hypothalamic-pituitary axis from returning to pretreatment state. The women who menstruated during non-sequential MTC treatment continued to have ovulatory cycles. In addition ovulation was restored in three women within 3 months (Fig. 7). The only patient in whom gonadal function did not return to normal during MTC therapy responded with intermittent elevated plasma œstradiol and fluctuating LH levels, but she stopped treatment after only one and a half cycles of therapy (Hagen et al., 1982b).

Partially in agreement with our data, Larsen (1981) was able to demonstrate an enhanced LH response to GnRH during 4 weeks of MTC treatment of 6 women with low weight amenorrhoea, but no significant changes in basal gonadotrophin and œstradiol levels were reported.

The mechanism of the long term stimulatory effect of MTC on plasma gonadotrophin and œstradiol concentrations cannot be determined from the present data. A possible placebo effect has not been evaluated but it is a possible, but unlikely, explanation for the observed effect. A psychological stimulus would probably have been seen early in the treatment period. Advis and Ojede (1978) reported that SPR induced hyperprolactinaemia in rats leads to an enhanced ovarian sensitivity to gonadotrophin stimulation. MTC has no acute effect on either œstradiol or progesterone levels in normal women (Andersen, 1979), neither is the follicular phase serum œstradiol levels altered by SPR (Robyn et al., 1977 ; Aono et al., 1978) or MTC (Andersen et al., 1982). In vivo studies suggest that if hyperprolactinaemia has a direct role in ovarian œstrogen production (Larsen and Honoré, 1980), it is inhibitory. Therefore, we find it unlikely that increased PRL levels or the drug itself could stimulate ovarian estrogen secretion, and thus exert a positive feedback effect on gonadotrophin secretion. A third, but remote, possibility is that MTC modulates gonadotrophin secretion by a direct action on the pituitary gland, but no DA receptors have been found on the gonadotrophs (Cronin et al., 1978 ; Nansel et al., 1979). The apparent discrepancies regarding the influence of MTC and SPR on gonadotrophin secretion may be the result of differences of doses and duration of treatment. One critical factor may be whether hyperprolactinaemia is induced or not. If it occurs, PRL may increase central dopaminergic tonus via the short-loop feedback and thus compete with a possible direct effect of the drugs on GnRH secretion.

It seems likely that amenorrhoea, in a proportion of HFA patients, is secondary to a raised hypothalamic dopaminergic tone since the hypogonadism responds to MTC. The reduction in DA-activity appears to allow GnRH to rise and circulating gonadotrophin levels to act on the gonad to stimulate steroidogenesis and thereby restore normal ovulatory cycles.

REFERENCES

Adams, T.E., Norman, R.L., Spies, H.G. *1981* — Gonadotropin-releasing hormone receptor binding and pituitary responsiveness in estradiol-primed monkeys. *Science, 213 :* 1388-1390.

Advis, J.P., Ojeda, S.R. *1978* — Hyperprolactinemia-induced precocious puberty in the female rat : Ovarian site of action. *Endocrinology, 103 :* 924-935.

Andersen, A.N., Hertz, J., Eskildsen, P.C., Schiøler, V. Micic, S. *1979* - Metoclopramide induced hyperprolactinaemia, effect on pituitary-ovarin axis. *In : Psychoneuroendocrinology in Reproduction*, Zichella, L. Pancheri, P. (eds), pp. 395-400. Amsterdam. Elsevier/North-Holland Biomedical Press.

Andersen, A.N., Schiøler, V., Hertz, J., Bennett, P. *1982* — Effect of metoclopramide induced hyperprolactinaemia on the gonadotrophic response to œstradiol and LRH. *Acta endocrinol. 100*, 1-9.

Aono, T., Shioji, T., Kinugasa, T., Onishi, T., Kurachi, K. *1978* — Clinical and endocrinological analyses of patients with galactorrhea and menstrual disorders due to sulpiride or metoclopramide. *J. Clin. Endocrinol. Metab., 47 :* 675-680.

Aono, T., Yasuda, M., Shioji, T., Kondo, K., Kurachi, K. *1978a* — Absence of inhibition by hyperprolactinaemia on ovarian response to exogenous gonadotrophin. *Acta Endocrinol. 89 :* 142-148.

Baird, D.T. *1978* — Pulsatile secretion of LH and ovarian estradiol during the follicular phase of the sheep estrous cycle. *Biol. Reprod., 18 :* 359-364.

Barraclough, C.A., Wise, P.M. *1982* — The role of catecholamines in the regulation of pituitary luteinizing hormone and follicle-stimulating hormone secretion. *Endocrine Rev. 3 :* 91-119.

Baumgarten, H.G., Bjørklun, A., Wuttke, W. *1978* — Neural control of pituitary LH, FSH and prolactin secretion : The role of serotonin. *In : Brain-Endocrine interaction. III. Neuronal hormone and reproduction.* Scott, D.E., Kozowski, G.P. and Weindl, A. (eds) pp. 327-343 Basel Karger.

Beck, W., Hancke, J.L., Wuttke, W. *1978* — Increased sensitivity of dopaminergic inhibition of luteinizing hormone release in immature and castrated female rats. *Endocrinology, 102 :* 837-843.

Belchetz, P.E., Plant, T.M., Nakai, Y., Keogh, E.J., Knobil, E. *1978* — Hypophysial responses to continuous and intermittent delivery of hypothalamic gonadotropin-releasing hormone. *Science, 202 :* 631-633.

Bergh, T., Nillius, S.J., Wide, L. *1978* — Bromocriptine treatment of 42 hyperprolactinaemic women with secondary amenorrhoea. *Acta Endocrinol., 88 :* 435-451.

Bhattacharya, A.N., Dierschke, D.J., Yamaji, T., Knobil, E. *1972* — The pharmacologic blockade of the circhoral mode of LH secretion in the ovariectomized rhesus monkey. *Endocrinology, 90 :* 778-786.

Blake, C.A. *1976* — Effect of intravenous infusion of catecholamines on rat plasma luteinizing hormone and prolactin concentration. *Endocrinology, 98 :* 99-104.

Buckman, M.T., Peake, G.T., Strivastava L. *1981* — Patterns of spontaneous LH release in normo- and hyperprolactinaemic women. *Acta Endocrinol. 97 :* 305-310.

Carmel, P.W., Araki, S., Ferin, M. *1976* — Pituitary stalk portal blood collection in rhesus monkeys : Evidence for pulsatile release of gonadotropin-releasing hormone (GnRH). *Endocrinology, 99 :* 243-248.

Chappel, S.C., Resko, J.A., Normal, R.L., Spies, H.G. *1981* — Studies in rhesus monkeys on the site where estrogen inhibits gonadotropins : Delivery of 17β-estradiol to the hypothalamus and pituitary gland. *J. Clin. Endocrinol. Metab., 52 :* 1-8.

Chiocchio, S.R., Chafuen, S., Tramezzani, J.H. *1980* — Changes in adenohypophysial dopamine related to prolactin release. *Endocrinology 106 :* 1682-1685.

Cramer, O.M., Parker, C.R., Jr., Porter J.C. *1979* — Estrogen inhibition of dopamine release into hypophysial portal blood. *Endocrinology, 104 :* 419-423.

Creese, I., Sibley, D.R., Leff, S., Hamblin, M. *1981* — Dopamine receptors : subtypes, localization and regulation. *Fed. Proc., 40 :* 147-152.

Cronin, M.J., Roberts, J.M., Weiner, R.I. *1978* — Dopamine and dihydroergocryptine binding to the anterior pituitary and other brain areas of the rat and sheep. *Endocrinology, 103 :* 302-309.

Dailey, R.A., Tsou, R.C., Tindall, G.T., Neill, J.D. *1978* — Direct hypophysial inhibition of luteinizing hormone release by dopamine in the rabbit. *Life Sci., 22 :* 1491-1498.

Del Pozo, E., Varga, L., Wyss, H., Tolis, G., Friesen, H., Wenner, R., Vetter, L., Uettwiler, A. *1974* — Clinical and hormonal response to bromocriptine (CB-154) in the galactorrhea syndromes. *J. Clin. Endocrinol. Metab., 39 :* 18-26.

Del Pozo, E., Goldstein, M., Friesen, H., Brun del Re, R., Eppenberger, U. *1975* — Lack of action of prolactin suppression on the regulation of the human menstrual cycle. *J. Obstet. Gynecol., 123 :* 719-723.

Djursing, H., Hagen, C., Christensen, F., Nickelsen, C. *1981* — Bromocriptine and œstrogen modulation of gonadotrophin release in normo- and hyperprolactinemic patients with amenorrhoea. *Clin. Endocrinol., 15 :* 125-132.

Djursing, H., Nyholm, H.C., Hagen, C., Carstensen, L., Mølsted Petersen, L. *1982* — Clinical and hormonal characteristics in women with anovulation and insulin treated diabetes mellitus. *Am. J. Obstet. Gynecol. 143 :* 876-882.

Drouva, S.V., Gallo, R.V. *1976* — Catecholamine involvement in episodic luteinizing hormone release in adult ovariectomized rats. *Endocrinology, 99 :* 651-658.

Evans, W.S., Rogol, A.D., MacLeod, R.M., Thorner, M.O. *1980* — Dopaminergic mechanisms and luteinizing hormone secretion. I. Acute administration of the dopamine agonist bromocriptine does not inhibit luteinizing hormone release in hyperprolactinemic women. *J. Clin. Endocrinol. Metab., 50 :* 103-107.

Faglia, G., Beck-Peccoz, P., Travaglini, P., Ambrosi, B., Rondena, M., Paracchi, A., Spada, A., Weber, G., Bara, R. & Bouzin, A. *1977* — Functional studies in hyperprolactinemic states. *In : Prolactin and Human Reproduction. Crosignani, P.G. and Robyn, C., (eds), pp. 225-238. New York, Academic Press.*

Falaschi, P., Frajese, G., Sciarra, F., Rocco, A., Conti, C. *1978* — Influence of hyperprolactinaemia due to metoclopramide on gonadal function in men. *Clin. Endocrinol., 8 :* 427-433.

Ferrin, M., Carmel, P.W., Zimmerman, E.A., Warren, M., Perez, R., Van de Wiele, R.L. *1974* — Location of intrahypothalamic estrogen-responsive sites influencing LH secretion in the female rhesus monkey. *Endocrinology, 95 :* 1059-1068.

Ferrari, C., Rampini, P., Malinverni, A., Scarduelli, C., Benco, R., Caldara, R., Barbieri, C., Testori, G., Crosignani, P.G. *1981* — Inhibition of luteinizing hormone release by dopamine infusion in healthy women and in various pathophysiological conditions. *Acta Endocrinol. 97 :* 436-440.

Fine, S.A., Frohman, L.A. *1978.* — Loss of central nervous system component of dopaminergic inhibition of prolactin secretion in patients with prolactin-secreting pituitary tumors. *Clin. Invest., 61 :* 973-980.

Fuxe, K., Løfstrøm, A., Agnati, L., Høkfelt L., Johansson, T., Eneroth, O., Gustavsson, J.-Å., Skett, P., Jeffcoate, S., Fraser, H. *1977.* — *In : Progress in Reproductive Neuroendocrinology, vol. 2,* Hubinot, P.O., L'Hermite, M. and Robyn, C., (eds) pp. 41-72.

Fuxe, K., Andersson, K., Agnati, L., Ferland, L., Hökfelt, T., Eneroth, P., Gustavsson, J.-A. *1980.* — Hypothalamic monoamine pathways and their possible role in disturbances of the secretion of hormones from the anterior pituitary gland. *In : Pituitary Microadenomas.* Faglia, G., Giovanelli, M.A., McLeod, R.M. (ed.), pp. 15-35. New York, Academic Press.

Gallo, R.V. *1980.* — Effect of manipulation of brain dopaminergic or serotoninergic systems on basal pulsatile LH release and perisuprachiasmatic-induced suppression of pulsatile LH release in ovariectomized rats. *Neuroendocrinology, 31 :* 161-167.

Glass, M.R., Shaw, R.W., Williams, J.W., Butt, W.R., Logan-Edwards, R., London, D.R. *1976.* — The control of gonadotrophin release in women with hyperprolactinaemic amenorrhoea : Effect of oestrogen and progesterone on the LH and FSH response to LHRH. *Clin. Endocrinol., 5 :* 521-530.

Goodman, R.L., Karsch, F.J. *1980.* — Pulsatile secretion of luteinizing hormone : Differential suppression by ovarian steroids. *Endocrinology, 107 :* 1286-1290.

Gudelsky, G. *1981.* — Tuberoinfundibular dopamine neurons and the regulation of prolactin secretion. *Psychoneuroendocrinology, 6 :* 3-16.

Gudelsky, G.A., Porter, J.C. *1980.* — Release of dopamine from tuberoinfundibular neurons into pituitary stalk blood after prolactin or haloperidol administration. *Endocrinology, 106 :* 526-529.

Gudelsky, G.A., Nansel, D.D., Porter, J.C. *1981.* — Role of estrogen in the dopaminergic control of prolactin secretion. *J. Clin. Endocrinol. Metab., 108 :* 440-444.

Hagen, C. *1978.* — Studies on the subunits of human glycoprotein hormones in relation to reproduction. *Scand. J. Clin. Lab. Invest. 37, suppl. 148 :* 1-19.

Hagen, C., Lindholm, J., Suenson, E. Riishede, J., Hummer, L., Jacobsen, H.-H. *1979.* — Relationship between plasma prolactin concentration and pituitary function in patients with a pituitary adenoma. *Clin. Endocrinol., 11 :* 671-679.

Hagen, C., Djursing, H., Andersen, A.N., Carstensen, L., Nyholm, H.C. *1981.* — Plasma PRL and gonadotrophin responses to TRH, metoclopramide and GnRH in insulin treated diabetic patients with amenorrhoea. *Neuroendocrine Letters, 3 :* 295.

Hagen, C., Djursing, H., Petersen, L., Fallentin, E. *1982a.* — The effect of metoclopramide on PRL, GH, LH and FSH fluctuations in normal women. (In preparation)

Hagen, C., Petersen, K., Djursing, H. *1982b.* — Metoclopramide therapy of functional amenorrhoea. *Xth World Congress of Gynecology and Obstetrics,* Abstract 2118.

Healy, D.L., Burger, H.G. *1977.* — Increased prolactin and thyrotrophin secretion following oral metoclopramide : Dose-response relationship. *Clin. Endocrinol., 7 :* 195-201.

Heritage, A.S., Stumpf, W.E., Sar, M., Grant, L.D. *1980.* — Brainstem catecholamine neurons are target sites for sex steroid hormones. *Science, 207 :* 1377-1379.

Huseman, C.A., Kugler, J.A., Schneider, I.G. *1980.* — Mechanism of dopaminergic suppression of gonadotropin secretion in men. *J. Clin. Endocrinol. Metab., 51* : 209-214.

Inaba, M., Kamata, K. *1979.* — Effect of estradiol-17β and other steroids on noradrenaline and dopamine binding to synaptic membrane fragments of rat brain. *J. Steroid Biochem., 11* : 1491-1497.

Jenner, P., Marsden, C.D. *1979.* — The substituted benzamides — a novel class of dopamine antagonists. *Life Sci., 25* : 479-486.

Judd, S.J., Lazarus, L., Smythe, G. *1976.* — Prolactin secretion by metoclopramide in man. *J. Clin. Endocrinol. Metab., 43* : 313-317.

Judd, S.J., Rakoff, J.S., Yen, S.S.C. *1978.* — Inhibition of gonadotropin and prolactin release by dopamine : Effect of endogenous estradiol levels. *J. Clin. Endocrinol. Metab., 47* : 494-498.

Judd, S.J., Rigg, L.A., Yen, S.S.C. *1979.* — The effects of ovariectomy and estrogen treatment on the dopamine inhibition of gonadotrophin and prolactin release. *J. Clin. Endocrinol. Metab., 49* : 182-184.

Kamberi, I.A., Mical, R.S., Porter, J.C. *1970.* — Effect of anterior pituitary perfusion and intraventricular injection of catecholamines and indoleamines on LH release. *Endocrinology, 87* : 1-12.

Kamberi, I.A., Mical, R.S., Porter, J.C. *1971.* — Effect of anterior pituitary perfusion and intraventricular injection of catecholamines on prolactin release. *Endocrinology, 88* : 1012-1020.

Kamberi, I.A., Mical, R.S. and Porter, J.C. *1971a.* — Effects of melatonin and serotonin on the release of FSH and prolactin. *Endocrinology, 88* : 1288-1293.

Kaptein, E.M., Kletzky, O.A., Spencer, C.A., Nicoloff, J.T. *1980.* — Effects of prolonged dopamine infusion on anterior pituitary function in normal males. *J. Clin. Endocrinol. Metab., 51* : 488-491.

Kebabian, J.W., Calne, D.B. *1979.* — Multiple receptors for dopamine. *Nature, 277* : 93-96.

Kitaoka, M., Takebe, K., Kobayashi, M., Nakazono, M., Kudo, M. *1980.* — Dose-dependency and reproducibility of the prolactin response to metoclopramide. *Hormone Metab. Res., 12* : 155-158.

Kletzky, O.A., Davajan, V., Mishell, D.R., Jr., Nicoloff, J.T., Mims, R., March, C.M., Nakamura, R.M. *1977.* — A sequential pituitary stimulation test in normal subjects and in patients with amenorrhea- galactorrhea with pituitary tumors. *J. Clin. Endocrinol. Metab., 45* : 631-640.

Knobil, E. *1974.* — On the control of gonadotropin secretion in the rhesus monkey. *Recent Prog. Horm. Res., 30* : 1-36.

Knobil, E. *1980.* — The neuroendocrine control of the menstrual cycle. *Rec. Prog. Horm. Res., 36* : 53-88.

Knobil, E., Plant, T.M., Wildt, L., Belchetz, P.E., Marshall, G. *1980.* — Control of the rhesus monkey menstrual cycle : Permissive role of hypothalamic gonadotropin-releasing hormone. *Science, 207* : 1371-1373.

Labrie, F., Ferland, L., Denizeau, F., Beaulieu, M. *1980.* — Sex steroids interact with dopamine at the hypothalamic and pituitary levels to modulate prolactin secretion. *J. Steroid Biochem., 12* : 323-330.

Lachelin, G.C.L., Abu-Fadil, S., Yen, S.S.C. *1977a.* Functional delineation of hyperprolactinemic-amenorrhea. *J. Clin. Endocrinol. Metab., 44* : 1163-1174.

Lachelin, G.C.L., Leblanc, H., Yen, S.S.C. *1977b.* — The inhibitory effect of dopamine agonists on LH release in women. *J. Clin. Endocrin. Metab., 44* : 728-732.

Larsen, S. *1981.* — Responses of luteinizing hormone, follicle-stimulating hormone, and prolactin to prolonged administration of a dopamine antagonist in normal women and women with low-weight amenorrhea. *Fertil. Steril., 35* : 642-646.

Larsen, S., Honoré, E. *1980.* — Estrogenic response in women with amenorrhea during treatment with human menopausal gonadotropin with and without the simultaneous administration of bromocriptine. *Fertil. Steril., 33* : 378-382.

Leblanc, H., Lachelin, G.C.L., Abu-Fadil, S. Yen, S.S.C. *1976.* — Effects of dopamine infusion on pituitary hormone secretion in humans. *J. Clin. Endocrinol. Metab., 43* : 668-674.

Leebaw, W.F., Lee, L.A., Woolf, P.D. *1978.* — Dopamine affects basal and augmented pituitary hormone secretion. *J. Clin. Endocrinol. Metab., 47* : 480-487.

L'Hermite, M., Delvoye, P., Nokin, J., Vekemans, M., Robyn, C. *1972.* — Human prolactin secretion, as studied by radioimmunoassay : some aspects of its regulation. *In : Prolactin and Carcinogenesis*, Bayns, A.R. & Griffiths, K. (eds), pp. 81-97. U.K. Alpha Omega Alpha Publishing.

L'Hermite, M., Delogne-Desnoeck, J., Michaux-Duchene, A., Robyn, C. *1978a.* — Alteration of feedback mechanism of estrogen on gonadotropin by sulpiride-induced hyperprolactinemia. *J. Clin. Endocrinol. Metabol., 47* : 1132-1136.

L'Hermite, M., Denayer, P., Golstein, J., Virasoro, E., Vanhaelst, L., Copinshi, G., Robyn, C. *1978b.* — Acute endocrine profile of sulpiride in the human. *Clin. Endocrinol., 9* : 195-204.

McCann, S.M., Moss, R.L. *1975.* — Putative neurotransmitters involved in discharging gonadotropin-releasing neurohormones and the action of LH-releasing hormone on the CNS. *Life Sci., 16* : 833-852.

310

McLeod, R.M., Lehmeyer, J.E. *1974.* — Studies on the mechanism of the dopamine-mediated inhibition of prolactin secretion. *Endocrinology, 94 :* 1077-1085.

McNeil, T.H., Sladek, J.R. *1978.* — Fluorescence-immunocytochemistry : Simultaneous localization of catecholamines and gonadotropin-releasing hormone. *Science, 200 :* 72-74.

Martin, W.H., Rogol, A.D., Kaiser, D.L., Thorner, M.O. *1981.* — Dopaminergic mechanisms and luteinizing hormone (LH) secretion. II. Differential effects of dopamine and bromocriptine on LH release in normal women. *J. Clin. Endocrinol. Metab., 52 :* 650-656.

Melis, G.B., Paoletti, A.M., Mais, V., Gambacciani, M., Guarnieri, G., Strigini, F., Fruzzetti, F., Fioretti, P. *1981.* — Inhibitory effect of the dopamine agonist bromocriptine on the postcastration gonadotropin rise in women. *J. Clin. Endocrinol. Metab., 53 :* 530-535.

Monroe, S.E., Levine, L., Chang, R.J., Keye, W.R., Jr., Yamamoto, M., Jaffe, R.B. *1981.* — Prolactin-secreting pituitary adenomas. V. Increased gonadotroph responsivity in hyperprolactinemic women with pituitary adenomas. *J. Clin. Endocrinol. Metab., 52 :* 1171-1178.

Moult, P.J.A., Rees, L.H., Besser, G.M. *1982.* — Pulsatile gonadotrophin secretion in hyperprolactinaemic amenorrhea and the response to bromocriptine therapy. *Clin. Endocrinol., 16 :* 153-162.

Müller, E.E., Camanni, F., Genazzani, A.R., Casanueva, F., Cocchi, D., Locatelli, V., Massara, F., Mantegazza, P. *1981.* — Dopamine-mimetic and antagonist drugs : Diagnostic and therapeutic applications in endocrine disorders. *Life Sci., 29 :* 867-883.

Nansel, D.D., Gudelsky, G.A., Porter, J.C., *1979.* — Subcellular localization of dopamine in the anterior pituitary gland of the rat : apparent association of dopamine with prolactin secretory granules. *Endocrinology, 105 :* 1073-1077.

Negro-Vilar, A., Ojeda, S.R., McCann, S.M. *1979.* — Catecholaminergic modulation of luteinizing hormone-releasing hormone release by median eminence terminals in vitro. *Endocrinology, 104 :* 1749-1757.

Okon, E., Koch, Y. *1976.* — Localisation of gonadotropin-releasing and thyrotropin-releasing hormones in human brain by radio-immunoassay. *Nature, 263 :* 345-347.

Oldendorf, W.H. *1971* —Brain uptake of radiolabeled amino acids, amines and hexoses after arterial injection. *Am. J. Physiol., 221 :* 1629-1639.

Olson, G.A., Olson, R.D., Kastin, A.J., Coy, D.H. *1981* — Endogenous opiates : 1980. *Peptides, 2 :* 349-369.

Ondo, J.G. *1974* — Gamme-aminobutyric acid effects on pituitary gonadotropin secretion. *Science, 186 :* 738-739.

Pinter, E.J., Tolis, G., Friesen, H.G. *1975* — L-dopa, growth hormone and adipokinesis in the lean and the obese. *Int. J. Clin. Pharmacol., 12 :* 277-280.

Plant, T.M., Krey, L.C., Moossy, J., McCormack, J.T., Hess, D.L., Knobil, E. *1978* — The arcuate nucleus and the control of gonadotropin and prolactin secretion in the female rhesus monkey (Macaca mulatta). *Endocrinology, 102 :* 52-62.

Polansky, S., Muechler, E. & Sorrentino, S. *1976* — The effect of L-dopa and clomiphene citrate on peripheral plasma levels of luteinizing hormone-releasing factor. *Obstetrics Gynecol., 48 :* 79-83.

Pontiroli, A.E., Alberetto, M., Pellicciotta, G., e Silva, E., Pasqua, A., Girardi A.M., Pozza, G. *1980* — Interaction of dopaminergic and antiserotoninergic drugs in the control of prolactin and LH release in normal women. *Acta Endocrinol. 93 :* 271-276.

Pucci, E., Franchi, F., Kicovic, P.M., Sgrilli, R., Barletta, D., Argenio, G.F., Casperi, M., Bernini, G.P., Luisi, M. *1981* — Amplification of LH response to LHRH by dopamine infusion in eugonadal women. *J. Endocrinol. Invest., 4 :* 55-58.

Quigley, M.E., Judd, S.J., Gilliland, G.B.,Yen, S.S.C. *1979* — Effect of a dopamine antagonist on the release of gonadotropin and prolactin in normal women and women with hyperprolactinemic anovulation. *J. Clin. Endocrinol. Metab., 48 :* 718-720.

Quigley, M.E., Sheehan, K.L., Casper, R.F., Yen, S.S.C. *1980* — Evidence for increased dopaminergic and opioid activity in patients with hypothalamic hypogonadotropic amenorrhea. *J. Clin. Endocrinol. Metab., 50 :* 949-954.

Raymond, V., Beaulieu, M., Labrie, F. *1978* — Potent antidopaminergic activity of estradiol at the pituitary level on prolactin release. *Science, 200 :* 1173-1175.

Rebar, R.W., Harman, S.M., Vaitukaitis, J.L. *1978* — Differential responsiveness to LRF after estrogen therapy in women with hypothalamic amenorrhea. *J. Clin. Endocrinol. Metab., 46 :* 48-54.

Reschini, E., Ferrari, C., Peracchi, M., Fadini, R., Meschia, M. Crosignani, P.G. *1980* — Effect of dopamine infusion on serum prolactin concentration in normal and hyperprolactinaemic subjects; *Clin. Endocrinol., 13 : 519-523.*

Robyn, C., Delvoye, P., Van Exter, C., Vekemans, M., Caufriez, A., de Nayer, P., Delogne-Desnoeck, J., L'Hermite, M. *1977* — Physiological and pharmacological factors influencing prolactin secretion and their relation to human reproduction. *In : Prolactin and Human Reproduction.* Crosignani, P.G. and Robyn, C. (eds) pp. 71-96, New York, Academic Press.

311

Rush, M.E., Ashiru, O.A., Blake, C.A. *1980* — Hypothalamic-pituitary interactions during the periovulatory secretion of follicle-stimulating hormone in the rat. *Endocrinology, 107 :* 649-655.

Santen, R.J., Bardin, C.W. *1973* — Episodic luteinizing hormone secretion in man. *J. Clin. Invest., 52 :* 2617-2628.

Sarda, A.K., Barnes, M.A., Nair, R.M.G. *1981* — Inter-relationship between changing patterns of LHRH and gonadotrophins in the menstrual cycle. *Clin. Endocrinol., 15 :* 265-273.

Sarkar, D.K., Fink, G. *1981* — Gonadotropin-releasing hormone surge : Possible modulation through postsynaptic α-adrenoreceptors and two pharmacologically distinct dopamine receptors. *Endocrinology, 108 :* 862-867.

Sawyer, C.H. *1975* — Some recent developments in brain-pituitary-ovarian physiology. *Neuroendocrinology, 17 :* 97-124.

Sawyer, C.H., Radford, H.M., Krieg, R.J., Carrer, H.F. *1978* — Control of pituitary-ovarian function by brain catecholamines and LH-releasing hormone. *In : Brain-Endocrine interaction. III. Neuronal hormone and reproduction.* Scott, D.E., Kizowski, G.P. and Weindl, A. (ed.), pp. 263-273. Basel, Karger.

Schmidt-Gollwitzer, M., Hardt, W., Bott, H., Nevinny-Stickel, J. *1979* — Untersuchungen zur Gonadotropin Sekretion nach intravenöser Gabe von Œstradiol bei norm— und hyperprolaktinämischen geschlechtsreifen Frauen. *Arch. Gynecol. 228 :* 592-594.

Schneider, H.P.G., McCann, S.M., *1969* — Possible role of dopamine as transmitter to promote discharge of LH-releasing factor. *Endocrinology, 85 :* 121-132.

Selmanoff, M. *1981* — The lateral and medial median eminence : Distribution of dopamine, norepinephrine, and luteinizing hormone-releasing hormone and the effect of prolactin on catecholamine turnover. *Endocrinology, 108 :* 1 716-1 722.

Selmanoff, M.K., Pramik-Holdaway, M.J., Weiner, R.I. *1976* — Concentrations of dopamine and noreprinephrine in discrete hypothalamic nuclei during the rat estrous cycle. *Endocrinology, 99 :* 326-329.

Shaar, C.J., Clemens, J.A. *1974* — The role of catecholamines in the release of anterior pituitary prolactin in vitro. *Endocrinology, 95 :* 1 202-1 212.

Shaw, R.W., Butt, W.R., London, D.R., Marshall, J.C. *1975* — The œstrogen provocation test : A method of assessing the hypothalamic-pituitary axis in patients with amenorrhoea. *Clin. Endocrinology, 4 :* 267-276.

Snyder, S.H., Goodman, R.R. *1980* — Multiple neurotransmitter receptors. *J. Neurochem. 35 :* 5-15.

Sowers, J.R., McCallum, R.W., Hershman, J.M., Carlson, H.E., Sturdevant, R.A.L., Meyer, N. *1976* — Comparison of metoclopramide with other dynamic tests of prolactin secretion. *J. Clin. Endocrinol. Metab. 43 :* 679-681.

Spellacy, W.N., Cantor, B., Kalra, P.S., Buhi, W.C., Bird, S.A. *1978* — The effect of varying prolactin levels on pituitary luteinizing hormone and follicle-stimulating hormone response to gonadotropin-releasing hormone. *Am. J. Obstet. Gynecol., 132 :* 157-163.

Spitz, I.M., Trestian, S., Cohen, H., Arnon, N., LeRoith, D. *1979* — Failure of metoclopramide to influence LH, FSH and TSH secretion or their response to releasing hormones. *Acta Endocrinol. 92 :* 640-647.

Strauch, G., Valcke, J.C., Mahoudeau, J.A., Bricaire, H. *1977* — Hormonal changes induced by bromocriptine (CB-154) at the early stage of treatment. *J. Clin. Endocrinol. Metab. 44 :* 588-590.

Thorner, M.O., Besser, G.M., Hagen, C., McNeilly, A.S. *1974* — Introduction of a new stimulation test for prolactin : the sulpiride test ; a comparison with other dynamic function tests. *J. Endocrinol., 43 :* p.lxxxii.

Thorner, M.O., McNeilly, A.S., Hagen, C., Besser, G.M. *1974a* — Long-term treatment of galactorrhoea and hypogonadism with bromocriptine. *Br. Med. J. i,* 419-422.

Thorner, M.O., Flückiger, E., Calne, D.B. *1980* — *Bromocriptine. A clinical and pharmacological review*, pp. 1-99, New York, Raven Press.

Tolis, G., Pinter, E.J., Friesen, H.G. *1975* — The acute effect of 2-bromo-a-ergocryptine (CB-154) on anterior pituitary hormones and free fatty acids in man. *Int. J. Clin. Pharmacol. 12 :* 281-283.

Tormey, W.P., Buckley, M.P., Taaffe, W., O'Kelly, D.A., Darragh, A. *1981* — Prolactin responsiveness to repeated decremental doses of sulpiride. *Horm. Metab. Res. 13 :* 454-455.

Travaglini, P., Montanari, C., Ballabio, R.E., Scarperrotta, R.C., Faglia, G. *1981* — Effects of increased central dopaminergic tonus on gonadotropin secretion. *J. Endocrinol. Invest., 4 :* 237-240.

Vijayan, E., McCann, S.M. *1978* — Re-evaluation of the role of catecholamines in control of gonadotropin and prolactin release. *Neuroendocrinology, 25 :* 150-165.

White, M.C., Rosenstock, J., Banks, L., Bydde, G., Mashiter, K., Joplin, G.F. *1981* — Increased dopaminergic activity in women with prolactinomas. *Neuroendocrine Letters, 3 :* 329.

Wise, P.M., Rance, N., Barraclough, C.A. *1981* — Effects of estradiol and progesterone on catecholamine turnover rates in discrete hypothalamic regions in overiectomized rats. *Endocrinology, 108 :* 2186-2193.

Wurtman, R.J., Larin, F., Mostafapour, S., Fernstrom, J.D. *1974* — Brain catechol synthesis : Control by brain tyrosine concentration. *Science, 185 :* 183-184.

312

Yen, S.S.C., Lein, A. *1976* — The apparent paradox of the negative and positive feedback control system on gonadotropin secretion. *Am. J. Obstet. Gynecol., 126 :* 942-950.

Yen, S.S.C., Lasley, B.L., Wang, C.F., Leblanc, H., Siler, T.M. *1975* — The operating characteristics of the hypothalamic-pituitary system during the menstrual cycle and observations of biological action of somatostatin. *Recent Prog. Horm. Res. 31 :* 321-357.

Zárate, A., Canales, E.S., Soria, J., Maneiro, P.J., MacGregor, C. *1973* — Effects of acute administration of L-dopa on serum concentrations of follicle-stimulating hormone (FSH) and luteinizing hormone (LH) in patients with the amenorrhea-galactorrhea syndrome. *Neuroendocrinology, 12 :* 362-365.

DISCUSSION

D. Lefaucheur

I wanted to ask if you think that LH is predominantly, as you have shown, under a positive control of LHRH and negative control from peripheral steroids and that FSH is predominantly under negative control from inhibine ?

C. Hagen

I take your point, but I do not think that the inhibine story is that well elucidated. The molecular weight, exact molecular structure and other biochemical and physiological parameters for inhibine have only been partially discovered. Secondly, the rise in FSH and the later rise in LH around the time of the rise in estradiol is similar to the pituitary gonadal event during puberty, which suggests to me that these patients are going through a new puberty.

K. Fuxe

I very much enjoyed your paper which really gives further support for the view, that there may be an inhibitory dopaminergic regulation of the LHRH secretion of human beings. With regard to the choice of blockers, the problem is of course that we have not yet been able to fully characterize what type of dopamine receptor population we have in the median eminence and I would like to hear your reasons for choosing metoclopramide and if you have had any ideas about testing further types of dopamine receptor blocking agents ?

C. Hagen

There was not much of a choice, because metoclopramide was the only drug which was registered in Denmark at the time of the study. Do you have any suggestions for another drug which would be more specific or better in this respect ?

K. Fuxe

No, I think that we do not have enough knowledge. Now we ourselves have started with receptor autoradiography to really characterize the median eminence dopamine receptor. So far, the biochemistry of that area in classical binding experiments is insufficient to allow us to really make any firm recommendation. We will just have to wait for a little while and hope to give some suggestions to you later on.

P. Grof

I was wondering whether you could elaborate on the confusing issue of bromocryptine and hyperprolactinaemic women ? Also, do you see many affective changes in the hyperprolactinaemic women ? The endocrinologists in these situations generally recommend treatment with bromocryptine and what happens, is that there is usually an improvement, but it is somewhat short-lasting and the patients seem to slip back. I would be interested in your thoughts about that.

C. Hagen

First of all, we do not see any psychological changes in women with hyperprolactinaemia. Secondly, I think we are talking about 2 groups of patients. The patients I was referring to had hyperprolactinaemia (prolactin above 50 ng/ml) not due to drugs or any other known factor, which usually harbours a pituitary tumor, whereas your patients have hyperprolactinaemia due to changes in central dopamine activity without a pituitary tumor. My experience with this last group of patients is very limited. I have no experience in treating patients with medically-induced hyperprolactinaemia, but I cannot see why it should not be possible. I do not know what happens to the effect of the psychotropic drug administered.

P. Grof

In the cases I mentioned there were no psychotropic drugs involved prior to the administration of bromocryptine. These ladies actually happen to be extraordinarily refractory to antidepressants and they are hypersensitive to side effects. So, if one tries some psychoactive drugs, one usually gives up pretty quickly and the ladies end up without psychiatric drugs until bromocryptine is tried.

C. Hagen

I have no comment on that.

P. Grof

In a way, this issue may tie up partly with Dr. Post's presentation on the dopamine role in affective disorders.

314

Dopamine in the symptoms and treatment of affective illness

R.M. Post[1], and D.C. Jimerson[2]

1) Biological Psychiatry Branch, and 2) Laboratory of Clinical Science, National Institute of Mental Health, Bethesda, U.S.A.

Summary : Although the catecholamine hypothesis of affective illness was formulated largely based on indirect pharmacological data from drugs that affected both norepinephrine (NE) and dopamine (DA), but until recently only NE mechanisms have been considered in detail. However, pharmacological, biochemical, endocrinological and direct evidence suggests that dopaminergic mechanisms may also be involved. Dopaminergic agonists such as piribedil and bromocriptine have been reported to have antidepressant effects. Moreover, a variety of commonly used antidepressants appear to induce DA autoreceptor subsensitivity measured physiologically (Antelman et al.) or biochemically (Gessa et al.). Apomorphine also produces greater prolactin inhibition in depressed compared to normal male volunteer subjects. Depressed patients with lower levels of the DA metabolite homovanillic acid (HVA) have been reported to respond better to several types of antidepressant treatments (piribedil, nomifensine, levodopa, and sleep deprivation) and to have a differential longitudinal course of affective symptoms.
Since DA has also been implicated in changes in motor activity, cognitive function, arousal, and self-stimulation reward in animals, its possible role in alterations in human affective disorder and its drug treatment should be reconsidered.

Introduction

Several different lines of evidence implicate dopaminergic alterations in affective illness. In this manuscript, we briefly review this evidence and discuss how the newly discovered treatment of manic-depressive illness, carbamazepine, might affect dopaminergic systems. Evidence suggestive of dopaminergic involvement in affective illness includes : 1) indirect pharmacological data ; 2) treatment response using dopamine agonists and antagonists ; 3) increasing evidence that commonly used psychotropic agents may alter dopaminergic function (there is evidence that major antidepressant modalities desensitize dopaminergic autoreceptors) ; and 4) measurement of dopaminergic function in man using the cerebrospinal fluid dopamine metabolite, homovanillic acid (HVA), and endocrine markers such as prolactin thought to be in part under dopaminergic regulation.

Dopamine agonists in depression

Indirectly acting dopamine agonists such as levodopa and direct dopamine agonists such as piribedil and bromocriptine have been reported to have antidepressant effects in a small series of patients. Van Praag and Korf (1975) reported antidepressant effects, particularly in retarded depressed patients with levodopa. Goodwin and associates (1970) found that levodopa treatment might increase agitation and psychosis in unipolar depressed patients and might be associated with the

315

switch into hypomania in bipolar patients. They concluded that levodopa was not a satisfactory antidepressant treatment modality, although it could be associated with psychomotor activation in selected patients.

Angrist et al. (1975), Post et al. (1978, 1979), and Shopsin and Gershon (1978) studied antidepressant effects of the dopamine agonist, piribedil. In contrast to Shopsin and Gershon (1978) who noted consistent dysphoric activation of patients treated with higher doses of piribedil, Post and associates (1978, 1979) observed mild to moderate antidepressant effects in the majority of patients (12 of the first 16 patients). Following placebo substitution, these patients tended to show relapses to the prior level of clinical depression, although, in several instances, depressed patients treated with piribedil showed marked antidepressant effects and clinical remission which persisted following piribedil discontinuation. Dysphoric activation and the induction of manic episodes (Gerner et al., 1976) were observed in isolated instances in only three patients. Exacerbation of depression was not observed at initial low doses of piribedil as has been noted following administration of the dopamine agonist apomorphine (Tesarova, 1972). Low doses of piribedil have been associated with antimanic effects in 3 of 4 patients studied (Post et al., 1976).

It is of interest in the studies of van Praag and Korf (1975) and Post et al. (1978) that those patients with lower levels of HVA in cerebrospinal fluid responded best to levodopa or piribedil treatment. These findings are consistent with those of van Scheyen et al. (1977) who found that lower levels of HVA in cisternal spinal fluid predicted better response to the dopamine-active antidepressant nomifensine.

Recent studies using another dopamine agonist, bromocriptine, have also reported that it was associated with improvement in depression. Colonna et al. (1979) observed marked antidepressant responses in 3, and mild responses in 5 of 12 patients in an open study. In blind studies, Waehrens and Gerlach (1981) and Nordin et al. (1981) reported improvement in 11 of 13 and 9 of 12 depressed patients respectively.

Antidepressant efficacy has been reported for several newer atypical drugs with effects on dopamine reuptake, release, or other indirect actions. Among these agents, nomifensine and buproprion are thought to have relatively selective effects on central dopamine systems (Cooper et al., 1980).

Effects of antidepressant treatment modalities on dopaminergic mechanisms

Until recently, most theories of the mechanism of action of antidepressants have implicated noradrenergic or serotonergic effects. However, evidence is accumulating that a variety of antidepressant modalities (including tricyclics, monoamine oxidase inhibitors, and electroconvulsive therapy) may affect dopaminergic function and produce desensitization of dopamine autoreceptors. Serra et al. (1979) have demonstrated that treatment of rats with tricyclic antidepressant agents attenuated apomorphine-induced decreases in brain HVA. These workers have also shown that this effect occurs following monoamine oxidase or electroconvulsive treatment. These biochemical data, consistent with a desensitization of dopaminergic autoreceptors, are paralleled by recent electrophysiological studies of Chiodo and Antelman (1980a, 1980b, 1981). These investigators found that tricyclic antidepressants, monoamine oxidase inhibitors, and

316

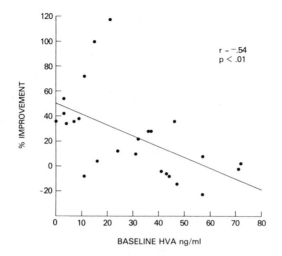

Fig. 1 - Low pretreatment HVA in cerebrospinal fluid and antidepressant response to sleep deprivation.

ECT all decreased responsivity of dopaminergic neurons in the zona compacta of the substantia nigra to low doses of parenterally administered apomorphine. These electrophysiological data thus suggest that dopaminergic autoreceptors may be desensitized with chronic antidepressant treatment. Chiodo and Antelman (1980a) noted that a chronic time course was necessary before the dopaminergic autoreceptor desensitization occurred. However, a single ECT followed by a delay was as effective in desensitizing dopamine autoreceptors as was chronic ECT administration. These data suggest that the period of time elapsed following initiation of treatment was as important in this instance as maintenance of the chronic treatment. The clinical relevance and application of these observations remain to be directly clinically tested however.

The biochemical and electrophysiological observations noted are consistent with the behavioral observations of increased responsivity to dopamine agonists following chronic ECT (Modigh, 1975, 1976 ; Deakin et al., 1981). The predicted activation of central dopaminergic pathways by antidepressant treatment has further been demonstrated by Fibiger and Phillips (1981). They studied intracranial self-stimulation in the rat and documented increased responsiveness in the mesolimbic dopamine pathway following long-term treatment with desimipramine.

In addition to classical antidepressant modalities which are thought to affect dopaminergic mechanisms, other new procedures with antidepressant efficacy may also affect dopamine. For example, the non pharmacological approach of one night's sleep deprivation often results in moderate to marked antidepressant effects in approximately one-half of severely depressed patients studied. Gerner et al. (1979) observed that a greater antidepressant response to sleep deprivation was associated with lower levels of HVA in cerebrospinal fluid obtained during a baseline medication-free interval (Fig. 1). It is of interest that in healthy volunteers, sleep deprivation has been reported to decrease growth hormone response to

317

apomorphine ; the prolactin response was unaltered (Lal et al., 1981). In laboratory animals, REM sleep deprivation, which has also been reported to be associated with antidepressant effects in depressed patients (Vogel et al., 1977), decreased the sensitivity of pre-synaptic dopamine receptors utilizing indirect behavioral measures (Serra et al., 1981). Thus, these clinical and laboratory studies of sleep deprivation and REM deprivation and possible relationship to low HVA in cerebrospinal fluid provide additional evidence consistent with the view that classical antidepressants may alter central dopaminergic mechanisms.

Antimanic and antidopaminergic effects

The well known antimanic effects of traditional neuroleptics (Randrup et al., 1975) is thought to be mediated through blockade of dopamine receptors (Snyder et al., 1974). Moreover, the relatively specific dopamine receptor antagonist, pimozide, has antimanic effects that roughly parallel those of the more traditional neuroleptics, thioridazine and chlorpromazine (Post et al., 1980b). While pimozide has effects on other neurotransmitter systems, including norepinephrine, considerable evidence suggests that its antidopaminergic effects might be associated with its efficacy in treating mania.

It is also possible that antidepressant and antimanic effects of lithium carbonate may be related to effects on dopaminergic mechanisms. Klawans et al. (1977) and Pert et al. (1978) have suggested that the effects of lithium carbonate treatment could be mediated through its ability to prevent the development of post-synaptic dopamine receptor supersensitivity as demonstrated in the neuroleptic withdrawal supersensitivity model. In the studies of Pert et al. (1978), there was behavioral and biochemical evidence that dopamine receptor supersensitivity was blocked by lithium co-treatment, suggesting the possibility that stabilization of dopamine receptors could be associated with their therapeutic effects of lithium carbonate. It is of considerable interest that Ross et al. (1981) and Coffey et al. (1982) have reported that lithium carbonate ameliorates the « on-off » phenomenon observed following chronic treatment of Parkinson's disease with levodopa or dopamine agonists. These findings suggest the possibility that lithium may be stabilizing dopamine receptor function in not only the cyclic mood and behavioral manifestations of affective illness, but also in the cyclic motor oscillations of the « on-off » syndrome. It is also noteworthy that another treatment of both phases of affective illness, ECT, has been reported useful in the treatment of the « on-off » syndrome in some studies (Balldin et al., 1980) but not others (Ward et al., 1980).

Possible effects of carbamazepine on dopaminergic mechanisms

Recent evidence from double-blind clinical trials suggest that carbamazepine may have acute antimanic and antidepressant effects as well as prophylactic effects in the treatment of affective illness (Ballenger and Post, 1978, 1980 ; Post et al., 1981, 1982 ; Okuma et al., 1979, 1981). As illustrated in Figure 2, there is a roughly similar time course of onset of antimanic effects of carbamazepine compared to similarly diagnosed and rated patients treated with the neuroleptic, pimozide, or with lithium carbonate. These findings of the antimanic effect of carbamazepine are consistent with double-blind observations in individual patients of repeated im-

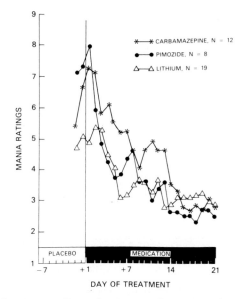

Fig. 2 - Time course of antimanic effects of carbamazepine compared to lithium and pimozide.

provement during administration of active compound and exacerbations of symptomatology when placebo is substituted (Ballenger and Post, 1978, 1980 ; Post et al., 1981, 1982). In this fashion, we have obtained unequivocal clinical evidence of response to carbamazepine in some patients who showed no evidence of prior response to traditional psychotropic agents, including lithium carbonate. Our preliminary evidence is also suggestive of antidepressant effects of carbamazepine. Of the first 25 patients to enter our study, 48 % showed evidence of antidepressant response. Thus, it appears that while lithium and carbamazepine may share a similar spectrum of clinical efficacy in affective illness, individual patients may respond to one but not the other treatment modality. Our emerging evidence, as well as that of Okuma et al. (1981), is consistent with the idea that carbamazepine may become a clinically useful alternative treatment modality for the acute and prophylactic management of affective illness.

The mechanisms underlying the clinical efficacy of carbamazepine are not known. Possible effects on noradrenergic, serotonergic, and GABA-minergic neurotransmitters as well as on opioid and vasopressinergic peptide systems are discussed in detail elsewhere (Post et al., 1983). In this manuscript, we discuss the possible effects of carbamazepine on dopaminergic mechanisms. Although the time course of antimanic response is similar to that of the neuroleptics, there is no direct or indirect evidence that carbamazepine blocks dopamine receptors. In animals, carbamazepine does not significantly block cocaine or amphetamine-induced hyperactivity (Koella et al., 1976 ; Post et al., 1983). Reynolds (1975) has reviewed the neurological side effects of carbamazepine in man and has indicated that the drug does not produce Parkinsonian side effects such as those usually associated

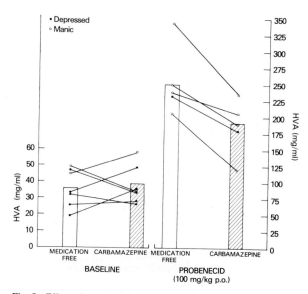

Fig. 3 - Effect of carbamazepine on cerebrospinal fluid HVA in affectively ill patients.

with classical neuroleptic administration. There are also no reports of the development of tardive dyskinesia even with long-term carbamazepine treatment of patients with seizure disorders and trigeminal neuralgia.

Consistent with this behavioral evidence that carbamazepine does not block dopamine receptors are the biochemical observations that the compound does not significantly increase HVA in rat brain (Morselli et al., 1977 ; Elhwuegi, 1978) or human spinal fluid (Post et al., 1983). As illustrated in Figure 3, there is no significant effect of carbamazepine on baseline levels of HVA in cerebrospinal fluid. Moreover, probenecid-induced accumulations of HVA (thought to represent a better measure of dopamine turnover in man) are actually significantly reduced on carbamazepine compared to patients studied during medication-free evaluation. Although the significant reductions in probenecid-induced accumulations on carbamazepine remain to be thoroughly documented in a larger series of patients, these apparent reductions are consistent with the direction of change that one might observe following treatment with a dopamine agonist. For example, administration of the dopamine agonist, piribedil, also significantly decreases cerebrospinal fluid HVA in man (Post et al., 1978).

Classical neuroleptic agents produce moderate to marked increases in prolactin in plasma or cerebrospinal fluid. This increase in prolactin levels has been used as a biochemical research tool as well as a marker for clinical compliance. In contrast to the robust increases in prolactin observed with neuroleptics, prolactin changes on carbamazepine are statistically significant, but usually of small magnitude and not clinically substantial. London et al. (1980) reported borderline elevation of basal prolactin levels on carbamazepine compared to placebo. Increased prolactin response to TRH or arginine stimulation tests has also been observed

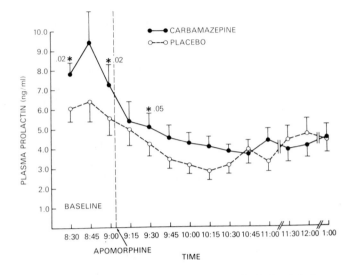

Fig. 4 - Effect of carbamazepine on plasma prolactin levels before and after apomorphine.

(London et al., 1980 ; Gold et al., 1981). As illustrated in Figure 4, basal prolactin levels were significantly elevated on carbamazepine compared to placebo treatment in affectively ill patients in studies in collaboration with N. Cutler, P.W. Gold, G. Brown and J.C. Ballenger. Apomorphine administration significantly reduced prolactin levels in patients both on and off carbamazepine. There is also no significant effect of chronic treatment with the dopamine agonist, piribedil, on apomorphine-induced suppression of prolactin secretion.

Thus, the behavioral, biochemical, and endocrine profile of effects of carbamazepine does not currently clarify the nature of its possible effects on dopaminergic mechanisms. There is no indirect evidence that it blocks dopamine receptors as do neuroleptics. Its minor degree of prolactin elevation is of interest in relation to the recent report that, compared to male normal volunteers, depressed patients had a trend toward lower baseline prolactin levels and significantly lower levels after apomorphine (0.75 mg) (Jimerson et al., 1981). These neuroendocrine findings would also be consistent with the recent observation of state-dependent tardive dyskinesia in rapidly cycling manic-depressive patients. Tardive dyskinesia, thought to be mediated in part by dopaminergic supersensitivity, was consistently worsened in depressed compared to manic phases of the illness (Cutler et al., 1981). It is noteworthy that carbamazepine not only was effective in ameliorating the severe and rapid cycling affective illness in these patients, but following its prolonged administration there was suggestive evidence that the tardive dyskinesias were also improved (Cutler and Post, in press). These preliminary observations suggest the usefulness of controlled clinical trials of carbamazepine in patients with tardive dyskinesia. Carbamazepine has been reported to decrease GABA turnover (Bernasconi and Martin, 1979) even though it does not alter levels of brain GABA in

321

animals or cerebrospinal fluid GABA in man (Post et al., 1980a). It remains for further investigation to ascertain whether any of carbamazepine's indirect effects on dopaminergic indices are mediated through its effects on GABA metabolism.

The interesting clinical spectrum of efficacy of carbamazepine in seizure disorders, affective illness, and paroxysmal pain syndromes might provide additional clues for its possible biochemical and physiological mechanisms of action. We have also been particularly interested in determining whether its particular anticonvulsant efficacy in patients with temporal lobe epilepsy and in animal models of limbic seizures such as amygdala-kindling (Albright and Burnham, 1980) is related to its psychotropic efficacy in patients with affective illness. It is of interest that another anticonvulsant, valproic acid, which is also highly effective in inhibiting the amygdala-kindled compared to cortical-kindled focus (Albright and Burnham, 1980), has recently been reported by Emrich and associates (1980) to be useful in the treatment of a small number of patients with lithium-resistant rapidly cycling affective illness. Whether other anticonvulsant compounds prove to be of clinical use in the treatment of affective illness remains for further clinical investigation. Our first patient to be crossed over in a double-blind fashion to other anticonvulsants including valproic acid and phenytoin demonstrated no evidence of clinical response to either agent, although she was an unequivocal responder to carbamazepine (Post et al., 1983).

The findings that some anticonvulsant agents may be useful in the treatment of affective illness raise the question of why the major motor seizures of electroconvulsive therapy are highly effective in treating manic-depressive illness. One conceptual approach to the paradox that both seizures and anticonvulsant agents may be effective in the treatment of affective illness is derived from our recent studies suggesting that electroconvulsive seizures (ECS) in the rat may exert marked anticonvulsant and antikindling effects (Post et al., 1981b). We noted that ECS seizures compared to sham ECS administered six hours prior to amygdala stimulation markedly suppressed the development of kindling. Moreover, we observed in the second study that seven daily ECS, but not a single ECS with a six-day delay, substantially suppressed amygdala-kindled seizures for up to five days following this course of treatment. These data suggest the possibility that major motor seizures of ECS may, like carbamazepine, be capable of exerting a potent stabilizing influence on limbic system excitability and inhibit amygdala-kindled seizures. The mechanism underlying these findings remains to be further explored, but the fact that a single ECS was not as effective as multiple ECS in this paradigm suggests that dopamine autoreceptor subsensitivity, which develops after a single ECS with a delay (Chiodo and Antelman, 1980a), may not be associated with this effect.

Conclusions

While we have particularly highlighted the possible role for altered dopaminergic receptor mechanisms in affective illness in this paper, we are not suggesting that only dopaminergic mechanisms are importantly involved in the mechanisms of action of psychotropic drugs that are used in the treatment of depression and mania. Cogent evidence is currently available that noradrenergic, serotonergic, and GABA-minergic alterations may also underlie some of the symptoms of affective illness and be related to mechanism of action of efficacious treatment modalities. Thus, we are merely highlighting the evidence that dopaminergic alterations may also play an important role and should not be excluded from consideration in neurotransmitter theories of affective illness. Measurement of the dopamine metabolite homovanillic acid (HVA) in affectively ill patients provides some supportive evidence for dopaminergic alterations in some patients. As reviewed elsewhere (Post et al., 1980), the majority of baseline and probenecid-induced accumulation studies in depressed patients reveal reductions compared to controls. It is possible that these decreases in HVA reflect primary alterations in pre-synaptic neurotransmitter function, although it is also possible that they could reflect secondary or compensatory changes in response to altered receptor supersensitivity changes. As direct and indirect clinical measurements of dopamine receptor function become available in man, such as neuroendocrine responsivity, apomorphine-induced hypothermia (Cutler et al., 1979), and measurements of dopamine receptors on peripheral blood elements, it will be of particular interest to measure altered neurotransmitter and receptor function simultaneously.

Neurotransmitter and receptor approaches to study the illness and its pharmacological treatment continue to suggest the possibility that multiple neurotransmitter mechanisms, including dopaminergic alterations, might be involved. These data thus highlight the importance of ascertaining in clinical populations the relative specificity of antidepressant response to manipulation of one or another neurotransmitter system. Do the patients who respond to dopamine-active manipulations also respond to those that affect serotonergic and noradrenergic mechanisms, or do these patients form separate subgroups ? The answer to this and related questions are obviously of importance in conceptualizing mechanisms underlying the pathophysiology of affective illness.

Other areas for future investigation might include the use of relatively selective pre-synaptic dopamine agonists in the treatment of affective syndromes, careful studies of clinical correlates of patients with altered dopaminergic function, and further elucidation of the mechanisms underlying the dopaminergic effects of atypical treatments of affective illness such as carbamazepine, as well as the typical psychotropic agents such as antidepressants and lithium carbonate.

REFERENCES

Albright, P.S., Burnham, W.M. 1980 — Development of a new pharmacological seizure model : effects of anticonvulsants on cortical- and amygdala-kindled seizures in the rat. Epilepsia, 21 : 681-689.

Angrist, B., Thompson, H., Shopsin, B., Gershon, S. 1975 — Clinical studies with dopamine-receptor stimulants. Psychopharmacologia, 44 : 273-280.

Antelman, S.M., Chiodo, L.A. 1981 — Dopamine autoreceptor subsensitivity : a mechanism common to the treatment of depression and the induction of amphetamine psychosis. Biol. Psychiatry, 16 : 717-727.

Balldin, J., Eden, S., Granerus, A.K., Modigh, K., Svanborg, A., Walinder, J., Wallin, L. 1980 — Electroconvulsive therapy in Parkinson's syndrome with « on-off » phenomenon. J. Neural Transm., 47 : 11-21.

Ballenger, J.C., Post, R.M. 1978 — Therapeutic effects of carbamazepine in affective illness : a preliminary report. Commun. Psychopharmacol., 2 : 159-175.

Ballenger, J.C., Post, R.M. 1980 — Carbamazepine (Tegretol) in manic-depressive illness : a new treatment. Am. J. Psychiatry, 137 : 782-790.

Bernasconi, R., Martin, P. 1979 — Effects of antiepileptic drugs on the GABA turnover rate. Naunyn. Schmiedebergs Arch. Pharmacol. (suppl.) 307 : R63, Abstract # 251.

Chiodo, L.A., Antelman, S.M. *1980a* — Electroconvulsive shock : progressive dopamine autoreceptor subsensitivity independent of repeated treatment. *Science, 210* : 799-801.

Chiodo, L.A., Antelman, S.M. *1980b* — Repeated tricyclic antidepressants induce a progressive « switch » in the electrophysiological response to dopamine neurons to autoreceptor stimulation. *Eur. J. Pharmacol., 66* : 255-256.

Coffey, C.E., Ross, D.R., Olanow, C.W. — Treatment of the « on-off » phenomenon in Parkinsonism with lithium carbonate. *Ann Neurol.* (in press).

Colonna, L., Petit, M., Lepine, J.P. *1979* — Bromocriptine in affective disorders : a pilot study. *J. Affective Disord., 1* : 173-177.

Cooper, B.R., Hester, T.J., Maxwell, R.A. *1980* — Behavioral and biochemical effects of the antidepressant bupropion (wellbutrin) : Evidence for selective blockade of dopamine uptake *in vivo*. *J. Pharmacol. Exp. Ther., 215* : 127-134.

Cutler, N.R., Post, R.M. *1982* — State-related cyclical dyskinesias in manic-depressive illness. *J. Clin. Psychopharmacol.,* (in press).

Cutler, N.R., Post, R.M., Bunney, W.E., Jr. *1979* — Apomorphine hypothermia : an index of central dopamine receptor function in man. *Commun. Psychopharmacol., 3* : 375-382.

Cutler, N.R., Post, R.M., Rey, A.C., Bunney, W.E., Jr. *1981* — Depression-dependent dyskinesias in two cases of manic-depressive illness. *N. Engl. J. Med., 304* : 1088-1089.

Deakin, J.F.W., Owen, F., Cross, A.J., Dashwood, M.J. *1981* — Studies on possible mechanisms of action of electroconvulsive therapy : effects of repeated electrically induced seizures on rat brain receptors for monoamines and other neurotransmitters. *Psychopharmacology, 73* : 345-349.

Elhwuegi, A. *1978* — Antiepileptic drugs and monoamine metabolism in the brain. *Br. J. Pharmacol., 64* : 407P.

Emrich, H.M., von Zerssen, D., Kissling, W., Moller, H.-J., Windorfer, A. *1980* — Effect of sodium valproate in mania. The GABA-hypothesis of affective disorders. *Arch. Psychiatr. Nervenkr., 229* : 1-16.

Fibiger, H.C., Phillips, A.C. *1981* — Increased intracranial self-stimulation in rats after long-term administration of desipramine. *Science, 214* : 683-685.

Gerner, R.H., Post, R.M., Bunney, W.E., Jr. *1976* — A dopaminergic mechanism in mania. *Am. J. Psychiatry, 133* : 1177-1180.

Gerner, R.H., Post, R.M., Gillin, J.C., Bunney, W.E., Jr. *1979* — Biological and behavioral effects of one night's sleep deprivation in depressed patients and normals. *J. Psychiatr. Res., 15* : 21-40.

Gold, P., Ballenger, J.C., Post, R.M., Brown, G. *1980* — Unpublished observations.

Goodwin, F.K., Brodie, H.K.H., Murphy, D.L., Bunney, W.E., Jr. *1970* — L-DOPA, catecholamines, and behavior : a clinical and biochemical study in depressed patients. *Biol. Psychiatry, 2* : 341-366.

Jimerson, D.C., Cutler, N.R., Post, R.M., Rey, A., Gold, P.W., Brown, G.M., Bunney, W.E., Jr. *1980* — Prolactin alterations in depression and the effects of piribedil treatment. Presented at Annual Mtg., Society for Biological Psychiatry, Boston.

Klawans, H.L., Weiner, W.J. and Naudieda, P.A. *1977* — The effect of lithium on an animal model of tardive dyskinesia. *Prog. Neuropsychopharmacol., 1* : 53-60.

Kœlla, W.P., Levin, P., Baltzer, V. *1975* — The pharmacology of carbamazepine and some other anti-epileptic drugs. *In : Epileptic Seizures-Behavior-Pain*, W. Birkmayer (ed.), Berne, Hans Huber.

Lal, S., Thavundayil, J., Nair, N.P.V., Etienne, P., Rastogi, R., Schwartz, G., Pulman, J., Guyda, H. *1981* — Effect of sleep deprivation on dopamine receptor function in normal subjects. *J. Neural. Transm., 50* : 39-45.

London, D.R. *1980* — Hormonal effects of anticonvulsant drugs. *In : Advances in Epileptology*, R. Carger, F. Angeleri and J.K. Penry (eds.) pp. 399-405. New York, Raven Press.

Modigh, K. *1975* — Electroconvulsive shock and post-synaptic catecholamine effects : increased psychomotor stimulant action of apomorphine and clonidine in reserpine pretreated mice by repeated ECS. *J. Neural Transm., 36* : 19-32.

Modigh, K. *1976.* — Long-term effects of electroconvulsive shock therapy on synthesis turnover and uptake of brain monoamines. *Psychopharmacology, 49 :* 179-185.

Morselli, P.L., Calderini, G., Consolaziones, A., Riva, E., Altamura, C. *1977.* — Effect of carbamazepine on brain mediators in control and cobalt-treated rats. *In : Advances in Epileptology*, R. Carger, F. Angeleri and J.K. Penry (eds.), pp. 176-182, New York, Raven Press.

Nordin, C., Siwers, B., Bertilsson, L. *1981.* — Bromocriptine treatment of depressive disorders : clinical and biochemical effects. *Acta Psychiatr. Scand., 64 :* 25-33.

Okuma, T., Inanaga, K., Otsuki, S., Sarai, K., Takahashi, R., Hazama, H., Mori, A., Watanabe, M. *1979.* — Comparison of the antimanic efficacy of carbamazepine and chlorpromazine : a double-blind controlled study. *Psychopharmacology, 66 :* 211-217.

324

Okuma, T., Inanaga, K., Otsuki, S., Sarai, K., Takahashi, R., Hazama, H., Mori, A., Watanbe, M. *1981.* — A preliminary double-blind study of the efficacy of carbamazepine in prophylaxis of manic-depressive illness. *Psychopharmacology, 73 :* 95-96.

Pert, A., Rosenblatt, J.E., Sivit, C., Pert, C.B., Bunney, W.E., Jr. *1978.* — Long-term treatment with lithium prevents the development of dopamine receptor supersensitivity. *Science, 201 :* 171-173.

Post, R.M., Gerner, R.H., Carman, J.S., Bunney, W.E., Jr. *1976.* — Effects of low doses of a dopamine receptor stimulator in mania. *Lancet, 1 :* 203-204.

Post R.M., Gerner, R.H., Carman, J.S., Gillin, J.C., Jimerson, D.C., Goodwin, F.K., Bunney, W.E., Jr. *1978.* — Effects of a dopamine agonist piribedil in depressed patients : relationship of pretreatment homovanillic acid to antidepressant response. *Arch. Gen. Psychiatry, 35 :* 609-615.

Post, R.M., Gerner, R.H., Jimerson, D.C., Carman, J.S., Rey, A.C., Bunney, W.E., Jr. *1979.* — The effects of piribedil on mood, sleep, endocrine function and amine metabolism in depressed patients. *Psychologie Méd., 11 :* 143-154.

Post, R.M., Ballenger, J.C., Hare, T.A., Bunney, W.E., Jr. *1980a.* — Lack of effect of carbamazepine on gamma-aminobutyric acid levels in cerebrospinal fluid. *Neurology, 30 :* 1008-1011.

Post, R.M., Jimerson, D.C., Bunney, W.E., Jr., Goodwin, F.K. *1980b.* — Dopamine and mania : behavioral and biochemical effects of the dopamine receptor blocker pimozide. *Psychopharmacology, 67 :* 297-305.

Post, R.M., Putnam, F.W., Contel, N.R. *1981.* — Electroconvulsive shock inhibits amygdala kindling. Presented at the Annual Meeting, Society for Neuroscience, Los Angeles, October, 1981. *Abstracts of the 11th Annual Meeting of the Society for Neuroscience, 7 :* 587, Abstract # 187.13.

Post, R.M., Ballenger, J.C., Goodwin F.K. *1980.* — Cerebrospinal fluid studies of neurotransmitter function in manic depressive illness. *In : The Neurobiology of Cerebrospinal Fluid, vol. I,* J. Wood (ed.), pp. 685-717. New York, Plenum Press.

Post, R.M., Ballenger, J.C., Uhde, T.W., Chatterji, D.C., Bunney, W.E., Jr. *1982.* — Efficacy of the temporal-lobe limbic anticonvulsant carbamazepine in manic and depressive illness. *In : Proceedings of the 3rd World Congress of Biological Psychiatry,* B. Jansson, C. Perris and G. Struwe (eds.), Amsterdam, Elsevier, in press.

Post, R.M., Ballenger, J.C., Uhde, T.W., Bunney, W.E., Jr. *1983.* — Efficacy of carbamazepine in manic-depressive illness : implications for underlying mechanisms. *In : Neurobiology of the Mood Disorders,* R.M. Post and K.C. Ballenger (eds.), Baltimore, Williams and Wilkins, in press.

Post, R.M., Contel, N.R., Goldman, B. — Unpublished observations.

Randrup, A., Munkvad, I., Fog, R., Gerlach, J., Molander, L., Kjellberg, B., Scheel-Kruger, J. *1975.* — Mania, depression, and brain dopamine. *Curr. Dev. Psychopharmacol, 2 :* 205-248.

Reynolds, E.H. *1975.* — Neurotoxicity of carbamazepine. *In : Complex Partial Seizures and Their Treatment : Advances in Neurology, Vol. II,* J.K. Penry and D.D. Daly (eds.), pp. 345-353, New York, Raven Press.

Ross, D.R., Coffey, C.E., Ferren, E.L., Walker, J.I., Olanow, C.W. *1981.* — « On-off » syndrome treated with lithium carbonate : A case report. *Am. J. Psychiatry, 138 :* 1626-1627.

Serra, G., Argiolas, A., Klimek, V., Fadda, F., Gessa, G.L. *1979.* — Chronic treatment with antidepressants prevents the inhibitory effects of small doses of apomorphine on dopamine synthesis and motor activity. *Life Sci., 25 :* 415-424.

Serra, G., Melis, M.R., Argiolas, A., Fadda, F., Gessa, G.L. *1981.* — REM sleep deprivation induces subsensitivity of dopamine receptors mediating sedation in rats. *Eur. J. Pharmacol., 72 :* 131-135.

Shopsin, B. *1978.* — Dopamine receptor stimulation in the treatment of depression : piribedil (ET-495). *Neuropsychobiology, 4 :* 1-14.

Snyder, S.H., Banerjee, S.P., Yamamura, H.I., Greenberg, D. *1974.* — Drugs, neurotransmitters and schizophrenia. *Science, 184 :* 1243-1254.

Tesarova, O. *1972.* — Experimental depression caused by apomorphine and phenoharmane. *Pharmakopsychiatrie, 5 :* 13-19.

Van Praag, H.M., Korf, J. *1975.* — Serotonin metabolism in depression : clinical application of the probenecid test. *Int. Pharmacopsychiatry, 9 :* 35-51.

Van Scheyen, J.D., van Praag, H.M., Korf, J. *1977.* — Controlled study comparing nomifensine and clomipramine in unipolar depression using the probenecid technique. *Br. J. Clin. Pharmacol., 4 :* 1179S-1184S.

Vogel, G.W., McAbee, R., Barker, K., Thurmond, A. *1977.* — Endogenous depression improvement and REM pressure. *Arch. Gen. Psychiatry, 34 :* 96-97.

Waehrens, J., Gerlach, J. *1981.* — Bromocriptine and imipramine in endogenous depression : a double-blind controlled trial in outpatients. *J. Affective Dis., 3 :* 193-202.

Ward, C., Stern, G.M., Pratt, R.T.C., McKenna, P. *1980.* — Electroconvulsive therapy in Parkinsonian patients with the « on-off » syndrome. *J. Neural Transm., 49 :* 133-135.

DISCUSSION

M. Ackenheil

From the many data you presented, all of which we do not have time to discuss, I would like to ask three questions : Firstly, you mentioned a patient with tardive dyskinesia, without stating for how long he was treated with neuroleptics before, therefore, I would like to ask, if this really was a tardive dyskinesia, or if in his depressive phase he experienced movement disorders ? Spontaneous dyskinesia can occur without medication, as was reported in a study of an English group, Owen and colleagues, who found that dyskinetic movement disorders could be seen in patients who never had been previously treated with neuroleptics. According to this, dyskinetic movement disorders occur in patients without any medication, therefore, would it be possible that this was a movement disorder in relation to his depressive phase.

R.-M. Post

This patient was treated with high doses of neuroleptics, several thousand gram equivalents of chlorpromazine over a 10 to 15 year period in the State Hospital, so we presume that this was tardive dyskinesia. We are aware of the point that you raised, that spontaneous dyskinesias have been observed in patients never treated with neuroleptics and it is possible that this is not a tardive dyskinesia. Clinically, it looked like classical tardive dyskinesia and with this patient and with the other patients with very long-term neuroleptic history we presumed that it was a tardive dyskinesia. In any event, whether spontaneous or tardive, it very markedly fluctuated with depression and mania in this particular state-related fashion.

M. Ackenheil

I would assume that you agree with me, that it is not a concordant finding in depressions. Patients long-term treated with neuroleptics sometimes have depressive symptoms, but the incidence of tardive dyskinesia is normally not related to depressive phases.

R.-M. Post

They are several studies, which suggest that depressed patients may be at increased risk of tardive dyskinesia with neuroleptics. There are also several reports that improvement in depression with either tricyclics or ECT also improves the dyskinesia, so there may be an evolving story there.

M. Ackenheil

The other point concerned the neuroendocrine study with apomorphine and the prolactin suppression response. In studies with apomorphine, we also found the prolactin suppression response in schizophrenics, but did not investigate depressive patients. However, it is well known that the prolactin suppression response is not a very good index for the dopamine receptor sensitivity, the GH response would be a better index. Therefore, I would like to know which GH secretion you found in your patients after apomorphine ?

R.-M. Post
It was normal.

M. Ackenheil

It was normal thus, one could say that there was no change in the dopamine receptors.

R.-M. Post

No. I agree that the neuroendocrine evidence as well as some of the other evidence remains ambiguous, but the GH response is under the control of several neurotransmitters and if there is a consistent difference between the prolactin change and GH change, that may actually be interesting in looking at the underlying differences in neurotransmitter mechanisms in those 2 systems.

M. Ackenheil

So the problem is, even in patients in which big differences in GH response could be found, no changes in prolactin suppression were measurable, because prolactin suppression is dependent on

326

base line levels. Normally, prolactin is very low and only slight changes occur. To come to my last point, are there really studies existing, in which noradrenaline re-uptake inhibitors have been compared with dopamine agonists and in such studies, is the dopamine agonist therapeutically better than the tricyclics?

R.-M. Post

There is only one study and more need to be made. I think that the question also raises the very interesting issue of sub-groups and whether or not there is a sub-group of depressed patients who might respond to a dopamine active treatment, when they do not respond to more classical treatment. I think the evidence is quite early, as you are indicating.

P. Grof

It is very refreshing to listen to your presentation. I think it is a very original contribution. It seems to me that our thinking about affective disorders has been stuck for too long on noradrenaline. Such direction was very useful in the mid sixties' and stimulated a tremendous amount of research and contributed to the good name of biological psychiatry, but as time goes on, it is becoming more and more limiting. The kind of conceptual re-thinking that you are offering is, at this point, even more important for further progress than new data, because it will allow us to see much more the complexity of the picture. I think your contribution can really help us out of the depression-noradrenaline groove, where the thinking seems to be stuck. Just a couple of quick comments : The effect of carbamazepine in affective disorders : I was wondering whether you know that there was a study by Japanese authors around 1970 using high doses of imipramine in treating mania. Those doses would be perhaps more comparable with the dosage of carbamazepine that one is using. There is perhaps a similarity there and if you had a dose-dependent effect on receptors, this could contribute to an explanation of the effect. I do not think the study with high imipramine dosage has ever been replicated. Maybe someone in the audience knows of another study finding high doses of imipramine (300 — 600 mg per day) effective in mania, but it is a very interesting observation, particularly as the early carbamazepine work also came from Japan.

R.-M. Post

In terms of the imipramine response, we were aware of those reports and also looked at the literature and found that Don Klein (I am not sure if it was quite as high doses) did treat several patients with imipramine and was not able to replicate those findings. In addition, the emerging literature now on treatment of bipolar patients with tricyclic prophylaxis shows that it will clearly increase the liability for manic recurrences. Prophylaxis is not the same as acute treatment of the episode, but it looks like a classical tricyclic may not be capable of doing the same thing as carbamazepine, but I think it would be very interesting to repeat those early observations of the Japanese workers. I was not aware of that other apomorphine study, but in our volunteers we did see sedation, comparable degrees of sedation in both our depressed patients and our volunteers, and actually as the apomorphine effect wore off, we did see a rebound feeling of elation, so that there may be some mood changes acutely with that endocrine response.

J. Mendlewicz

I was very interested in your sleep deprivation data. If I understood correctly, that was total sleep deprivation?

R.-M. Post

Yes, for one night.

J. Mendlewicz

Do you have any data on the correlation between pre-treatment level of CSF HVA and treatment with sleep deprivation? Not for one night, but the whole sleep deprivation treatment in depression.

R.-M. Post

No, we did not do that. Several of the patients had repeated sleep deprivations and we found that with repetition most often the second and third sleep deprivation was not as effective as the first. In the data that I presented, the correlation between the low HVA response and the antidepressant response was to the first sleep deprivation.

B.-E. Leonard

I was very interested in your carbamazepine findings also. Two things : I noticed on your slide, you said that there was no change in 5-HIAA. I think there is some evidence from animal studies, that the drug affects serotonin metabolism (Julien et al., Adv. Neurol. 11, 263 ; Purdy et al., Epilepsia, 18, 251, 1977). More importantly, there is a finding in the clinical literature by Dewhurst (Nature 219, 506, 1968) that methysergide is effective in the treatment of mania. Now, that was an open trial admittedly, but this could fit in with the serotonergic effect of carbamazepine. I wonder if you have any comment on this ?

R.-M. Post

Morselli's group did not find 5-HIAA changes and Crunelli et al. have looked at carbamazepine's anticonvulsant effects in relation to serotonergic manipulations and raphe lesions and did not find a major serotonergic component to the anti-convulsant effects of carbamazepine. Those data and our 5-HIAA data in patients' spinal fluid were what I was referring to in terms of lack of major evidence of serotonergic changes.

U. Corsini

I would like to add a couple of points : One was on apomorphine's depressant effect. We have some experience on this point and we found that apomorphine at low dosages in humans induces a real depressive state. It is difficult to evaluate well, because of the short-lasting effect of the compound, but I think that Tesarova's findings, at least in our experience, have been confirmed. The second point adding to the dopamine hypothesis of depression is about sulpiride. I think that also sulpiride may be a good point for the dopamine hypothesis of depression, since sulpiride is supposed to be a dopamine receptor blocker or in some dosages, at least low dosages, to be a rather specific dopamine auto-receptor blocker, and in low dosage it has been shown that it has a clear-cut antidepressant effect, as we were able to show several times and as has been shown by several other authors too. So, I think that also sulpiride and the orthomethoxy-benzamides in general, but specifically sulpiride, may be considered also a good proof for the dopaminergic hypothesis of depression.

R.-M. Post

Yes, I think it would be very interesting to examine the suggestive evidence for antidepressant effects of sulpiride and other neuroleptics more systematically under controlled conditions and in terms of your first point about low doses increasing depression ; in our piribedil trial, as we were building the dose slowly initally, in order to avoid the side effects of nausea, we specifically looked into that low dose period, to see whether we were exacerbating depression in the beginning of the piribedil trial and found no evidence for that. We then achieved higher doses of piribedil similar to those used in Parkinson's disease, which were presumably working at post-synaptic sites, but in the low dose phase we found no evidence of increased depression, at least with piribedil.

N. Matussek

Only 2 questions : Piribedil, I think, also increases the noradrenaline turnover, which has been shown by some groups in animal experiments ? My second question is : Have you the impression (since you talk about sub-groups) or some data, saying that primary or secondary depressed patients differed in the HVA values ?

R.-M. Post

We have tried to systematically exclude patients who did not meet RDC criteria for primary major affective illness. We looked at the issue of a range atypically of depression within our whole group meeting criteria and HVA did not differentiate those 2 groups. However, almost all of the patients met criteria for RDC endogenous depression. On the first point I would agree that piribedil and its active metabolite are less clean than dopamine agonists and they do have effects on noradrenergic mechanisms, particularly in the very high doses employed in animal studies. I believe Fuxe has also demonstrated some changes in noradrenaline turnover in his studies as well, so that piribedil again is not that clean a drug and only a relatively selective dopamine agonist agent.

Laboratory indicators of recurrence risk in affective disorders

P. Grof, E. Grof, G.M. Brown

Affective Disorders Program and Departments of Psychiatry and Neurosciences, McMaster University, Hamilton, Ontario, Canada.

Summary : A major shift has taken place over the past two decades : Many affective disorders are now investigated and treated on long-term basis. If we want to adjust our management to the episodic recurrent nature of the disorders, it becomes imperative to search for laboratory indicators of recurrence liability. Several neuroendocrine responses appear to show some promise in this respect : elevated prolactin response to hypoglycemia, decreased response of TSH to TRH, and dexamethasone suppression test. To-date promising observations are based mainly on anecdotal reports. There is a need to investigate these responses in a systematic, integrated way and some principles of such exploration are briefly outlined.

In the past twenty years, psychiatry has changed dramatically. The advances are particularly visible in the treatment and research of affective disorders. While two decades ago, psychiatrists concentrated their treatment and research almost completely on the acute phase of the patient's illness, interest has in recent years shifted markedly to long-term issues. There are two main reasons for this shift : First, we have become more effective in preventing the episodes of affective illness and, second, the recurrent nature of affective disorders has been widely acknowledged. Thus, the interest of clinicians has focused on long-term treatment as an important strategy. Similarly, the emphasis in research on affective disorders has gradually shifted from exploring state-dependent variables during the acute illness to stressing trait-variables and markers of affective illness.

Clearly, there is good justification for this development, yet it also poses certain new problems. Long-term treatment in the current practice means chronic treatment. However, affective disorders are essentially intermittent in nature and it does not make much sense to treat episodic conditions in a chronic manner. In addition, most of the long-term side-effects are very clearly related to long-term uninterrupted administration of psychoactive substances. To wit, there is a significant correlation between the length of lithium administration and the extent of urinary concentration defect. Another example of a side-effect resulting from long-term treatment is, of course, tardive dyskinesia produced by neuroleptics. For episodic disorders it would make good sense to give medication only prior to and during the upcoming episode, as long as the drug is clearly needed. The paradigm for such approach may be the strategy Dr. Chazot mentioned in this symposium : His team gives lithium salts starting about four weeks prior to the time of risk for cluster headaches. It would make good sense to take a similar approach to the treatment of affective disorders.

Unfortunately, at present we can manage very few affective disorders in this intermittent manner. The main reason for treating affective disorders chronically is our inability to tell when the next recurrence will come. Clearly, studies on the clinical course of affective disorders, such as drug discontinuation studies, have shown that recurrences in a group of patients follow predictable patterns and do not tend to happen at a certain fixed point in time after the discontinuation of lithium. However, these findings do not help in predicting reliably a recurrence in an individual case. The only predictors of recurrences available to us at present are predictors of a clinical nature. Such predictors are to be found in the individual history of each patient.

First of all, one can state obviously that the patient with many frequent episodes in the past is likely to have another episode soon again, and is badly in need of effective preventative treatment. In addition, the most sensitive indicators of a high recurrence risk are high frequency of recent episodes, short length of recent free intervals, high number of previous episodes and the patient's age. In research, these clinical indicators achieve an impressive predictability of subsequent episodes, and have an acceptable statistical validity. Good quality data for such predictors can be frequently obtained in a research follow-up of patients. In practice, however, the clinician is, for several reasons, much less likely to obtain reliable data necessary for valid predictions. Clinical thinking is much more accustomed to performing a laboratory test and leaning heavily on laboratory results in clinical decisions.

If we had laboratory indicators of recurrence liability which would give a warning signal for a relapse before the clinical manifestations start developing, it would become possible to tailor the preventative treatment to the individual patterns of the disease. There has been a general paucity of studies into this problem. In the past, several indicators have been proposed as warning signs of an upcoming episode but none survived a closer scrutiny. However, recent research studies raised some hope in this respect and indicate that certain neuroendocrine responses may become detectibly altered prior to a recurrence. We will briefly review some of the pertinent findings of others as well as our own. The promising neuroendocrine responses appear to be : 1) cortisol response to dexamethasone suppression, 2) TSH response to TRH stimulation, 3) prolactin response to hypoglycemia.

Cortisol response

The ground work for the use of dexamethasone suppression test in this context was done by several investigators (Carroll, 1972b ; Albala et al., 1980 and 1981 ; de la Fuente, 1980 ; Goldberg, 1980a and 1980b ; Greden et al., 1980 and 1981) who showed that abnormal dexamethasone tests normalize with clinical improvement, that dexamethasone suppression tests may become positive even before the development of recurrence and that the failure of dexamethasone suppression tests to convert to normal is associated with early relapse (Carroll, 1972a ; Goldberg, 1980a ; Greden et al., 1980). Thus, Greden et al. (1981) were able to conclude recently that dexamethasone suppression was well suited for early prediction of impending relapse among previously diagnosed patients. The basis for this statement comes mainly from anecdotal observations and systematic work has not yet been completed.

TSH response

Similar observations have been gathered for the TSH response to TRH. It has been shown that reduced response returns to normal after clinical recovery (Mendlewicz et al., 1979) and that following the TRH stimulation a low TSH response may be associated with bad prognosis (Kirkegaard et al., 1975). In particular, a relapse appears impending if there is gradual decrease in the sequence of TSH responses (Langer et al. 1980, 1981).

Prolactin response

Less is known about the possible value of prolactin response. In general, in depression it has been found that prolactin response may be reduced to TRH (Gregoire et al., 1977, D'Agata et al., 1979) as well as to hypoglycemia (Kleesiek et al., 1980 ; Grof, E. et al., 1982) and also that the rhythm of prolactin responses may be altered (Nathan et al., 1980).

With regards to prolactin response to hypoglycemia, we have data on 24 subjects, 14 bipolar patients and 10 healthy controls. The background of the testing : In essence, a modified triple bolus challenge is given with angiocatheter inserted at 8:00 a.m., insulin stimulation given at 9:00 a.m., TSH and LHRH given at 11:00 a.m. Sampling takes place every 15 minutes and the responses of growth hormone, prolactin, cortisol, TSH, LH and blood sugar are determined. All patients we have tested in this context were suffering from bipolar primary affective disorder and met the RDC criteria. In addition, the diagnosis was confirmed by long-term follow up of each patient over several years. The subjects were all males, in order to avoid the confounding influence of the menstrual cycle. To allow a valid interpretation of the neuroendocrine findings, none of the subjects were obese, none suffered from a serious organic illness and none had a history of endocrine disorder. The average age was 46 years and at the time of testing the patients had been on lithium on the average for 7 years, with a mean standardized serum lithium level = 0.77 mEq/l. After the testing the treatment decisions were made on clinical grounds. The most interesting finding so far has been that of the 14 tested patients, 4 relapsed within the subsequent 3 months and showed a different prolactin response. The comparison of relapsing and nonrelapsing patients showed that relapsing and nonrelapsing patients did not differ in the GH response to insulin hypoglycemia and prolactin response to TRH, but they did behave differently in their prolactin response to hypoglycemia. This difference in response occurred in spite of the lack of difference in the degree of hypoglycemia. The association between low prolactin responses and the freedom from relapses was statistically significant (chi-square test).

Because of these promising findings in the pilot study we have decided to explore these questions systematically. In an integrated way we studied the hypothesis that the recurrence liability of affective disorders is associated 1) with an elevated prolactin response to insulin-induced hypoglycemia, 2) with decreased

331

response of TSH to TRH and 3) with the escape of plasma cortisol levels from dexamethasone suppression.

Ideally, the problem of the association between neuroendocrine responses and recurrence liability should be studied by serial testing of a representative sample of untreated patients with frequent recurrences. However, such a research strategy is not acceptable ethically and we have therefore initiated an alternative design with two groups of patients, both of them including carefully selected male and postmenopausal female bipolar patients.

We are doing longitudinal studies on 1) a group of patients with poorly stabilized illness to give us data about the predictive value of the responses ; 2) a well stabilized group of patients on and off medication, to give us data about the representativeness of the findings in unstable patients and about the effects of medication itself.

Positive findings in this area could provide laboratory tests which would improve the monitoring and managing of affective illness, and could result in an individually tailored, more effective treatment with less side effects. Moreover, with this approach valuable insights can be gained about the mechanisms of action of psychopharmacological treatment and the nature of the process leading to affective recurrences.

REFERENCES

Albala, A.A., Greden, J.F., Carroll B.J. *1980* — Serial dexamethasone suppression tests in affective disorders. *Am. J. Psychiatry, 137* : 383.

Albala, A.A., Greden, J.F., Tarika, J., Carroll, B.J. *1981* — Changes in serial dexamethasone suppression tests among unipolar depressives receiving electroconvulsive treatment. *Biol. Psychiatry (in press)*.

Carroll, B.J. *1972a* — The hypothalamic-pituitary axis : functions, control mechanisms and methods of study. *In : Depressive Illness*, B. Davies, B.J. Carroll and R.M. Mowbray (eds) pp. 23-68. Springfield. Charles C. Thomas.

Carroll, B.J. *1972b* — Control of plasma cortisol level in depression : Studies with the dexamethasone suppression test. *In : Depressive Illness*, B. Davies, B.J. Carroll and R.M. Mowbray, (eds) pp. 87-148. Springfield, Charles C. Thomas.

D'Agata, R., Paci, C., Buongiorno, G., Guilizia, S., Marchett, B., Gerendi, I., Polosa, P., Rapisarda, V., Scapagnini, U. *1979* — Abnormal response of prolactin to TRH stimulus in depression : *In : Neuroendocrine correlates in neurology and psychiatry*, Muller, E., and Anoli, A. (eds) pp. 273-281. (Amsterdam), Elsevier/North Holland.

De La Fuente, J.R., Rosenbaum, A.H. *1980* — Neuroendocrine dysfunction and blood levels of tricyclic antidepressants. *Am. J. Psychiatry, 137* : 1260-1261.

Goldberg, I.K. *1980a* — Dexamethasone suppression tests in depression and response to treatment. *Lancet, 2* : 91.

Goldberg, I.K. *1980b* — Dexamethasone suppression tests as an indicator of safe withdrawal of antidepressant therapy. *Lancet, 1* : 376.

Greden, J.F., Albala, A., Haskett, R.F., Carroll, B.J. *1980* — Normalization of dexamethasone suppression test : A laboratory index of recovery from endogenous depression. *Biol. Psychiatry, 15* : 449-458.

Greden, J.F., Devigne, J.P., Albala, A., Tarika, J., Butterham, M., Eiser, A., Carroll, B.J. *1981* — Postdexamethasone plasma cortisol levels among lithium-treated rapidly cycling bipolar patients. *In : The Prediction of Lithium Response*, H. Dufour (ed), Paris, Economica.

Gregoire, F., Brauman, H., De Buck, R., Corvilain, J. *1977* — Hormone release in depressed patients before and after recovery. *Psychoneuroendocrinology, 2* : 303-312.

Grof, E., Brown, G.M., Grof, P. *1982* — Neuroendocrine responses as an indicator of recurrence liability in primary affective illness. *Br. J. Psychiat., 140* : 320-334.

Kirkegaard, C., Norlem, N., Lauridsen, U., Bjorum, N. *1975* — Prognostic value of thyroptropin-releasing hormone stimulation test in endogenous depressions. *Acta. Psychiatr. Scand., 52* : 170-177.

Kleesiek, K., Czernik A., Eberhard, A., *1980* — Klinisch-chemische Diagnostik depressiver Syndrome. *J. Clin. Chem. Clin. Biochem., 18* : 867-877.

332

Langer, G., Schonbeck, G., Koinig, G., Reiter, H., Schussler, M., Reiter, H., *1980* — Neuroendocrine status of depressed patients at admission and during antidepressant drug therapy (clomipramine). *Neuropsychobiology, 6* : 153.

Langer, G., Schonbeck, G., Koinig, G., Aschauer, H., *1981* — Neuroendocrine mechanisms in therapeutic effects of antidepressant drugs : The « Thyroid-Axis » hypothesis. *3rd. World Congress Biological Psychiatry, Stockholm.* Presentation, Abstracts, S-211.

Mendlewicz, J. *1979* — TSH responses to TRH in women with bipolar depression. *Lancet, 2* : 1079.

Nathan, R.S., Sachar, E.J., Asnis, G., Halbreich, U., Tabrizi, M.A. *1980* — Diurnal variation in response of plasma prolactin cortisol and growth hormone to insulin-induced hypoglycemia in normal men. *J. Clin. Endocrinol. Metab., 49,2* : 321-335.

DISCUSSION

C. Hagen
You are doubtless well aware, that the prolactin response and prolactin levels differ according to sex, age, menstrual cycle and previous and current treatment with sex hormones. Have you considered these aspects ?

P. Grof
I apologize that I omitted to mention that these patients and controls were all males. They were all physically healthy, they had no history of endocrine disease, there was no obesity and at least within this group, when we tried to co-variate for age we did not have any significant differences in the findings. We got around the issues you mentioned by dealing with males only. I think probably the pilot work has to be done this way. However, there is a point in the research developments where you will have to move into female populations and that is obviously going to be a major headache !

C. Hagen
Could you please comment on where you think insulin hypoglycaemia works, because I think that it is well known that it is very effective stimulus to a lot of endocrine systems, but I still think that it is rather difficult to say what exactly happens. Is it intra-cellular hypoglycaemia ? Is it the stimulus of serotonin, noradrenaline or is it dopamine ? What happens when you do this test ?

P. Grof
The stimulus itself is certainly hypoglycaemia, but as to the precise mechanism beyond hypoglycaemia, I could only quote the theories mentioned in the literature.

D. Lefaucheur
Mr. Soulairac found in many patients that there are clinical signs of disturbance of hypothalamo-hypophyseal function, which begins usually just before the relapse. For instance, some patients begin to complain of a polyuro-polydypsic syndrome just before the recurrence, so probably abnormalities of antidiuretic hormone could be investigated systematically ?

P. Grof
Yes, I think that is a good point. It could be included. The other issue connected with it is the big issue : Whether changes usually take place quite early or whether they happen just a week or 2 weeks prior to the episode, in which case these techniques would not be terribly valuable in a long-term treatment. I think that needs to be discovered. Some of the early findings from the systematic study now suggest that the elevated prolactin response may be more characteristic of patients with very active, frequently recurrent illness, rather than specifically episode-related. In other words, the elevated response could be characteristic of that particular patient with active illness, but not related directly to a specific relapse.

Cortisol dexamethasone suppression as a neuroendocrine test in the diagnosis of affective disorders

J. Mendlewicz[1], G. Charles[2], J.M. Franckson[3]

1) Department of Psychiatry, Brussels University Clinics, Erasme Hospital, Free University of Brussels, Belgium.
2) C.G.T.R. Department of Neurosciences, Montignies le Tilleul, Belgium.
3) Department of Medical Chemistry, Free University of Brussels, Belgium.

Summary : We have studied plasma cortisol suppression after dexamethasone administration in patients suffering from a major depressive disorder (54 patients with primary depression and 41 with secondary depression) and 18 non depressed controls. Our study shows the presence of early morning hypersecretion of plasma cortisol and cortisol non suppression after dexamethasone mainly in patients with primary depression. Comparing depressed patients suffering from primary depression to patients with secondary depression, we find the sensitivity of the dexamethasone suppression test (DST) to be 79 % in primary depressed patients, its specificity also being 79 % and the diagnostic confidence of a positive test to be 82 %.
In our study, there were no differences in the performances of the DST between unipolar and bipolar patients. Non suppression to dexamethasone was observed in 81 % of patients with psychotic depression as compared to only 37 % of patients with non psychotic depression. As previously shown by Carroll et al., 1981, age, sex and severity of depression did not influence the results of the DST.
The menopausal status in depressed female patients was of no influence on the DST results and recent intake of benzodiazepines had no effect on the dexamethasone test in all groups studied. There was no association between cortisol non suppression to dexamethasone and any genetic subgroup of affective disorder. Our study confirms the excellent performances of the dexamethasone suppression test and its validity as a laboratory marker for the neuroendocrine diagnosis of depression.

Introduction

Depression is one of the most frequent illnesses in psychiatric practice, its diagnosis remaining confusing because of the lack of agreement about the nosological classification of depressed patients.

Therefore, the current search for biochemical markers of affective illnesses provides a promising tool for developing laboratory methods potentially useful in the biochemical diagnosis of depression.

Hypothalamic pituitary adrenal hyperactivity has been postulated to be the main neuroendocrine abnormality in endogenous depression (Carroll et al., 1968).

Disturbances of cortisol secretion have been observed in some depressed patients with high 17 hydroxycorticosteroid urinary excretion (Board et al., 1957 ; Gibbons, 1964 ; Bunney et al., 1969) or high cortisol plasma levels (Gibbons, 1964 ; Sachar et al., 1970). Abnormal cortisol circadian rhythm with increased nocturnal secretion has also been described in depression (Doig et al., 1966 ; Sachar et al., 1973).

335

Failure to suppress cortisol secretion after dexamethasone administration has recently been described as a specific episode-related (state dependent) biological marker of endogenous depression (Carroll et al., 1968 ; Stokes, 1972 ; Carroll, 1976 ; Carroll et al., 1976 ; Carroll et al., 1980).

According to some studies, dexamethasone resistance is observed in about 50 % or more of endogenous depressions (Carroll et al., 1968 ; Carroll et al., 1976 ; Brown et al., 1979 ; Schlesser et al., 1980 ; Nuller and Ostroumova, 1980 ; Carroll et al., 1981 ; Charles et al., 1981) while normal dexamethasone suppression occurs in reactive depressions, in mania and schizophrenia (Schlesser et al., 1980 ; Carroll et al., 1976b ; Carroll et al., 1981).

However, other studies failed to confirm the magnitude of these results.

These discrepancies may be due to methodological differences in dexamethasone dosage, timing and frequency of plasma sampling, assay for cortisol determination, selection and diagnosis of patients as well as non specific factors such as previous or concomitant drug intake or intercurrent somatic disorders. Because of the conflicting results and the ongoing interest in the use of the dexamethasone suppression test (DST) in depressive illness, we have undertaken the present study in order to estimate the diagnostic value of the DST in clinical and genetic subgroups of patients with affective disorders and psychiatric controls.

Sample and methods

All 113 patients included in the present study were consecutively hospitalized in our Department of Psychiatry during the period of December 1, 1979 to August 30, 1980. The clinical diagnosis was made according to the Research Diagnostic Criteria of Spitzer et al. (1978) and family history data were also collected from the patients and some relatives according to a previously described methodology (Mendlewicz et al., 1975). Among those 113 patients, 95 depressed patients were suffering from a major depressive disorder according to Spitzer et al. (1978) and 18 non depressed subjects (6 schizophrenics, 11 manic or hypomanic bipolars and 1 normal control) were considered as non depressed controls. Severity of depressed mood was assessed by using the Hamilton Rating Scale (Hamilton, 1960).

The 95 patients with major depressive disorder were classified into primary depression (N=54, 31 females and 23 males, aged from 31 to 68 years) and secondary depression (N=41, 21 females and 20 males, aged from 19 to 67 years).

The 54 patients with primary depression were further subdivided into 29 patients suffering from recurrent unipolar illness (17 females, 12 males, aged from 33 to 68 years) and 25 patients with bipolar illness (14 females, 11 males, aged from 31 to 66 years).

Patients presenting somatic problems as evidenced by routine and laboratory tests, as well as pregnant women and obese subjects, were excluded from the present study.

Alcoholics and drug dependant patients were also discarded from the study. All patients were free of neuroleptics and M.A.O.I. for at least one month before the investigation, and free of tricyclic antidepressants at least seven days prior to the study.

Patients using lithium salts and hormonal contraceptives were not included in this study.

After obtaining informed consent, patients were kept on complete wash-out for seven days. Sixteen patients (10 females, 6 males) all suffering from a major depressive disorder had to be given small amounts of benzodiazepines during this period for anxiety symptoms and major sleep difficulties (eight patients on bromazepam and eight patients on flunitrazepam).

On day 8, a single intramuscular dose of 1 mg dexamethasone was given to the patient at 11.30 p.m.

Suppression of cortisol secretion was estimated by determining the cortisol plasma levels at 4 p.m. the day after the injection of dexamethasone.

In order to evaluate cortisol basal levels, a plasma sample was also collected at 8 a.m. the day before the dexamethasone test for cortisol measurements.

Plasma cortisol was measured without knowledge of the clinical diagnosis using the gamma coat cortisol radioimmunoassay kit for clinical assays (Rymer, 1978). Determinations were carried out in duplicate. The intra assay cœfficient of variation was below 4 % ; the inter-assay cœfficient of variation averaged 5 %.

Abnormal test response, i.e. non suppression of cortisol was defined according to the criteria of Carroll et al. 1981 : a postdexamethasone cortisol plasma level at 4 p.m. equal to or greater than 50 μg/l. Statistical comparisons were performed using the Anova test and the X^2 test (with Yates correction when appropriate). Plasma cortisol values are expressed as means $\pm$ SEM.

Results

Figure 1 illustrates cortisol plasma levels at 8 a.m. before dexamethasone in depressed patients and controls.

Morning cortisol plasma levels are significantly higher in unipolar (208 μg/l $\pm$ 58) and bipolar (196 μg/l $\pm$ 57) depressed patients as compared to depressed patients with secondary depression (158 μg/l $\pm$ 48, t = 3.91, t = 2.25 ; $p < 0.01$, $p < 0.05$).

Depressed patients suffering from primary depression (unipolar and bipolar) as a group show significantly higher 8 a.m. cortisol plasma levels (202 μg/l $\pm$ 57) than patients with secondary depression (t = 3.51 ; $p < 0.01$) and controls (t = 3.26 ; $p < 0.01$).

Conversely, there is no significant difference in 8 a.m. cortisol plasma levels between patients with secondary depression and controls nor between patients with unipolar and bipolar depression. These results, indicating spontaneous early morning hypersecretion of cortisol in primary depression, are in line with previous studies demonstrating the presence of cortisol hypersecretion in endogenous depression (Sachar et al., 1970 ; Carroll et al., 1976 ; Schlesser et al., 1980 ; Charles et al., 1981).

Figure 2 illustrates 4 p.m. plasma cortisol values after dexamethasone in depressed patients with major depressive disorders and non depressed controls. Patients with primary depression (unipolar and bipolar) have significantly higher 4 p.m. post-dexamethasone plasma cortisol values (87 μg/l $\pm$ 45) than patients with

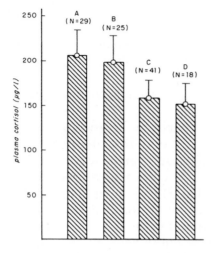

Fig. 1 — Plasma cortisol values at 8 a.m. before dexamethasone in patients with unipolar (A), bipolar (B), secondary depression (C) and non depressed controls (D).

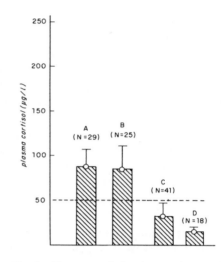

Fig. 2 — Plasma cortisol values at 4 p.m. after dexamethasone in patients with unipolar (A), bipolar (B), secondary depression (C) and non depressed controls (D).

secondary depression (32 μg/l ± 35 ; t = 5.81 ; p<0.001) and controls (12 μg/l ± 5 ; t = 6.48, p<0.001).

Among the primary depressives, bipolar and unipolar patients are equally non suppressors to dexamethasone (87 μg/l ± 51 ; 87 μg/l ± 40) when compared to secondary depressives (t = 5.70 ; p<0.001 ; t = 5.97 ; p<0.001) and controls (t = 6.36 ; p<0.001 ; t = 6.55 ; p<0.001).

Furthermore, there was no significant difference in cortisol dexamethasone suppression between bipolar and unipolar patients nor between patients with secondary depression and controls. The distribution of 4 p.m. postdexamethasone plasma cortisol concentrations in primary (N = 54) and secondary (N = 41) depression and controls (N = 18) is also illustrated in Figure 3.

Logarithmic transformation of the plasma cortisol concentrations are used in Figure 3 because of the non normal distribution of plasma cortisol values. Most of the 41 patients with a diagnosis of secondary depression and the 18 controls have plasma cortisol concentrations below 50 μg/l, and these values have a unimodal distribution. This is not the case for patients with primary depression for whom cortisol values tend to be higher than 50 μg/l.

We also present the performances (sensitivity, specificity, predictive value) of the dexamethasone suppression test in our sample.

Sensitivity is defined as the frequency of positive results (non suppression to dexamethasone) in patients with primary depression. Specificity is the frequency of negative results (normal suppression to dexamethasone) in secondary depressions.

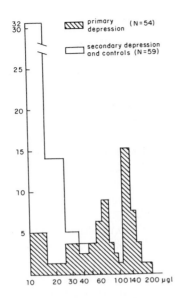

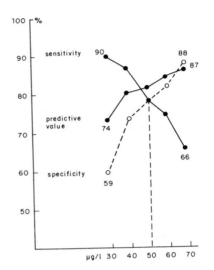

Fig. 3 — Distribution of 4 p.m. postdexa-methasone plasma cortisol values (log transform-ed in μg/l) in 54 patients with primary depression (shaded area) and 41 patients with secondary depression and controls (white area).

Fig. 4 — Sensitivity, specificity and predictive value (positive test) of dexamethasone suppres-sion test in relation to plasma cortisol values (μg/l) in 54 patients with primary depression and 41 patients with secondary depression.

The predictive value of a positive test indicates the frequency of primary depres-sion in all depressed subjects with positive results.

Figure 4 illustrates the sensitivity of the dexamethasone suppression test (DST) in relation to postdexamethasone plasma cortisol concentration at 4 p.m. (μg/l) among 54 patients with primary depression (sensitivity) and 41 patients with secon-dary depression (specificity), using a class interval of 10 μg/l for plasma cortisol. The overall sensitivity of the DST in our patients with primary depression ranges from 90 % at a plasma cortisol criterion value of 30 μg/l to 66 % at a criterion value of 70 μg/l. Specificity increases from 59 % at a cortisol value of 30 μg/l to 74 % at a value of 40 μg/l to reach a maximum value of 88 % for a cortisol criterion of 70 μg/l.

The predictive value of a positive test (or diagnostic confidence) is also il-lustrated in Figure 4 for different values of the postdexamethasone plasma concen-tration of cortisol at 4 p.m.

The predictive values of the DST are comparable to its specificity ranging from 74 % at a cortisol criterion value of 30 μg/l, to 87 % for a value of 70 μg/l.

Figure 4 indicates that the sensitivity and specificity curves intersect at a cor-tisol value of 50 μg/l.

This cortisol criterion value gives an overall test sensitivity of 79 % and specificity of 79 %. The diagnostic confidence for primary depression associated with a plasma concentration of 50 μg/l is 82 %.

The performances of the DST are also indicated separately for bipolar depres-sion and unipolar depression with reference to secondary depression. The sensitivity value of the DST is 76 % for bipolar depression and 82 % for unipolar depression while the predictive value of a positive test is 72 % for unipolar depression and 67 % for bipolar depression.

Thus, in our study, there were no real differences in the DST performances between bipolar and unipolar illness ; a finding in disagreement with Schlesser et al. (1980) who find the DST to be much more sensitive in bipolar depression. Our 95 patients with major depressive disorder were further examined for the presence or absence of psychotic symptoms such as delusions or hallucinations. Thirty seven patients (21 females, 16 males aged between 33 and 68 years) were suffering from psychotic depression while the 58 others had no evidence of psychotic depression.

The postdexamethasone 4 p.m. cortisol plasma values were significantly higher in the group of psychotic depression (93 $\mu g/l$ ± 43) as compared to non psychotic depression (48 $\mu g/l$ ± 49, t = 4.65 ; p<0.001).

Psychotic depressives also have significantly higher 4 p.m. cortisol values than controls (t = 7.93 ; p<0.001), while this is not the case for non psychotic depressed patients. The sensitivity of the DST at a 4 p.m. cortisol criterion value of 50 $\mu g/l$ is 81 % for psychotic depressives and 37 % for non psychotic depressed patients. Specificity at the same cortisol value is 70 % while the predictive or diagnostic value of a positive test is only 58 %. These results show the DST to be highly sensitive in psychotic depression, but less specific and with poor diagnostic confidence in the differential diagnosis of psychotic and non psychotic depression. In addition, we find no correlation with severity of depression as assessed by the Hamilton rating scores (Hamilton, 1966) and postdexamethasone 4 p.m. cortisol plasma values. (r = 0.2, p = NS).

No correlation could be shown between age or sex and 4 p.m. postdexamethasone cortisol levels in all groups studied (patients with major depressive disorders, with primary or secondary depression and controls). The age and sex distributions were also comparable in all subgroups. These results are in agreement with Carroll et al. (1981).

The potential influence of the menopausal status on the DST was also examined in female patients with primary (N = 31), secondary depression (N = 21) and female controls (N = 12). No statistical difference could be found in postdexamethasone 4 p.m. cortisol plasma values between postmenopausal (101 $\mu g/l$ ± 36.9) and premenopausal (85 $\mu g/l$ ± 60.4) women in the subgroups of primary depression (t = 0.9 ; p = NS), secondary depression (21.5 $\mu g/l$ ± 19.3, 30.0 $\mu g/l$ ± 40.0, t = 0.89 ; p = NS) and controls (10.0 $\mu g/l$ ± 3.0 ; t = 0.15 ; p = NS).

These results indicate that the menopausal status has no influence on the results of the DST in depressed and non depressed female patients.

As stated before in the method section, 8 depressed patients (4 primary, 4 secondary depression) were treated with bromazepam (0.33 mg/kg/day ± 0.27) during the wash-out period before the DST, and an additionnal 8 patients (4 primary, 4 secondary depression) were given flunitrazepam (0.06 mg/kg/day ± 0.01) during the same period. There was no difference in 4 p.m. cortisol values between treated (N = 16, 62.8 $\mu g/l$ ± 46) and untreated patients (N = 79, 63.2 $\mu g/l$ ± 49 ; t = 0.02 ; p = NS).

Among the patients treated with benzodiazepines, there was no difference in 4 p.m. cortisol values between patients with primary or secondary depression or with regard to the type of benzodiazepine (bromazepam or flunitrazepam) used (62.5 μg/l $\pm$ 36, 63.1 μg/l $\pm$ 57, t = 0.03 ; p = NS).

These results are consistent with those of Carroll et al., (1981) and indicate that recent intake of small or moderate amounts of benzodiazepines do not seem to have a significant effect on the DST results.

Table I shows the 4 p.m. cortisol values in relation to diagnostic subgroups and the presence or absence of a family history of affective illness in first degree relatives of our patients with major depressive disorders. Among the familial affective disorders were included documented secondary cases of suicide, unipolar and bipolar depression according to the RDC criteria (Spitzer et al., 1978).

Table 1 : *Plasma cortisol values at 4 p.m. (μg/l) after dexamethasone in relation to diagnostic subgroups and family history of affective illness in first degree relatives of patients with major depressive disorders.*

| Diagnosis | Family history of affective illness | | p value |
	positive (N=27)	negative (N=66)	
Unipolar depression (N=29)	85.5 ± 39.9	87.7 ± 42.2	N.S
Bipolar depression (N=23)	92.5 ± 58.6	90.0 ± 42.0	N.S
Secondary depression (N=41)	23.0 ± 23.9	33.5 ± 36.8	N.S
TOTAL	77 ± 52.8	58.5 ± 47.5	N.S.

Two bipolar patients were excluded from the genetic analysis because of lack of reliable data.

There was no significant difference in 4 p.m. cortisol values after dexamethasone in each diagnostic subgroup (unipolar, bipolar, secondary depressives) according to the presence or absence of affectively ill secondary cases in first degree relatives (Table 1). This was also the case for the overall group of depressed patients with major depressive disorders and for non depressed controls. Using 50 μg/l as our 4 p.m. postdexamethasone cortisol criterion value, we find 18 out of 27 patients with a positive family history to be non suppressors (sensitivity = 66 %) compared to 34 out of 66 patients with no history of affective disorders in first degree relatives (sensitivity = 52 %).

This difference is not significant (X^2 = 0.49 ; p = NS) and indicates that psychiatric genetic loading may be of less importance in analyzing the response rate of the DST in samples of psychiatric patients.

This is also true for each diagnostic subgroup, since no significant difference could be demonstrated for the DST results in unipolar, bipolar and secondary depressives in relation to family history of affective illness.

If we consider unipolar patients only (N = 29) and classify them according to the genetic criteria of Winokur (1979), we are unable to find any significant difference in 4 p.m. cortisol values between the three groups studied (familial pure depressive disease, N = 7, 95.7 μg/l $\pm$ 34.8 ; sporadic depressive disease, N = 19, 87.4 μg/l $\pm$ 41.8 ; depression spectrum disease, N = 3, 61.7 μg/l $\pm$ 12.6).

Using 50 $\mu g/l$ as the 4 p.m. cortisol criterion value, the sensitivity of the DST is 85 % in unipolar patients with familial pure depressive disease, 84 % in patients with sporadic depressive disease and 66 % in patients with a diagnosis of depression spectrum disease. These results are in line with those of Carroll et al., 1980, Hwu et al., 1981, indicating that the DST is not as good a discriminant of Winokur's genetic subtypes of depression as was postulated by Schlesser et al., 1980.

Discussion

Our study confirms the presence of early morning (8 a.m.) plasma cortisol hypersecretion in patients with primary depression (unipolar and bipolar) as compared to secondary depression and non depressed controls. Similar data have recently been published by Fang et al. (1981) who demonstrated that elevated cortisol basal levels before or after dexamethasone were not related to high plasma ACTH levels. The interpretation of cortisol basal level studies in psychiatric disorders is, however, difficult because non-specific factors such as stress may influence plasma cortisol basal values. Using 50 $\mu g/l$ as the cortisol criterion value postdexamethasone, the application of the DST reveals striking differences among patients with major depressive disorders. Selected patients diagnosed as bipolar and unipolar depression (primary depressives) show a high rate of cortisol non suppression to dexamethasone compared to patients with secondary depression and controls. The sensitivity of the DST is 79 % in patients with primary depression, its specificity is 79 % and the diagnostic confidence (or predictive value) of a positive test is 82 %.

There are no differences in the DST performances between bipolar and unipolar patients in our study, thus not confirming the finding of Schlesser et al., 1980, of a greater sensitivity of the DST in bipolar than unipolar patients. Our results are in general agreement with those of Carroll et al. (1976), Brown et al. (1979), Schlesser et al. (1980), Nuller and Ostroumova (1980), Carroll et al. (1981), Charles et al., (1981) and demonstrate the value of the DST in discriminating between primary and secondary depression among a group of depressed patients suffering from a major depressive disorder according to the criteria of Spitzer et al. (1978).

Like Carroll et al. (1981) we did not find a correlation between severity of depression assessed by the Hamilton rating scale (1960) and cortisol dexamethasone suppression or non suppression in patients with major depressive disorders. These data indicate that the high incidence of DST non suppression observed in patients with primary depression is not related to global severity of depressed mood. In contrast, non suppression to dexamethasone is present in 81 % of patients with psychotic symptoms and only 37 % of patients without psychotic symptoms but the specificity and predictive value of a positive test are lower (70 % and 58 %). These results are in agreement with those of Carroll et al. (1980) and Rudorfer et al. (1982) who also find such differences between psychotic and non psychotic patients. However, because of the relative lack of specificity and diagnostic confidence of the DST in distinguishing psychotic from non psychotic depressives, it may be less relevant to use it in this classification unless it is supported by other criteria such as the RDC (Spitzer et al., 1978) as indicated in our study, or Carroll's criteria for melancholia (Carroll et al., 1981).

342

As previously shown by Carroll et al. (1981), age and sex do not appear to be of any influence on the DST results in this investigation. In addition, our results demonstrate the menopausal status in depressed female patients to be of no influence on the results of the DST. The effect of psychotropic drugs has been studied on the DST with negative results (no effect) for tricyclic antidepressants (Amsterdam et al., 1981), and low dose benzodiazepines (Carroll et al., 1981).

High doses of benzodiazepines tend to produce false negative results (cortisol suppression postdexamethasone) (Langer et al., 1979). In our study, recent intake of moderate amounts of two benzodiazepines (bromazepam and flunitrazepam) had no effect on the DST results regardless of the diagnosis of the patients. This observation is consistent with the known lack of effect of benzodiazepines on liver microsomal enzymes (Hafeli et al., 1981).

Carroll et al. (1980) have shown an association between the presence of a positive family history of depression and abnormal DST response in melancholic patients.

In our study, there is no such association between the presence of affective illnesses in first degree relatives of our depressed patients and non suppression to dexamethasone regardless of the clinical diagnosis (unipolar — bipolar or secondary depression). When applying Winokur's criteria (1979) to genetically classify our unipolar patients, we were unable to find any significant differences in DST results between familial pure depressive disease, sporadic and depression spectrum disease. These results agree with those of Carroll et al. (1980) Hwu et al. (1981) and Rudorfer et al. (1982) and do not support the finding of a higher rate of DST non suppression among patients with familial pure depressive disease than in patients with depression spectrum disease (Schlesser et al., 1981 ; Coryell et al., 1982).

The interpretation of these conflicting genetic data should be undertaken with great care because of the small number of patients studied in each diagnostic subgroup in our study and others, and because of the relative lack of sophistication in genetic methodology (no blind family study).

In conclusion, evidence from our study confirms the validity of the DST as a laboratory marker of primary depression.

Our present results indicate high sensitivity (79 %), high specificity (79 %) and high diagnostic confidence (82 %) of cortisol non suppression after dexamethasone in depressed patients with unipolar and bipolar depression. We have recently reported high reproducibility of non suppression to dexamethasone in untreated depressed patients whose mood remained unchanged before antidepressant treatment (Charles et al., in press).

Carroll demonstrated that abnormal DST results are not psychological stress responses (Carroll, 1972, 1976).

The present investigation also shows that DST results are not influenced by such factors as age, sex, menopausal status, severity of depression and recent administration of benzodiazepines. Clinical remission following antidepressant therapy with tricyclics or ECT is associated with a normalization of the DST (Brown et al., 1979 ; Carroll, 1972 ; Carroll et al., 1968 ; Dysken et al. 1979 ; Albala et al., 1981).

All these results emphasize the potential value of the DST as a neuroendocrine laboratory tool providing an indirect indication of abnormal limbic system activity in some patients with affective disorders. Whether these patients benefit more from pharmacotherapy or psychotherapy or a combination of both treatments deserves further investigations.

REFERENCES

Albala, A.A., Greden, J.F., Tarika, J., Carroll, B.J. *1981.* — Changes in serial dexamethasone suppression tests among unipolar depressives receiving electroconvulsive treatment. *Biol. Psychiat.,* 16, 551-560.

Amsterdam, M.D., Winokur, A., Caroff, S. *1981* — Effect of tricyclic antidepressants on the dexamethasone suppression test. *Am. J. Psychiat., 138 :* 1245-1246.

Board, F.A., Wadeson, R., Persky, H. *1957* — Depressive affect and endocrine functions. *Arch. Neurol. Psychiat., 78 :* 612-620.

Brown, W.A., Jonhson, R., Mayfield, D. *1979* — The 24-hour dexamethasone suppression test in a clinical setting : relationship to diagnosis, symptoms and response to treatment. *Am. J. Psychiat., 136 :* 543-547.

Bunney, W.E., Fawcett, J.A., Davis, J-M., Gifford, S. *1969* — Further evaluation of urinary 17 — hydroxycorticosteroïds in suicidal patients. *Arch. Gen. Psychiat., 21 :* 138-150.

Carroll, B.J. *1972* — The hypothalamic — pituitary — adrenal axis in depression. *In : Depressive illness : some research studies.* B. Davies, B.J., Carroll and R.M. Mowbray (ed), pp. 23-28 Springfield, C.C. Thomas.

Carroll, B.J. *1976* — Limbic system — pituitary — adrenal cortex regulation in depression and schizophrenia. *Psychosomat. Med., 38 :* 106-121.

Carroll, B.J., Martin, F.I.R., Davies, B.M. *1968* — Resistance to suppression by dexamethasone of plasma 11 — OHCS levels in severe depressive illness. *Br. Med. J., 2 :* 285-287.

Carroll, B.J., Curtis, G.C., Mendels, J. *1976* — Neuroendocrine regulation in depression ; ii. Discrimination of depressed from non-depressed patients. *Arch. Gen. Psychiat., 33 :* 1051-1058.

Carroll, B.J., Greden, J.F., Feinberg, M., James, M., Haskett, R.F., Steiner, M., Tarika, J. *1980* — Neuroendocrine dysfunction in genetic subtypes of primary unipolar depression. *Psychiat. Res., 2 :* 251-258.

Carroll, B.J., Feinberg, M., Greden, J.F., Tarika, J., Albala, A.A., Haskett, R.F., James, N., Kronfol., Z., Lohr, N., Steinert, M., De Vigne, J.P., Young, E. *1981* — A specific laboratory test for the diagnosis of melancholia : standardisation, validation and clinical utility. *Arch. Gen. Psychiat., 38 :* 15-22.

Charles, G., Vandewalle, J., Meunier, J.C., Wilmotte, J., Noel, G., Fossoul, C., Mardens, Y., Mendlewicz, J. *1981* — Plasma and urinary cortisol levels after dexamethasone in affective disorders. *J. Affective Disorders., 3 :* 397-406.

Charles, G., Wilmotte, J., Quenon, M., Mendlewicz, J. *1982* — Reproducibility of the dexamethasone suppression test in depression. *Biol. Psychiat.,* in press.

Coryell, W., Gaffney, G., Burkhardt, P.E. *1982.* — The dexamethasone suppression test and familial subtypes of depression — a naturalistic replication. *Biol. Psychiat., 17 :* 33-40.

Doig, R.J., Mummery, R.F., Wills, M.R., Elkes, A. *1966* — Plasma cortisol levels in depression. *Br. J. Psychiat., 112 :* 1263-1267.

Dysken, M.W., Pandey, G.N., Chang, S.S. *1979* — Serial postdexamethasone cortisol levels in a patient undergoing ECT. *Am. J. Psychiat., 136 :* 1328-1329.

Fang, V.S., Tricou, B-J., Robertson, A., Metzer, H.Y. *1981* — Plasma ACTH and cortisol levels in depressed patients : relation to dexamethasone suppression test. *Life Sci., 29 :* 931-938.

Gibbons, J.L. *1964* — Cortisol secretion rate in depressive illness. *Arch. Gen. Psychiat., 10 :* 572-575.

Hafeli, W., Pieri, L., Pole, P., Schaffner, R. *1981* — General pharmacology and neuropharmacology of benzodiazepines derivates. *Handbook of experimental pharmacology* pp. 85-96 — Berlin, Springer Verlag.

Hamilton, M. *1960* — A rating scale for depression. *J. Neurol. Neurosurg. Psychiat., 23 :* 56-62.

Hwu, H., Rudorfer, M.V., Clayton, P.J. *1981* — Dexamethasone suppression test and subtypes of depression. *Arch. Gen. Psychiat., 38 :* 363-367.

Langer, G., Schonbeck, G., Koinig, G., Lesch, O., Schussler, M. *1979* — Hyperactivity of hypothalamic — pituitary — adrenal axis in endogenous depression. *Lancet, 2 :* 524.

Mendlewicz, J., Fleiss, J.L., Cataldo, M., Rainer, J.D. *1975* — The accuracy of the family history method in family studies of affective illness. *Arch. Gen. Psychiat., 32 :* 309-314.

Nuller, J.L., Ostroumova, M.N. *1980* — Resistance to inhibiting effect of dexamethasone in patients with endogenous depression. *Acta. Psychiat. Scand., 61 :* 169-177.

Rudorfer, M.V., Hwu, H.G., Clayton, P.J. *1982* — Dexamethasone suppression test in primary depression : significance of family history and psychosis. *Biol. Psychiat., 17 :* 41-48.

Rymer, J.C. *1978* — Estimation of plasma cortisol by radio-competition or radioimmunoassay. Use of commercial kits. *Ann. Biol. Clin., 36 :* 509-514.

Sachar, E.J., Hellman, L., Fukushima, D.K., Gallagher, T.F. *1970* — Cortisol production in depressive illness, *Arch. Gen. Psychiat., 23 :* 289-298.

Sachar, E.J., Hellman, L., Roffwarg, H.P., Halpern, F.S., Fukushima, D.K., Gallagher, T.F. *1970* — Disrupted 24-hour patterns of cortisol secretion in psychotic depression. *Arch. Gen. Psychiat., 28 :* 19-24.

Schlesser, M.A., Winokur, G., Sherman, B.M. *1980* — Hypothalamic — pituitary — adrenal axis activity in depressive illness : its relationship to classification. *Arch. Gen. Psychiat., 37 :* 737-743.

Spitzer, R.L., Endicott, J., Robbins, E. *1978* — Research diagnostic criteria : rationale and reliability. *Arch. Gen. Psychiat., 35 :* 773-782.

Winokur, G. *1979* — Unipolar depression. Is it divisible into autonomous subtypes ? *Arch. Gen. Psychiat., 36 :* 47-52.

DISCUSSION

P. Grof
I know that you have done a number of interesting genetic studies and I was wondering whether you have any data that pertains to the families ? Have you looked at your twins, for example, from this point of view ?

J. Mendlewicz
Yes, we are doing a study right now. In fact, it is very interesting, because a couple of weeks ago we were able to have a couple of 14-year old, manic depressive twins hospitalized in our unit. One was manic and the other depressed. They had never been treated with any psychotropic drugs, they were altogether clean of drugs and the dexamethasone suppression results were concordant. In the one who was manic, there was clearly no suppression to DST and we repeated it 3 times and the same was true for the one who was depressed. We have data on relatives suffering from depressive disorders, secondary cases, and it looks like there is some familial trend, but I cannot really be too positive about it, because these are really very preliminary data.

P. Grof
The second question was related to the finding you reported, that you did not have a correlation with therapeutic response. I was wondering whether you have some thoughts on why that happened, because that is a bit disturbing to me. If the test was separating clearly primary and secondary depression, all clinical experience suggests that there is a different responsiveness to treatments between primary and secondary depression. I was wondering if there may be something specific about your sample, e.g. the type of secondary depressions you had, or whether you have some other thoughts why the result came out that way ?

J. Mendlewicz
We know that the treatment with tricyclics (we used amitriptyline) does not interfere, does not modify the results of the tests and this has been shown recently by Mendel's group. The reason is difficult to interpret, because usually you deal with small samples. You also know that the tricyclics are not such good antidepressants, they only work in about 60 — 70 % of the patients, so it may reflect the limitations of the tricyclics more than the validity of the test. For the ECT, it is more interesting, because there is a much more clear-cut picture. The treatment seems to work in about 80 % of patients with endogenous depression, primary depression and there may be predictive value in using the DST.

P. Grof
Perhaps the number of ECT treated patients was not large enough to produce a significant correlation. Could you say more about your secondary depressions ? What kind of patients were they ? Were they primarily neurotics, alcoholics or what kind of secondary depressions ?

J. Mendlewicz
The patients were suffering from a well-defined, neurotic disorder with symptoms according to the RDC criteria, so some of them were suffering from obsessional neuroses, some of them from phobic neuroses. There were only 2 or 3 with phobic neuroses and a large group of schizophrenics, who had a clear-cut diagnosis of schizophrenia, paranoid type.

P. Grof
The last point might relate to the interesting finding that you mentioned, that there is no link between the hyper-secreters and the results of DST. We noticed that the DST dose interferes with other neuroendocrine tests, in particular it may influence for example GH responses. If one does DST testing, one should be very careful during the subsequent neuroendocrine tests.

J. Mendlewicz
We always start with the sleep EEG study first and then we carry on with the suppression test, always after the circadian studies and the sleep EEG studies.

N. Matussek
In our hospital Holsboer (F. Holsboer, R. Leibl, E. Hofschuster : Repeated dexamethasone suppression test during depressive illness : normalization of test result compared with clinical improvement. J. Affect. Dis. 4, 93-101, 1982) has shown that endogenously depressed patients under tricyclics and ECT suppress the cortisol secretion in the DST 3 to 4 weeks before clinical improvement. Comparing the test between different groups makes it maybe a little bit more complicated. However, it should be kept in mind that it could be of predictive value with regard to treatment, also with tricyclics.

J. Mendlewicz
This seems to be true, but I do not know if it is 3 weeks before.

N. Matussek
Holsboer found it three and a half weeks prior to clinical improvement.

J. Mendlewicz
Indeed, it seems to normalize before the clinical improvement.

N. Matussek
One more question : Did you find a correlation between the Hamilton Rating Score and the DST response in your primary affective disorder patients ?

J. Mendlewicz
None.

N. Matussek
That was found in a study in Munich (F. Holsboer, W. Bender, O. Benkert, H. Klein, M. Schmauß : Diagnostic value of DST in depression. Lancet 27th September, 1980, 706).

J. Mendlewicz
You found the same.

N. Matussek
No, they found a correlation between higher Hamilton Rating Scores and the escape.

C. Hagen
Could I just make a comment and then a question ? The comment is that, from an endocrinological

point of view, the short DST which you used is what we usually call a « screening test », because some people will not suppress in this short test, but will suppress on the longer tests, so could the difference between the hyper-secreters and suppressors not lie in the fact that you are doing the full test ? The other thing I want to ask, is it possible that cortisol is involved in this type of depression. The reason for asking is that e.g. in Cushings' syndrome there are various psychotic disturbances.

J. Mendlewicz

There are indeed quite a number of reports mentioning behavioral aspects of corticosteroids or psychiatric obligation of Cushings' syndrome and these are not quite clear. There are reports of mania, of depression, anxiety disorder, of psychotic hallucinating states, it seems to be perhaps more affective disturbances in general, so it may very well be that cortisol has something to do with mood and that hyper-cortisol secretion may be involved in depression. After all, maybe depression is not a central disorder, but a peripheral one.

L. Meyzen

My question is about Cushings' symptoms. You mentioned that endogenously depressed patients have high cortisol levels without any signs of Cushings' symptoms, so do we have any idea of this fact and could we think of any abnormalities of the transport protein of cortisol ? I mean, such as increase of that protein, or are there any abnormalities of the sensitivity of cortisol receptor cells ?

J. Mendlewicz

First of all, one should not have the impression that depressed patients are permanently in the state of hypercortisism, this seems to be true only during the depressed phase and if you looked at the cortisol 24-hour secretion, as we did, during remission it is not like Cushings'. You have sort of peaks during the depressive episodes and they are not cortisol hyper-secreters for most of their lives, so that could be one reason why there is no clinical sign. The other thing I do not know, is if there is perhaps a disturbance in transport mechanisms, I do not know.

R.M. Post

Just in terms of another drug that will interfere with the DST, Priveteran in Carroll's group and Rubinonow in our group have observed that carbamazepine clearly will induce escape from DST. And just another comment in terms of symptomatology of depression and relationship to the system : We did not find a good correlation between 24-hour urinary cortisol and dexamethasone suppression either. 24-hour urinary cortisol secretion did not correlate with severity of depression, but did with the degree of cognitive disturbance measured on the Halstead Categories test. The patients with higher 24-hour urinary free cortisol had much poorer abstracting and cognitive ability, thus cortisol may have an interesting relationship to the cognitive processing disturbance if not to the severity of the depression.

J. Mendlewicz

That is very interesting. Does this work like other drugs to liver microsomal induction, or how do you explain the effect of carbamazepine ?

R.M. Post

We are looking to see whether it effects the dexamethasone level itself, as it does induce liver microsomal enzymes. There may also be a direct effect, since there is evidence that carbamazepine increases your 24-hour urinary free cortisol excretion, which could be on a central basis.

The possible role of glutamate in schizophrenia : Human and animal studies

J.-S. Kim

Department of Neurology, University of Ulm, Schwendi/Ulm, Germany

Summary : Glutamate concentration was measured in cerebrospinal fluid (CSF) of schizophrenic patients and in non-psychiatric controls. The mean CSF glutamate level in the schizophrenic patients was found to be about half the control. Preliminary data indicate that the low CSF glutamate is not due to neuroleptic treatment. It is hypothesized that the glutamate decrease is due to an impaired function of glutamatergic neurons in schizophrenia. Dopaminergic mechanisms inhibit glutamate release from cortico-striatal terminals. Thus, the glutamate theory of schizophrenia is compatible with the beneficial effect of neuroleptics which block dopaminergic receptors. In a subsequent study, the hypothesis of glutamatergic underactivity in schizophrenia was investigated, using amphetamine as a model. In rats, chronic amphetamine administration resulted in a significant decrease of the glutamate content in the CSF and concomitant increase of glutamate levels in some brain areas. Conversely, chronic sulpiride treatment resulted in a significant increase of glutamate content in the CSF and concomitant decrease of glutamate levels in some brain areas. These findings are discussed with respect to the new ideas about the role of glutamate in schizophrenia.

Introduction

Glutamate is one of the most widely distributed excitatory substances in the brain, where it may function as an important transmitter.

Besides its possible importance as a transmitter at certain synapses in the CNS, glutamate has other functions including incorporation into proteins and peptides, being involved in fatty acid synthesis, contributing along with glutamine, to the regulation of ammonia levels, and control of osmotic or anionic balance (Johnson, 1972). Glutamate is, of course, the immediate precursor of GABA and the precursor of Krebs cycle intermediates. The principal source of glutamate in the brain is derived from the aerobic breakdown of glucose via the Krebs cycle. However, according to Shank and Aprison (1979), the transmitter pool of glutamate is thought to have its metabolic origin in both glucose and glutamine. In rat brain, a high content of glutamate was found in the striatum, frontal cortex and the hippocampus, whereas a low level of glutamate was found in the globus pallidus and the substantia nigra (Kim, unpublished data). It is interesting that there was a reverse relationship between glutamate and GABA levels.

Since 1977, glutamate has been proposed as the excitatory transmitter for the cortico-striatal pathway. The evidence can be summarized as follows : Firstly, the glutamate content is higher in the striatum than in other brain regions. Secondly, the destruction of the frontal cortex results in a fall of glutamate concentration in the ipsilateral striatum, whereas other aminoacids (Kim et al., 1977), dopamine, noradrenaline, serotonin and the cholinergic system remain unchanged (Kim,

349

1978). Furthermore, the high affinity of glutamate uptake into the synaptosomal fraction of the striatum is markedly reduced after frontal cortex ablation (Divac et al., 1977 ; Mc Geer et al., 1977). Thirdly, the decreased release of tritiated glutamate in the striatum is synthesized from tritiated glutamine following cortical lesion (Reubi and Cuénod, 1979). Fourthly, the specific calcium-dependent release of endogenous glutamate from striatum is reduced by destruction of the frontal cortex (Rowlands and Roberts, 1980a). Fifthly, the excitatory responses of striatal neurons to direct cortical stimulation, and to iontophoretically applied glutamate are suppressed by the L-glutamate diethylester (Spencer, 1976).

Similarly the distribution of glutamate-containing neurons in mammalian brain has been rapidly expanded on within the last few years. Thus, Fonnum et al. (1981) reported that apart from the cortico-striatal pathway, the cortico-mesolimbic system, the cortico-thalamic projection, the cortico-amygdala connection and the cortico-tectal fibres are also glutamatergic. In addition, a number of glutamate-containing neurons have been reported in fornix fimbria fibers from hippocampus-subiculum (Fonnum et al., 1981). Recent data suggest that glutamate is a neurotransmitter of corticofugal fibers to many subcortical areas and most of the terminal sites of the glutamatergic projections are also supplied with dopaminergic afferents.

The activation of dopamine receptors inhibits glutamate release from cortico-striatal terminals, and blockade of dopamine receptors by haloperidol or sulpiride antagonizes the dopamine inhibition of glutamate release (Rowlands and Roberts, 1980b ; Mitchell, 1980). Furthermore, neither picrotoxin, nor atropine, antagonized the response, indicating that GABAergic or cholinergic mechanisms were not involved in glutamate release (Rowlands and Roberts, 1980b). Moreover, after unilateral lesions of the frontal cortex, tritiated haloperidol or tritiated spiroperone binding in the striatum was decreased, suggesting that some of the specific dopamine receptors may be present on the pre-synaptic terminals and modulate the release of glutamate from those terminals (Garau et al., 1978 ; Schwarcz et al., 1978). On the other hand, behavioral studies indicate that frontal cortex lesions result in perseverative or stereotyped behavior in animals as well as in human patients suffering from frontal lobe tumor. More importantly, the experimental lesions of the caudate nucleus cause disturbances of complex behavior analogous to those produced by the frontal cortex lesions (Divac, 1972). In this connection, it is worthwhile to note that in the chronic schizophrenics, the regional cerebral blood was found to be more from the hypofrontal than the postcentral regions (Ingvar, 1980). More interestingly, Farkas (1979) has found by using positron emission tomography that schizophrenic patients have markedly diminished glucose utilization in the frontal cortex. Furthermore, following neuroleptic treatment the mental state of the patient improved and the frontal glucose utilization returned to normal. These and other findings led us to examine CSF glutamate in schizophrenic patients. We also studied the effects of amphetamine or sulpiride on the glutamate contents in the CSF and various brain areas in rats.

The purpose of this paper, therefore, is to focus on the possible role of glutamate in schizophrenia. The studies described below have been published in detail (Kim et al., 1980a ; Kim et al., 1980b ; Kim et al., 1981 ; Kim and Kornhuber, 1982).

350

CSF studies in man

Patients and methods

All participants were matched as closely as possible for age (Table 1). At the time of the study, only two of the patients were drug free, two were receiving diazepam and sixteen were on treatment with neuroleptic drugs.

The duration of illness varied from 1 to 40 years (mean, 13 years). The controls were subjects admitted to hospital for neurological assessment, but in whom no abnormality was detectable and 3 healthy volunteers.

Lumbar punctures were performed at 10.00 h in patients who had been recumbent and fasting for at least 12 hours, in order to avoid errors due to circadian rhythm, diet and activity. The CSF was taken in a sitting position, without anaesthesia. About 10 ml were collected in a glass tube, immediately frozen at —80° C with a mixture of dry ice and acetone, and then stored in a deep-freezer at —80° C until analysis. Blood was taken at the same time as the CSF.

Glutamate was measured by means of the enzymatic fluorometric method of Graham and Aprison (1966) with some modifications. This method is based on the measurement of the NADH formed as glutamate and is converted to α-ketoglutarate by glutamate dehydrogenase. In our experience the enzymatic fluorometric assay for glutamate is accurate and reproducible. Recovery of glutamate added to CSF after deproteinization and assay was 94 %. Samples stored up to 12 months showed no significant changes in glutamate level. No significant change in glutamate concentration was found in CSF left at room temperature for up to 6 hours. Glutamine had no effect on the glutamate assay. In contrast, unsatisfactory results were obtained using an automatic aminoacid analyzer to quantitate glutamate (Pye et al., 1978). The glutamine was determined by the fluorometric method as described previously (Liu and Khaya-Bashi, 1980). All samples were assayed in triplicate.

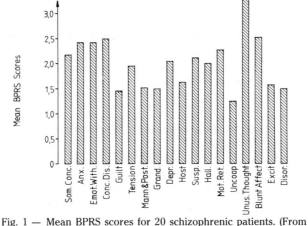

Fig. 1 — Mean BPRS scores for 20 schizophrenic patients. (From Kim and Kornhuber, 1982).

Figure 1 shows the psychopathological states of 20 schizophrenic patients by means of the Brief Psychiatric Rating Scale (BPRS). The diagnostic criteria of Schneider (1971) were applied.

351

Table 1 — *CSF and serum glutamate (GLU) in schizophrenic patients and controls* (from Kim et al. 1980a)

Groups	Number and sex of patients	Mean Age (yr) ± SEM	Mean CSF Glu. (nmol/ml) ± SEM	Mean Serum Glu. (nmol/ml) ± SEM
Control	44 (20M, 24F)	47,3 ± 2,4	25,8 ± 0,7	128,1 ± 9,1
Schizophrenia	20 (2M, 18F)	45,0 ± 4,1	13,4 ± 0,6*	112,1 ± 6,3
acute : 4				
chronic : 16				

*$p < 0.001$

Results and discussion

The mean concentrations of CSF and serum glutamate in each group of subjects are shown in Table 1. Glutamate levels in the lumbar CSF of schizophrenic patients were significantly lower than CSF glutamate from the control group ($p < 0.001$). In the serum, on the other hand, there was no difference between schizophrenic patients and controls (Table 1) and there was no correlation with CSF glutamate. Moreover, in the group of schizophrenic patients the correlation between CSF glutamate and duration of illness and scores of BPRS was not significant. There were no significant correlations between CSF glutamate levels and age or sex in any group. Furthermore, CSF glutamine was not different between the two groups. In the control subjects, the CSF glutamine was 657,5 ± 14,5 (SEM) nmol/ml, whereas in schizophrenic patients the CSF glutamine was 647,1 ± 25,9 nmol/ml.

Recently, Perry (1982) reported no differences between control individuals and schizophrenic patients in terms of CSF glutamate levels. The reason for the discrepancy between the results of the present study and Perry's work is not apparent. However, it is noteworthy that Perry used an automatic acid analyzer, which is susceptible to interference by various factors (Pye et al., 1978). Moreover, Perry's method is not sensitive enough for highly accurate measurement of the low concentrations of glutamate in human CSF (Perry et al., 1968). Another possible reason for the discrepancy is the selection of patients. Normal control values will be important for future studies. Further studies will hopefully clarify the discrepancy.

It is unlikely that the decrease of glutamate in CSF of schizophrenic patients is due to neuroleptic treatment. The activation of dopamine receptors inhibits calcium-dependent glutamate release from cortico-striatal terminals (Rowlands and Roberts, 1980b).

Blockade of dopamine receptors by neuroleptic drugs, therefore, is expected to enhance the release of glutamate.

Decreased CSF glutamate concentration in schizophrenia could be interpreted in two ways (Fig. 2). If increased dopaminergic activity in the brain is a primary abnormality in this condition, then decreased activity of glutamate neurons may occur as a compensatory mechanism. This could conceivably be reflected in decreased CSF glutamate levels. However, there is no convincing, direct evidence for central dopaminergic hyperactivity in schizophrenia. Alternatively, decreased CSF glutamate levels could reflect primary underactivity glutamatergic neurons. In both cases of primary defect, the therapeutic action of neuroleptic drugs might be explained by the blocking of dopaminergic receptors, resulting in disinhibition of

352

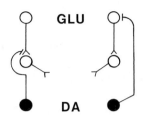

Fig. 2 — Hypothetical schemas of interactions in schizophrenia between dopaminergic (DA) and glutamatergic (GLU) neurons. The DA neurons are assumed to inhibit GLU neurons. (From Kim et al., 1980a).

glutamate release. We believe an impaired function of the glutamatergic neurons to be more likely for the following reasons :

1. Although no consistent neuropathological abnormality has been defined in schizophrenia, cortical ganglion cell loss occurs most frequently in frontal and temporal lobes, and principally in the supragranular layers (especially layer III) of schizophrenic patients (Pope, 1974).

2. Using computed tomography, Weinberger and Wyatt (1980) found subtle degeneration of brain tissue in chronic schizophrenia. It includes dilatation of several fissures on the surface of the brain, enlargement of cerebral ventricles and in some cases even atrophy of the cerebellar vermis.

3. In the initial stage of Huntington's chorea, there is often a schizophreniform psychosis (Brothers, 1964). The essential pathology of Huntington's disease consists of a slow degeneration of the corpus striatum and frontal cortex, particulary in the third and fifth layers (Bruyn et al., 1979). Currently, we have also found a significant reduction of CSF glutamate content in Huntington's disease (Kim et al., 1980a).

4. Lastly, the finding that neuroleptic drugs seem to have little influence on the CSF glutamate in our cases.

Animal studies : Effects of chronic amphetamine or sulpiride treatment on the glutamate concentration in CSF and brain

Amphetamine psychosis is the best model psychosis for understanding schizophrenia. In man, chronic amphetamine administration produces a schizophreniform psychosis, whereas in animals a behavioral stereotypy is evoked. Amphetamine is taken up by brain tissue, where it releases dopamine (Heikkila et al., 1975) from its storage sites in the nerve terminals and prevents its inactivation by synaptic reuptake (Taylor and Snyder, 1970). Thus, it appears an attractive idea that amphetamine psychosis may be related to a dopaminergic hyperactivity. However, besides its effects on brain dopamine, amphetamine is known to act in an analogous manner on brain noradrenaline. On the basis of a CSF dopamine turn-over study in man with amphetamine (Angrist et al., 1974) and animal experiments using both isomers of amphetamine (Creese and Iversen, 1975), a dopaminergic overactivity is more likely to be the cause of the behavioral effects of amphetamine. Dopamine, in turn, inhibits the release of glutamate.

On the other hand, the substituted benzamide, sulpiride, has been shown to possess antipsychotic effects in man, while producing less extrapyramidal side-effects than most commonly used neuroleptic drugs (Köhler et al., 1979). It has been

353

suggested that sulpiride is a selective cerebral dopamine antagonist which interacts specifically with D_2 adenylate cyclase independent dopamine receptors (Jenner and Marsden, 1979). Of particular interest in this respect is the recent finding that approximately one-third of the receptors associated with tritiated haloperidol binding in the striatum lie on a neuron of the cortico-striatal glutamatergic afferent fibers not associated with adenylate cyclase activity (Schwarcz et al., 1978).

Maybe sulpiride acts on the non-adenylate cyclase receptors of the cortical afferents, whereas classical neuroleptics act not only on these receptors, but also on the adenylate cyclase dependent receptor system on striatal interneurons (Jenner and Marsden, 1979).

In this study, therefore, the glutamate hypothesis of schizophrenia was evaluated by measuring the glutamate contents in the CSF and some brain areas in rats after treatment with amphetamine or sulpiride.

Materials and methods

Male Sprague-Dawley rats, weighing approximately 250 g, were housed individually with ad libitum access to food and water. The amphetamine group received daily s.c. injection of d-amphetamine sulfate at a dose of 5 mg/kg for 12 days, and samples were obtained 5 hours after the last injection. The sulpiride group received daily i.p. injection of sulpiride (Schürholz, Munich) at a dose of 50 mg/kg for 12 days, and samples were obtained 3 h after the last injection. The control group received an equal volume of saline solution.

To obtain rat CSF, the animals were anesthesized with Evipal, the atlanto-occipital membrane was exposed and 120-150 μl of CSF was taken from the cisterna magna by a microsyringe. After the CSF was obtained, the brain was removed quickly and dissected on ice. From the prefrontal cortex, rostral part of striatum, hippocampus and septum, 6-10 mg were removed from each brain for amphetamine study. The prefrontal cortex, rostral part of striatum, hippocampus and substantia nigra were removed for sulpiride study. The glutamate in the CSF and tissue samples was essentially measured by the method of Graham and Aprison (1966).

The GABA was determined by the fluorometric method as described previously (Kim et al., 1971).

Results and discussion

Figure 3 illustrates the effects of chronic amphetamine on the glutamate content in CSF and brain areas. As shown here, the CSF glutamate content was reduced by 32 % after long-term amphetamine treatment ($p < 0.001$).

In the brain, there are three major glutamate compartments : the glia, neuronal perikarya and the nerve endings. Although little is known about the source of the glutamate in the CSF, it may reflect, at least in part, release of glutamate from the brain. To pursue this question, we measured the glutamate contents in various brain areas after amphetamine treatment.

Twelve days after repeated amphetamine treatments, the glutamate levels were significantly increased in the frontal cortex ($p < 0.001$), striatum ($p < 0.001$) and hippocampus ($p < 0.001$), but not in septum (Kim et al., 1981 ; Figure 3). On the other hand, chronic sulpiride administration resulted in a significant increase of the

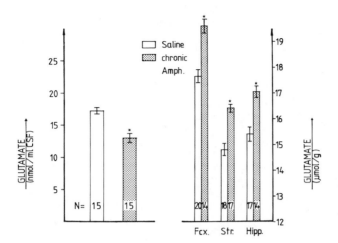

Fig. 3 — Effect of chronic d-amphetamine (5 mg/kg, s.c., 12 days and 5 hr) on the glutamate levels in rat CSF and the frontal cortex (Fcx), striatum (Str) and hippocampus (Hipp). Each bar indicates mean ± SEM. N : number of animals. *p < 0.001. (From Kim et al., 1981).

glutamate content in the CSF (+ 15 %, p < 0.05) and concomitant decrease of glutamate levels in the striatum (− 5 %, p < 0.02) and hippocampus (− 8 %, p < 0.02), but not in frontal cortex or in substantia nigra (Kim et al., unpublished data). In contrast, chronic amphetamine or chronic sulpiride had no effect on the GABA content in any of the brain areas examined.

The amphetamine study extended the previous findings of reduced CSF glutamate in schizophrenic patients. The present results could be explained as follows : Chronic amphetamine treatment causes dopaminergic overfunction, resulting in enhanced dopamine inhibition of glutamate release. This may reflect in increased glutamate levels in the frontal cortex, striatum and hippocampus and decreased glutamate content in CSF as shown in the study. Conversely, chronic sulpiride administration causes blocking of dopamine receptors, resulting in disinhibition by dopamine of glutamate release. This may reflect in decreased glutamate levels in the striatum and hippocampus and the increased glutamate content in the CSF. The glutamate hypothesis of schizophrenia is compatible with the present findings on amphetamine or sulpiride effects.

Conclusions

The dopamine hypothesis in schizophrenia is based mainly on pharmacological observations. However, the available biochemical data from schizophrenia patients indicate that there is no direct increase in dopamine activity. In this case, it is equally possible that there is normal function in the dopamine system in the schizophrenic brain, but hypoactivity of the glutamate system instead. Overall, the various results (human studies, the amphetamine data and the sulpiride results) tend to support the hypothesis that schizophrenia is mediated by glutamate. However, it must be said that this thesis is probably a simplification, because the

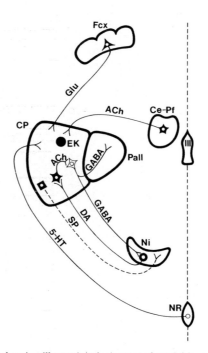

Fig. 4 — Schematic drawing illustrating the proposed model for some neuronal connections in the basal ganglia. Fcx = frontal cortex ; CP = caudate putamen ; Pall = pallidum ; Ce-Pf = centromedian-parafascicular complex ; Ni = substantia nigra ; NR = nucleus raphe ; Glu = glutamate ; ACh = acetylcholine ; GABA = θ-aminobutyric acid ; EK = enkephaline ; SP = substance P ; 5-HT = 5-hydroxytryptamine ; DA = dopamine.

brain consists not only of isolated neuronal groups, but also of interconnected circuits involving different transmitters which are regulated by various control mechanisms. For example, the striatum is regulated by at least seven transmitters with various afferent and efferent connections (Fig. 4).

Moreover, schizophrenia is quite possibly a heterogenous disorder, involving other transmitters, such as GABA, noradrenaline and serotonin.

Acknowledgements
I would like to thank Prof. H.H. Kornhuber for his support in these studies. I also acknowledge the valuable technical assistance of Mrs. A. Steingruber.

REFERENCES

Angrist, B., Sathananthan, G., Wilk, S., Gershon, S. *1974* — Amphetamine psychosis : behavioral and biochemical aspects. *J. Psychiat. Res., 11* : 13-23.

Brothers, C.R.D. *1964* — Huntington's chorea in Victoria and Tasmania. *J. Neurol. Sci., 1* : 405-420.

Bruyn, G.W., Bots, F. Th. A.M., Dom, R., *1979* — Huntington's chorea : current neuropathological status. *In : Advances in Neurology, Vol. 23,* T.N. Chase, N.S. Wexler, A. Barbeau (eds) pp. 83-93. New York, Raven Press.

Creese, I., Iversen, S.D. *1975* — The pharmacological and anatomical substrates of the amphetamine response in the rat. *Brain Res., 83* : 419-436.

Divac, I. *1972* — Neostriatum and functions of prefrontal cortex. *Acta Neurobiol. Exp., 32* : 461-477.

Divac, I., Fonnum, F., Storm-Mathisen, J. *1977* — High affinity uptake of glumatate in terminals of corticostriatal axons. *Nature, 266* : 377-378.

Farkas, T. *1979* — Application of fluorinated deoxyglucose and positron emission tomography in the study of psychiatric disorders. *Symposium on Cerebral Metabolism and Neural Function*, National Institute of Health, May 21-23.

Fonnum, F., Soreide, A., Kvale, I., Walker, J., Walaas, I. *1981* : Glutamate in cortical fibers. *In : Advances in Biochemical Psychopharmacology, Vol. 27*, G. Di Chiara, and G.L. Gessa (eds) pp. 29-41, New York, Raven Press.

Garau, L., Govoni, S., Stefanini, E., Trabucchi, M. Spano, P.F. *1978* — Dopamine receptors : pharmacological and anatomical evidences indicate that two distinct dopamine receptor populations are present in rat striatum. *Life Sci., 23* : 1745-1750.

Graham, T., Aprison, M.H. *1966* : Fluorometric determination of aspartate, glutamate and gamma-aminobutyrate in nerve tissue using enzymic method. *Ann. Biochem., 15* : 487-497.

Heikkila, R.E., Oransky, H., Mytilineou, C., Cohen, G. *1975* — Amphetamine : evaluation of d- and l-isomers as releasing agents and uptake inhibitors for ³H-dopamine and ³H-norepinephrine in slices of rat neostriatum and cerebral cortex. *J. Pharmacol. Exp. Ther., 194* : 47-56.

Ingvar, D.H. *1980* — Abnormal distribution of cerebral activity in chronic schizophrenia : a neurophysiological interpretation. *In : Perspectives in Schizophrenia Research*, C. Baxter, T. Melnechuk (eds), pp. 107-125. New York, Raven Press.

Jenner, P., Marsden, C.D. *1979* — The substituted benzamides — A novel class of dopamine antagonists. *Life Sci., 25* : 479-486.

Johnson, J. L. *1972* — Glutamic acid as a synaptic transmitter in the nervous system. A review. *Brain Res., 37* : 1-19.

Kim, J.S. *1978* — Transmitters for the afferent and efferent systems of the neostriatum and their possible interactions. *In : Advances in Biochemical Psychopharmacology, Vol. 19*, P.J. Roberts, G.N. Woodruff, and L.L. Iversen (eds), pp. 217-233. New York, Raven Press.

Kim, J.S., Kornhuber, H.H., *1982* — The glutamate theory in schizophrenia : Clinical and experimental evidence. *In : Psychobiology of schizophrenia*, N. Namba and H. Kaiya (eds), pp. 221-234. Oxford, New York, Pergamon Press.

Kim, J.S., Bak, I.J., Hassler, F., Okada, Y. *1971* — Role of GABA in the extrapyramidal motor system. 2. Some evidence for existence of a type of GABA-rich nigro-strial neurons. *Exp. Brain Res., 14* : 95-104.

Kim, J.S., Hassler, R., Haug, P., Paik, K.S. *1977* — Effect of frontal cortex ablation on striatal glutamic acid level in rat. *Brain Res., 132* : 370-374.

Kim, J.S., Kornhuber, H.H., Holzmüller, B., Schmid-Burgk, W., Mergner, T., Krzepinski, H. *1980a* — Reduction of cerebrospinal fluid glutamic acid in Huntington's chorea and in schizophrenic patients. *Arch. Psychiat. Nervenkr., 228* : 7-10.

Kim, J.S., Kornhuber, H.H., Schmid-Burgk, W., Holzmüller, B. *1980b* — Low cerebrospinal fluid glutamate in schizophrenic patients and a new hypothesis on schizophrenia. *Neurosci. Lett., 20* : 379-382.

Kim, J.S., Kornhuber, H.H., Brand, U., Menge, H.G. *1981* — Effects of chronic amphetamine treatment on the glutamate concentration in cerebrospinal fluid and brain : implication for a theory of schizophrenia. *Neurosci. Lett., 24* : 93-96.

Köhler, C., Ögren, S.O., Haglund, L., Ängeby, T. *1979* — Regional displacement by sulpiride of (³H)-spiperone binding in vivo. Biochemical and behavioral evidence for a preferential action on limbic and nigral dopamine receptors. *Neurosci. Lett., 13* : 51-56.

Liu, T.Z., Khayam-Bashi, H. *1980* — Fluorometric quantitation of glutamine in cerebrospinal fluid. *Clin. Chem., 26* : 700-701.

McGeer, P.L., McGeer, E.G., Scherer, U., Singh K. *1977* — A glutamatergic corticostriatal path ? *Brain Res., 128* : 369-373.

Mitchell, P.R. *1980* — Dopaminergic modulation of striatal (³H)-glutamic acid release. *Br. J. Pharmacol., 70* : 48-49.

Perry, T.L. *1982* — Normal cerebrospinal fluid and brain glutamate levels in schizophrenia do not support the hypothesis of glutamatergic neuronal dysfunction. *Neurosci. Lett., 28* : 81-85.

Perry, T.L., Stedman, D., Hansen, S. *1968* — A versatile lithium buffer elution system for single column automatic amino acid chromatography. *J. Chromatog., 38* : 460-466.

Pope, A. *1974* — Problems of interpretation in the chemical pathology of schizophrenia. *J. Psychiatr. Res., 11* : 265-272.

Pye, I.F., Stonier, C., McGale, E.H.F. *1978* — Double-enzymatic assay for determination of glutamine and glutamic acid in cerebrospinal fluid and plasma. *Anal. Chem., 50* : 951-953.

357

Reubi, J.C., Cuénod, M. *1979* — Glutamate release in vitro from corticostriatal terminals. *Brain Res., 176* : 185-188.

Rowlands, G.J., Roberts, P.J. *1980a* — Activation of dopamine receptors inhibits calcium-dependent glutamate release from cortico-striatal terminals in vitro. *Europ. J. Pharmacol., 62* : 241-242.

Rowlands, G.J., Roberts, P.J. *1980b* — Specific calcium-dependent release of endogenous glutamate from rat striatum is reduced by destruction of the corticostriatal tract. *Exp. Brain Res., 39* : 239-240.

Schneider, K. *1971* — *Klinische Psychopathologie.* 9th ed. Stuttgart, Georg Thieme.

Schwarcz, R., Creese, I., Coyle, J.T., Snyder, S.H. *1978* — Dopamine receptors localized on cerebral cortical afferents to rat corpus striatum. *Nature, 271* : 766-768.

Shank, R.P., Aprison, M.H. *1979* — Biochemical aspects of the neurotransmitter function of glutamate. *In :* *Glutamic acid,* L.J. Filer, Jr., S. Garattini, M.R. Kare, W.A. Reynolds, and R.J. Wurtman (eds) pp. 139-150. New York, Raven Press.

Spencer, H. J. *1976* — Antagonism of cortical excitation of striatal neurons by glutamic acid diethyl ester : evidence for glutamate acid as an excitatory transmitter in the rat striatum. *Brain Res., 102* : 91-101.

Taylor, K.M., Snyder, S.H. *1970* — Amphetamine : differentiation by d- and l-isomers of behavior involving brain norepinephrine or dopamine. *Science, 168* : 1487-1489.

Weinberger, D.R., Wyatt R.J. *1980* — Structural brain abnormalities in chronic schizophrenia : computed tomography findings. *In : Perspective in Schizophrenia Research,* C. Baxter, T. Melnechuk (ed.) pp. 29-38, New York, Raven Press.

DISCUSSION

B.E. Leonard

That was a very interesting paper. Can I ask two questions ? First of all, did you look at CSF GABA levels in your patients ? Secondly, could you tell us what dose of amphetamine and sulpiride you used and for how long were the animals treated ?

J.S. Kim

We did not measure GABA, because it is very difficult to measure the CSF GABA levels. Secondly, to dosage and treatment : The amphetamine group received daily an s.c. injection of d-amphetamine sulphate at a dose of 5 mg/kg for 12 days, and the sulpiride group received daily an i.p. injection of sulpiride at a dose of 50 mg/kg for 12 days.

N. Matussek

Do you know any studies in which glutamic acid has been given to schizophrenics and the effect thereof ? And secondly, what kind of schizophrenic patients did you mostly have in your studies ? Did you have more with minus or more with plus symptomatics ?

J.S. Kim

We are now on the way to these examinations, although glutamate does not pass well through the blood-brain barrier. As far as your second question is concerned, you have already seen the BPRS scores and we had 20 schizophrenic patients, 16 of whom were chronic, so we had more negative symptoms.

W.H. Vogel

I think that is a very nice finding and it shows that schizophrenia indeed is probably a very complex biochemical disorder. I have 2 questions to the methodology. The first one is, how did you measure glutamate in the CSF ? It has recently been shown, that there are quite a number of small peptides, which contain all kinds of amino acids including glutamate. These small peptides can very quickly hydrolize during drawing from the CSF and during determination of amino acids. They break down very quickly during technical procedures, so I would be interested in how you determined the glutamic acid ? And the second question is to the amphetamine studies. In our hands, if we give amphetamine on a chronic basis, our animals start losing weight. Did your animals lose weight, because if they start losing weight, that would, of course, then change their whole amino acid metabolism and just the loss in weight or the decreased food intake would reduce the glutamic acid ?

J.S. Kim
We measured CSF glutamate by means of the enzymatic fluorometric method using glutamate dehydrogenase. In our experience the method is accurate and reproducible. Recovery of glutamate added to CSF and assay was 94 %. To the second question : We did not actually measure body weight, but I agree that what you say is possible.

P. Grof
Did you by any chance look at the correlation between the duration of illness and the glutamate CSF levels ?

J.S. Kim
Yes, we did. However, there was no correlation.

Pharmacological classification
of central effects of neuroleptics

A. J. Puech[1], P. Rioux[2] and P. Simon[1]

1) Department of Pharmacology, 2) INSERM Research Unit, U88, University Hospital
Pitié-Salpêtrière, Paris, France

Summary : It is suggested that the negative and positive symptomatologies of schizophrenic patients are not only different but opposed states. Dopamine may be the underlying disturbance as suggested by clinical, pharmacological, therapeutic, and biological evidence :
— Overactivity of dopaminergic functions in patients with positive symptoms (e.g. : paranoid patients) is treated by dopaminergic blocking agents.
— Hypoactivity of dopaminergic function in patients with negative symptoms (e.g. : simple schizophrenia) is improved by low doses of neuroleptics able to enhance dopaminergic activity. Dopaminergic stimulants are also useful in this group of patients.
The hypothesis focuses on the fact that the role of opposed dopaminergic functioning in the two groups is restricted to symptomatology which is consistent with the therapeutic findings. Long-term deficit, occuring in chronic patients, may be a different process. The implications in the pharmacological field are presented.

Introduction

All the substances classified as neuroleptics have points in common : Clinically they are antipsychotic ; pharmacologically they antagonize apomorphine induced behavior ; biochemically they block dopaminergic receptors.

Neuroleptics do differ, however, so a system of classification is needed.

Clinically, Lambert and Revol (1960) first proposed that sedative neuroleptics could be distinguished from antipsychotic neuroleptics. Several authors (Delay and Deniker, 1971 ; Bobon et al., 1972) subclassified antipsychotic effects as antihallucinatory or disinhibitory.

Pharmacologically and biochemically, there are consistent differences among the relative potencies of neuroleptics to block dopaminergic and alpha-adrenergic receptors (Niemegeers and Janssen, 1979).

It seems that there is a relationship between sedative effects in man and alpha-adrenergic blocking properties in animals.

More recently, it has been demonstrated that there are several dopaminergic structures in the brain. It has been proposed that several types of dopaminergic receptors exist (Kebabian and Calne, 1979 ; Sokoloff et al., 1980). There is data to suggest that some neuroleptics may have a particular affinity for the nucleus accumbens (Bartholini, 1976) which could explain why some neuroleptics, such as sulpiride or clozapine, have less extrapyramidal effects when used as antipsychotics.

Although it appears that neuroleptics have two distinct therapeutic effects in man, antihallucinatory and disinhibitory, the animal model related to the disinhibitory effect has not yet been determined.

We have previously shown (Puech et al., 1978) that neuroleptics can be differentiated by their interactions with several apomorphine-induced behaviors. All the neuroleptics antagonize stereotyped behavior, climbing behavior and increased locomotor activity, but only some of them antagonize apomorphine-induced hypothermia.

Among the substances antagonizing apomorphine-induced hypothermia, some of them exert this effect at very low doses compared to the doses needed to antagonize other behaviors.

Some neuroleptics at very low doses potentiate apomorphine-induced hypermotility.

This paper presents data concerning the interaction of various neuroleptics which are chemically (phenothiazine, butyrophenone, diphenylbutylpiperidine and benzamides) and clinically different (sedative, antihallucinatory, disinhibitory) with four behaviors induced by apomorphine (stereotyped behavior, climbing behavior, hypermotility and hypothermia).

Materials and methods

The animals were isolated in small clear plastic boxes ($11 \times 7 \times 4.5$ cm) which were placed in slots in a frame (1.20 m long and 0.74 m high) equipped with a stainless-steel screen (5 mm² mesh). The mice could thus assume two different positions : Normal position in the bottom of the box or vertical against the walls or screen (« verticalization» or « climbing behavior »). This behavior was scored in a « all or none » manner. Stereotypy was graded 0-3 according to the following criteria :

0 = absence of stereotypy or any abnormal movement ;
1 = slight stereotyped head movements and intermittent sniffing ;
2 = intense head movements. Mild licking interspersed with sniffing ;
3 = intense licking and/or gnawing.

Rectal temperature was measured with a thermoelectric probe inserted to a constant depth.

The substances studied, including distilled water used as a control, were injected intraperitoneally 30 min before subcutaneous administration of apomorphine. Verticalization and stereotypies were evaluated « blindly » 20 min after apomorphine administration. Rectal temperatures were measured before each evalutation (homogeneous groups of six mice were constituted at this time) and again at the end of the experiment, i.e. 30 min after apomorphine administration. Changes in verticalization, stereotypies and rectal temperature were expressed as percent of control values in simultaneously studied mice receiving distilled water.

Results

The results are presented in Table 1. Three of the effects of apomorphine (stereotypy, verticalization and hypermotility) were antagonized by all the substances studied when sufficient doses were administered. The hypothermia in-

Table 1 - Effects of apomorphine

	Doses mg.kg^{-1} i.p.	Stereo- typed behavior	Vertical- ization	Hypo- thermia	Motor activity
Chlorpromazine	0.25	100	100	100	108
	0.5	100	100	100	85
	1	81	100	100	48
	2	31	67	100	6
	4	0	17	100	5
Clozapine	1	100	100	100	91
	2	100	100	100	81
	4	89	100	100	78
	8	61	100	100	60
	16	56	67	100	55
	32	33	56	100	45
DAN 2163	0.06	100	100	100	94
	0.125	100	100	100	91
	0.25	100	100	69	120
	0.25	100	100	67	113
	1	100	100	54	125
	2	100	100	51	85
	4	100	100	33	60
	8	100	83	33	46
	16	100	100	20	30
	32	30	50	41	22
	128	12	0	62	4
Flupentixol	0.03	100	100	89	100
	0.06	86	100	100	99
	0.125	82	75	48	141
	0.25	44	50	35	129
	0.5	0	0	17	62
	1	0	0	67	10
Fluphenazine	0.015	100	100	100	98
	0.03	100	100	74	115
	0.06	100	100	53	117
	0.125	53	67	39	147
	0.25	39	33	6	26
	0.5	0	17	26	13
	1	0	17	0	8
GRI. 1665	0.5				110
	1	100	100	77	148
	2	100	100	77	121
	4	81	100	40	110
	8	82	63	28	81
	16	100	86	13	83
	32	41	44	32	18
	64	29	63	36	13
	128	1	25	68	8

363

Table 1 - Effects of apomorphine

	Doses mg.kg^{-1} i.p.	Stereo- typed behavior	Vertical- ization	Hypo- thermia	Motor activity
Haloperidol	0.007	100	100	100	95
	0.015	100	100	100	118
	0.03	100	100	100	124
	0.06	100	100	95	105
	0.125	44	83	63	50
	0.25	0	17	25	16
Levomepromazine	0.015	100	100	100	113
	0.03	100	100	100	83
	0.06	100	100	100	92
	0.125	100	100	100	70
	0.25	100	100	100	77
	0.5	87	100	100	60
	1	50	83	100	32
	2	50	50	100	6
	4	0	0	100	4
Metoclopramide	0.5	100	100	100	90
	1	89	92	81	97
	2	83	92	72	78
	4	56	56	72	59
	8	44	0	50	33
	16	33	0	23	20
Pimozide	0.004	100	100	100	100
	0.007	100	100	100	124
	0.015	100	100	100	131
	0.03	100	100	100	178
	0.06	67	83	74	209
	0.125	94	100	68	179
	0.25	6	17	20	135
	0.5	21	62	28	107
	1	0	0	35	21
	2	0	0	19	12
Pipotiazine	0.125	100	100	65	111
	0.25	94	100	54	139
	0.5	73	34	32	136
	1	13	17	14	86
	2	7	0	24	27
Prochlorperazine	0.125	100	100	100	118
	0.25	83	100	100	94
	0.5	61	83	95	123
	1	39	67	45	45
	2	6	83	49	22
	4	0	17	45	12

Table 1 - Effects of apomorphine

	Doses mg.kg^{-1} i.p.	Stereo-typed behavior	Vertical-ization	Hypo-thermia	Motor activity
Sulpiride	1	100	100	100	127
	2	100	100	100	156
	4	100	100	84	159
	8	100	100	83	129
	16	100	100	44	97
	32	50	50	38	81
	64	0	30	26	19
Sultopride	0.125	100	100	100	91
	0.25	100	100	100	87
	0.5	100	100	100	104
	1	100	100	100	105
	2	100	100	50	88
	4	100	100	58	59
	8	36	45	31	43
	16	0	53	49	25
	32	0	51	26	10
TER. 1546	2				86
	4				131
	8	88	100	79	145
	16	94	100	38	98
	32	88	96	46	63
	64	21	40	46	41
	128	1	67	100	26
Thioproperazine	0.03	100	100	100	97
	0.06	100	100	86	113
	0.125	100	100	62	131
	0.25	87	100	20	88
	0.5	20	17	31	16
	1	0	0	31	16
Tiapride	1	100	100	100	104
	2	100	100	100	107
	4	100	100	100	128
	8	100	100	100	118
	16	96	100	68	74
	32	40	50	60	37
	63	0	50	40	9
	128	0	54	43	4
Thioridazine	0.25	100	100	114	
	0.5	100	100	100	93
	1	100	100	100	73
	2	80	100	76	96
	4	53	87	100	39
	8	13	33	100	9

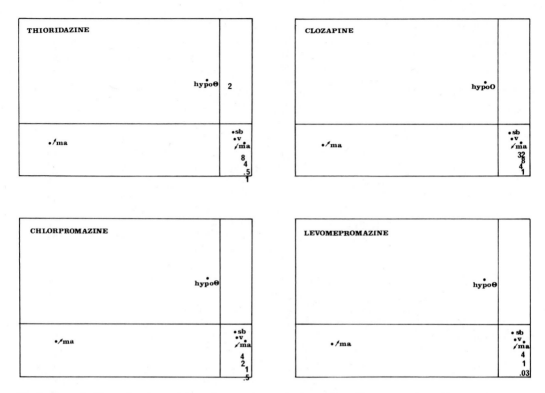

Fig. 1 - Group 1 : The active doses of these drugs project to the same place. They antagonize with the same intensity, stereotyped behavior, climbing behavior and hypermotility. They are not active on the two other tests.

duced by apomorphine, however, was only antagonized by some substances. Furthermore, apomorphine-induced hypermotility was potentiated by several neuroleptics. This phenomenon could be observed over a narrow range of doses for some drugs (haloperidol, thioproperazine, flupenthixol, pipotiazine, fluphenazine) or a larger range of doses in other cases (especially sulpiride and pimozide). It should be noted that all the substances which potentiated hypermotility also antagonized hypothermia, but the reverse is not true.

The effective doses of the various substances in the different tests may be dissociated. Four groups can be discerned.

Group 1 : Substances which antagonize stereotyped behavior, verticalization and hypermotility at similar doses without antagonizing hypothermia or potentiating hypermotility : Chlorpromazine, levomepromazine, clozapine, thioridazine ;

Group 2 : Substances which antagonize the four effects studied without potentiating hypermotility : Metoclopramide, prochlorperazine, sultopride ;

Group 3 and 4 : Substances which antagonize the four effects studied and which, in a certain dose range, potentiate hypermotility. Among these substances,

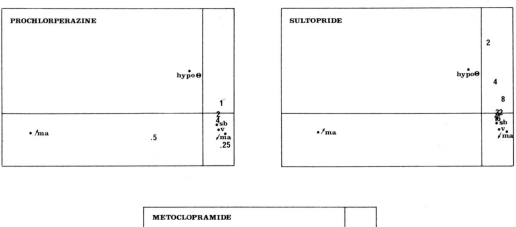

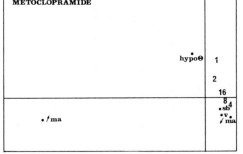

Fig. 2 - Group 2 : More of the active doses project between hypothermia and the three other tests because they are antagonistic in the four tests with approximately the same intensity.

two groups of drugs can be distinguished :

— those which antagonize the four effects in similar doses and which potentiate hypermotility at much lower dose levels (pimozide, sulpiride, haloperidol, tiapride, GRI 1665 and TER 1546) ;

— those which antagonize hypothermia and potentiate hypermotility in doses much smaller than those which antagonize stereotypies, verticalization and hypermotility (DAN 2163 [N (1-ethyl-2-pyrrolidinylmethyl)-x-methoxy-5-ethylsulfonyl benzamide hydrochloride], fluphenazine, flupenthixol, pipotiazine and thioproperazine)

These differences can be presented visually after factorial analysis of correspondence.

In Figures 1, 2, 3 and 4, points representing the tests and the active doses of the various substances are projected on a plane defined by two principal axes determined by factorial analysis.

The projections demonstrate the discriminative power of these tests.

Antagonism of stereotyped behavior, climbing behavior and hypermotility are only weakly discriminative.

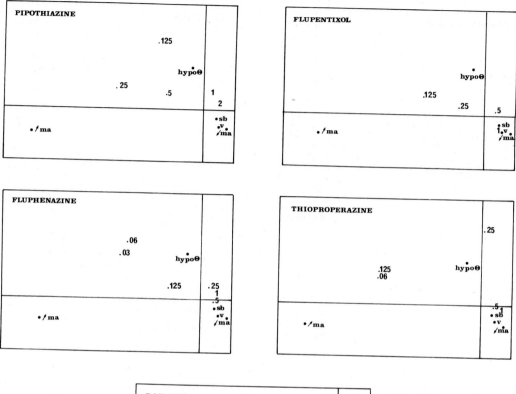

Fig. 3 - Group 3 : The lowest active doses project to the center, between antagonism of hypothermia and potentiation of hypermotility because at these doses they exert two effects but are not active in the three other tests. At higher doses, these substances project as group 2.

Antagonism of hypothermia and potentiation of hypermotility are, however, clearly differentiated from the other three tests. Neuroleptics can therefore be analysed and classified according to their behavior in three tests : Antagonism of stereotyped or climbing behavior , antagonism of hypothermia, and potentiation of hypermotility.

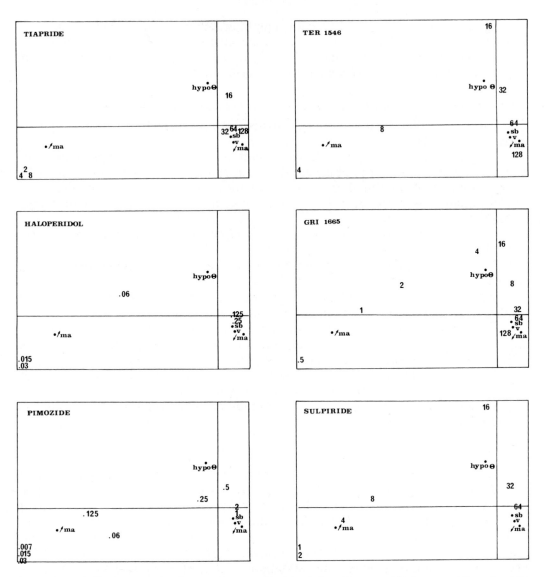

Fig. 4 - Group 4 : The lowest active doses project near the potentiation of hypermotility because at these doses the drugs exert only these effects. When the doses are increased, the drugs project as group 3, and at high doses project as group 2.

Discussion

Pharmacological classification of neuroleptics

The results of the interaction of 18 neuroleptics with four effects of apomorphine show that these tests are discriminative and allow classification of neuroleptics uniquely with respect to their dopaminergic properties.

369

Three tests, stereotyped behavior, climbing behavior and hypermotility, are approximately equivalent and thus do not permit clear classification of the drugs.

Antagonism of hypothermia and potentiation of hypermotility, however, differentiate the four groups of neuroleptics presented in the results.

Relationship between pharmacological classification and biochemical data

There are different dopaminergic structures and probably different types of dopaminergic receptors.

The fact that stereotyped behavior, climbing behavior and hypermotility induced by apomorphine are antagonized with approximately the same intensity by a large number of neuroleptics suggest that these three effects are mediated by similar dopaminergic receptors in structures equally accessible to the neuroleptics studied.

A very precise study has previously shown that a small number of neuroleptics can selectively antagonize climbing behavior.

The ED_{50} for antagonism of climbing behavior and stereotyped behavior by sulpiride are statistically different but very close (Sokoloff, this book).

Some neuroleptics antagonize apomorphine-induced hypothermia at doses smaller than those required to antagonize the other behaviors.

The hypothesis can be formulated that hypothermia is mediated by different dopaminergic receptors than the other behavior, or that the dopaminergic receptor is the same but is located in a structure with increased accessibility to the drug.

Some neuroleptics at very low doses potentiate apomorphine-induced hypermotility. We have presented these data in a previous paper.

Several explanations for the paradoxical effects of neuroleptics with respect to apomorphine can be offered.

Pre- and post-synaptic receptors

There is evidence for pre-synaptic dopaminergic receptors. Apomorphine is thought to stimulate these receptors at very low doses. At the same doses apomorphine induces a decrease in locomotor activity (Puech et al., 1974 ; Carlsson, 1975). This decrease could be related to the stimulation of the pre-synaptic receptors (Carlsson, 1975). The locomotor activity induced by 1 mg.kg^{-1} of apomorphine may be the sum of two components, stimulation of pre-synaptic receptors which decreases locomotor activity, and stimulation of post-synaptic receptors which decreases locomotor activity. Potentiation by neuroleptics of the locomotor activity could be due to the preferential blockade of pre-synaptic receptors by very low doses of some neuroleptics.

Two different structures regulating locomotor activity

The dopaminergic stimulation of nucleus accumbens increases locomotor activity.

The dopaminergic stimulation of mesocortical cortex decreases locomotor activity (Le Moal et al., 1977).

So the potentiation of apomorphine-induced locomotor activity could reflect a preferential blockade of mesolimbic dopaminergic receptors.

370

Prolactin hypothesis

Prolactin induces an increase in dopaminergic receptors. A very small dose of neuroleptic which increases prolactin secretion can increase the number of central dopaminergic receptors, thereby increasing the effects of apomorphine (Hruska et al., 1982).

Whatever the explanation, it seems important to consider the fact that in animal models some neuroleptics induce opposite effects depending on the dose.

Relationship between pharmacological classification and clinical effects

The main central therapeutic effects of neuroleptics are antihallucinatory, disinhibitory, sedative, antimanic and extrapyramidal.

Some correlations have previously been observed between pharmacological and clinical activity :

— sedative/adrenolytic
— antihallucinatory/dopaminolytic
— extrapyramidal/dopaminolytic.

Extrapyramidal effects are reasonably related to the antagonism of stereotyped behavior.

Antihallucinatory activity seems to be reflected by antagonism of either stereotyped behavior, climbing behavior, hypermotility or hypothermia. If it is correlated with antagonism of one of the first three behaviors, it will be difficult to select an antihallucinatory drug that does not have extrapyramidal effects at the same dose. If the antihallucinatory effect is reflected by antagonism of apomorphine-induced hypothermia, it should be possible to select antihallucinatory drugs that have few extrapyramidal effects if the drug is used at the minimum active dose.

Until now, few explanations for the disinhibitory effects of neuroleptics have been proposed.

There is quite a good correlation between substances potentiating apomorphine-induced hypermotility in mice and drugs described as disinhibitory in schizophrenic patients.

We propose that the disinhibitory property of neuroleptics might be related to the activation of a dopaminergic system by low doses of neuroleptics. The different mechanisms by which neuroleptics can activate the dopaminergic system are discussed above.

The clinical implications of this hypothesis are discussed in the same book by Lecrubier et al. (see page 375)

In short, productive symptomatology and defective symptomatology might be related to opposite dysfunction of dopaminergic systems. Productive symptomatology could be related to dopaminergic overactivity and improved by high doses of any neuroleptic which decreases dopaminergic activity.

Defective symptomatology could be related to dopaminergic hypoactivity and improved only by the same neuroleptic at low doses which increases dopaminergic activity.

REFERENCES

Bartholini, G. *1976* - Differential effect of neuroleptic drugs on dopamine turnover in the extrapyramidal and limbic system, *J. Pharm. Pharmacol, 26 :* 429.

Bobon, J., Pinchard, A., Collard J., Bobon D.P. *1972* - Clinical classification of neuroleptics, with special reference to their antimanic, antiautistic and ataraxic properties, *Compr. Psychiat., 13,* 123-131.

Carlsson, A. *1975* - Receptor-mediated control of dopamine metabolism. *In : Pre- and Postsynaptic Receptors,* E. Usdin and W.E. Bunney (ed.), New York, Marcel Dekker.

Delay, J., Deniker, P. *1971* - Essai de classification des agents psychotropes. *Psychopharmacologie,* 115-119.

Hruska, R.E., Pitman, K.T., Silbergeld, E.K., Ludmer, L.M. *1982* - Prolactin increases the density of striatal dopamine receptors in normal and hypophysectomized male rats. *Life Sci. 30 :* 547-553.

Kebabian, J.W., Calne D.B. *1979* - Multiple receptors for dopamine. *Nature, 277 :* 93-96.

Lambert, P.A., Revol L. *1960* - Classification psychopharmacologique et clinique des différentes indications thérapeutiques générales dans les psychoses, *Presse méd., 68,* 1509-1512.

Le Moal, M., Stinus, L., Simon, H., Tassin, J.P., Thierry, A.M., Blanc, G., Glowinski, J., Cardo, B., *1977* - Behavioral effects of a lesion in the ventral mesencephalic tegmentum. Evidence for involvement of A_{10} dopaminergic neurons. *Advances in Biochemical Psychopharmacology, vol. 16,* Costa E., and Gessa G.L. (ed.) pp. 237-245. New York, Raven Press.

Niemegeers, C.J.E., Janssen, P.A.J. *1979* - A systematic study of the pharmacological activities of dopamine antagonists, *Life Sci., 24,* 2201-2216.

Puech, A.J., Simon, P., Chermat, R., Boissier, J.R. *1974* - Profil neuropsychopharmacologique de l'apomorphine, *J. Pharmacol. (Paris) 5,* 241-254.

Puech, A.J., Simon, P. Boissier, J.R. *1978* - Benzamides and classical neuroleptics ; comparison of their actions using six apomorphine-induced effects. *Eur. J. Pharmacol., 50,* 291-300.

Sokoloff, P., Martres, M.P., Schwartz, J.C. *1980* - Three classes of dopamine receptors (D2, D3, D4) identified by binding studies with ^{3}H-apomorphine and ^{3}H-domperidone. *Naunyn Schmiedeberg's Arch. Pharmacol., 315,* 89-102.

DISCUSSION

M. Ackenheil

The effects of neuroleptics in a single dosage are sometimes time-dependent. Could it be possible that the different effects are due to time effects, perhaps you have rebound effects sometimes and one should consider this in such investigations ? Generally, I would believe that there are differences of this kind, but in my opinion one should consider these time effects too.

A.J. Puech

The administration of neuroleptics was at the same times, 30 minutes before apomorphine, but it is a well-known fact, that for some of these drugs it is not the best time. For example, for pimozide it is better to administer one or 2 hours before. However, we have verified that this profile is the same when the drug is administered half an hour before apomorphine, one hour, 2 hours and 4 hours and for 6 hours and we observe the same profile, so these different profiles are not related to time-dependence.

J. Mendlewicz

Are you aware of any evidence that pimozide at low doses may have a disinhibitory effect, working on the negative symptomatology ?

A.J. Puech

I think it is better to discuss this point after the presentation of Yves Lecrubier.

N. Matussek
Would you say that all drugs that influence the motor activity in this way have a better effect on the minus symptomatology ?

A.J. Puech
Yes, it is a possibility.

G. Bartholini
I wonder whether this « activation » of locomotor activity of some compounds as compared to other neuroleptics, reflects just a lack of sedative action ?

A.J. Puech
I did not present the results of drugs on locomotor activity, but there is no correlation. We have verified this point.

G. Bartholini
Yes, but all these neuroleptics sulpiride, haloperidol, pimozide and tiapride are devoid of sedative action.

A.J. Puech
Haloperidol is sedative.

G. Bartholini
I wonder whether, in the line of the question of Prof. Ackenheil, this is not a methodological artefact ? Firstly, I would express the data in terms of ED_{50}, which is the classical pharmacological way, rather than in milligramm, so that I cannot accept your explanation. Secondly, your results parallel, in a way, the data presented by Prof. Sedvall : You have shown that orthomethoxy-benzamides activate locomotion and in the trial of Prof. Sedvall, sulpiride should be associated with anxiolytics, whereas in the case of chlorpromazine, levopromazine and thioridazine you have a sedative action.

A.J. Puech
Do you think that all neuroleptics can potentiate hypermotility ?

G. Bartholini
No, only those devoid of alpha-adrenoreceptor blocking properties.

A.J. Puech
Do you think that all these drugs could be disinhibitory, if they are not sedatives ?

G. Bartholini
Possibly, because we see that those which do not block alpha-adrenoreceptor sites are not sedative and do potentiate motility, whereas the others which have alpha-adrenoreceptor blocking properties are sedative and do not potentiate motility. Maybe all of the neuroleptics potentiate motility, but for some of them this effect is masked by the blockade of noradrenergic transmission.

A.J. Puech
Do you think that the pharmacological effect can predict disinhibitory effect in man ?

G. Bartholini
Possibly.

P. Sokoloff
On what basis can you say that haloperidol or pimozide have a preferential effect on pre-synaptic dopamine receptors or in mesocortical regions ? I think there is no biochemical data showing that haloperidol or pimozide display a higher potency for a pre-synaptic receptor or in mesocortical regions.

373

A.J. Puech

I said that small doses of pimozide potentiate the hypermotility induced by apomorphine and that is my interpretation. Some biochemists said that there is a correlation between the hypomotility induced by apomorphine and effect on pre-synaptic receptors.

G. Bartholini

This is an answer more than a question. Haloperidol, for instance, in small doses seems to block preferentially pre-synaptic receptors. Indeed, it increases the turnover of dopamine after administration of gamma-butyrolactone, which turns down the firing rate of dopaminergic neurons, so that the activation by haloperidol cannot be due other than to pre-synaptic receptor blockade.

Neuroleptics and the bipolar dopaminergic hypothesis of schizophrenia

Y. Lecrubier, P. Douillet

Department of Psychiatry, University Hospital Pitié-Salpêtrière, Paris, France

Summary : It is suggested that the negative and positive symptomatologies of schizophrenic patients are not only different but opposed states. Dopamine may be the underlying disturbance as suggested by clinical, pharmacological, therapeutic and biological evidence :
— Overactivity of dopaminergic functions in patients with positive symptoms (e.g. : paranoid patients) is treated by dopaminergic blocking agents.
— Hypoactivity of dopaminergic functions in patients with negative symptoms (e.g. : simple schizophrenia) is improved by low doses of neuroleptics able to enhance dopaminergic activity. Dopaminergic stimulants are also useful in this group of patients.
The hypothesis focuses on the fact that the role of opposed dopaminergic functioning in the two groups is restricted to symptomatology which is consistent with the therapeutic findings. Long-term deficit, occuring in chronic patients, may be a different process. The implications in the clinical field are presented.

Introduction

During this symposium the implications of noradrenaline (NA) and dopamine (DA) in schizophrenia and in depressive states were widely discussed. The question arises whether the clinical classification, based mainly on diagnosis and nosology, can be related to these biochemical implications.

We can assume that pharmacological effects are due to modifications of discrete structures in the CNS responsible for behavioral changes. If the therapeutic effects of chemotherapy deal with the same or equivalent structures, they should also be evaluated in terms of behavioral changes i.e. patterns of symptoms and not in terms of nosology. The course of illness and to some extent the etiology and associated psychiatric symptoms are part of the nosological criteria and are unlikely to be related to the effects of neuroleptics in schizophrenia.

The major finding of the last thirty years of classical neuroleptic use in schizophrenia is not that they are antischizophrenic or antipsychotic agents but that they act on positive symptoms whatever the cause. The hypothesis that a dopaminergic blockade is responsible for the therapeutic properties of neuroleptics is very consistent with this behavioral effect (Carlsson et al., 1963). But another syndrome is known in schizophrenia as the schizophrenic deficit which consists of « negative symptoms ». This could be the basic symptom pattern in schizophrenia as proposed by Bleuler (1911) and Kraepelin (1913) : Poverty of speech, flattening of affect, psychomotor retardation, loss of initiative, energy and creative ability are amongst the easiest to assess. Classical neuroleptics like chlorpromazine show no effect on this pattern or may even worsen it (Riviera Calimlim et al., 1976). The therapeutic interpretation of these symptoms is made even more difficult as these symptoms may exist in different groups of schizophrenics for different reasons :

— presence in young patients at the onset of the illness, simple schizophrenia,
— deficit in chronic patients which may be due to an evolution of the disease process,
— deficit due to institutionalization in chronic patients,
— deficit due to a real depressive episode,
— deficit due to high doses of neuroleptics.

The first group appears the most appropriate for clinical and therapeutic research.

Some neuroleptics seem to improve this deficit when prescribed in low dosages as shown in several classifications (Deniker and Ginestet, 1973 ; Bobon et al., 1972). The neuroleptics displaying this original property are precisely those shown by Puech et al. (1978) to enhance dopaminergic transmission when administered in low doses to animals.

If we consider the two syndromes present in schizophrenia, the positive and negative symptoms are not only different, but to some extent opposite as shown in Table 1.

Table 1

Florid syndrome	Deficit syndrome
Delusions, hallucinations	Poverty of speech
Vigorously expressed	Flattened affect
	Loss of initiative
Agitation	Psychomotor retardation
Stereotyped behavior	Akinesia.Increased tone
Hyperkinetic movements	Catatonic behavior

Long before the neuroleptics were discovered, akinesia and increased tone were described as features of the deficit group while hypermotility and stereotypies were associated with the patients presenting positive symptoms, mainly paranoids.

Paradoxically, the deficit pattern mimics a dopaminergic deficiency and is precisely the behavior exhibited when the best dopaminergic blockers we know are administered in man i.e. the neuroleptics themselves (see their definition by Delay and Deniker, 1957).

This led us to propose the following hypothesis (Lecrubier et al., 1980a and 1980b) : In patients presenting positive symptoms there is a hyperdopaminergy blocked by classical dopaminergic blockers. In patients presenting negative symptoms a hypodopaminergy is the basis for these symptoms. Logically, it would be treated by neuroleptics able to enhance dopaminergic transmission, at least in some structures.

If the hypothesis is consistent certain implications on treatment and side effects depending on the type of symptomatology and the type of neuroleptic should follow.

Classically dopaminergic blockers like chlorpromazine are effective against

376

positive symptoms. However, there is no correlation between their dosage or their blood levels and a therapeutic effect on negative symptoms. In fact, high blood levels worsen these symptoms (Riviera Calimlim et al., 1976).

The disinhibitory neuroleptic at low dosages exhibits stimulant properties (Deniker and Ginestet, 1973), restoring initiative and interest. Pimozide has been shown to be superior to haloperidol in terms of social and mimic adaptation (Baro and Dom, 1976). In long term maintenance therapy pimozide has been shown to be superior to fluphenazine in stimulating activity, improving interpersonal relations and impairment (Falloon et al., 1978).

The same claims are made for sulpiride (Justin - Besançon et al., 1967), although few controlled studies are available (Sutter, 1971) at these low dosages. As one would expect from the hypothesis, low dosages of these neuroleptics are able to reactivate hallucinations, delusions or agitation (Marshall, 1971).

When prescribed in high doses, all neuroleptics seem to have similar effects mainly on positive symptoms as shown by Sedvall (this symposium) with sulpiride. Figure 1 summarizes the differences and similarities of both groups of neuroleptics depending on the pattern of symptoms exhibited by the patient.

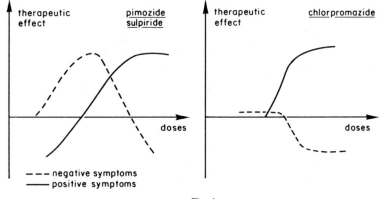

Fig. 1

The same contrast is found for side effects (Table 2) :

— The psychic side effects of chlorpromazine-like compounds are similar to most negative symptoms while low dosages of the other group of neuroleptics may reactivate positive symptomatology.

— As for neurological side effects, akinesia and increased tone are the logical effects of classical DA blockers. Some patients are more sensitive to this sort of side effect and are found to have lower urinary levels of dopamine (Crowley et al., 1976) or metabolites (Chase et al., 1970) following neuroleptic treatment.

The best therapeutic results are obtained in patients able to increase their dopamine turnover after neuroleptic administration as shown by Rüther et al., 1976 ; Van Praag et al., 1976. If prescribed at high doses, the other group of neuroleptics produces the same effects (Sedvall, this symposium) (Table 2).

377

Table 2 : *Side effects*

CPZ type	Disinhibitory type
＼of interest contact initiative	Efficacy on these symptoms
(efficacy on these symptoms)	Agitation
(efficacy on these symptoms)	Delusions hallucinations rebound
Sedation	Stimulation
Akinesia	(symptoms of the disease)
Increased tone	
(efficacy on these symptoms)	Acathisia.Hyperkinesia

On the other hand, low doses induce hyperkinesia, acathisia, and acute dyskinesia and fewer extrapyramidal syndromes or depressive states (Falloon et al., 1978). Sulpiride has been described as displaying antidepressant properties.

If patients with negative symptoms show decreased DA functioning in some structures, even if the striatum is not the most appropriate structure, one should carefully observe the neurological state of patients with purely negative symptomatology.

As will be shown, increased tone and akinesia are common in such a group. Although neuroleptics are supposed to induce such symptoms and if low doses of pimozide or sulpiride are able to enhance DA transmission, they should not worsen but improve this symptomatology.

In a preliminary study we included 11 young schizophrenics presenting a marked and purely negative symptomatology. Most of them had relapsed following cessation of treatment several months before ; two had no previous treatment and for two patients the wash-out period from previous neuroleptics was only two weeks.

All patients were treated with pimozide 2 mg (1 to 4) per day. The only association allowed was benzodiazepines (anxiolytic dosage). Patients were assessed before treatment and after 1 week of treatment by an independant neurologist using the extrapyramidal symptoms rating scale (EPRS) of Chouinard.

The psychiatrist in charge of the patient rated the patient with a global evaluation and a BPRS before treatment and 1 month later.

As can be seen from Table 3 mildly increased tone and akinesia are present in this very selected group of patients. We do not believe that this was due to the previous neuroleptic treatment stopped several months before as the two patients with no previous treatment (no 2 and no 7) presented a similar picture.

Table 4 shows that low doses of pimozide improve these symptoms which is paradoxical for a neuroleptic, but logical according to our hypothesis (Table 4).

After the therapeutic results were evaluated, it appeared that the existence of such neurological symptoms on admission was a good prognostic factor in terms of the treatment used (Table 5).

Classical dopaminergic stimulants have been used in schizophrenia. Quantitative effects are still under discussion, but there is good agreement for qualitative results in both groups of symptoms (Angrist et al., 1973 and 1980 ; Yaryura-Tobias et al., 1970 ; Gerlach et al., 1975 ; Inanaga et al., 1975) (Table 6).

Here again we find the same contrast in the patients symptomatology, suggest-

378

Table 3 : *Extrapyramidal symptom rating scale (Chouinard)*
11 young schizophrenics presenting a marked
and « pure » deficit state

Case :	1	2	3	4	5	6	7	8	9	10	11
Ptyalism	1	0	0	1	0	3	0	0	0	0	0
Tremor	2	0	0	0	0	0	0	1	0	0	0
Automatic expressive movements	3	4	2	2	3	3	3	4	2	2	4
Gait-posture	2	4	2	2	2	3	2	2	1	1	2
Bradykinesia	2	4	2	3	2	2	3	2	1	2	3
Rigidity Left	0	3	2	4	0	4	1	4	1	1	2
Right	2	4	3	5	1*	4	1	2	1	1	3

Range = 0 to 6   1 — 2 = very slight pathology
* patient 5 presented a waxy flexibility

Table 4 : *Effect of pimozide 1 week treatment on the extrapyramidal symptoms*
of 9 schizophrenics with a « pure » deficit state

	Before TT (n=9)	After TT (n=9)	% improvement
Automatic expressive movements	2,9	1,1**	62
Gait posture	2,2	0,9*	59
Bradykinesia	2,3	0,6**	74
Rigidity Left	2,5	0,5*	81
Right	2,1	0,4*	80

Pimozide 1 — 4 mg/day
Student t test   *p < .05
           **p < .01

Table 5 : *Individual therapeutic results after 1 month treatment and initial scores on the EPRS*

Case	1	2	3	4	5	6	7	8	9	10	11
Automatic expressive movements	3	4	2	2	3	3	3	4	2	2	4
Gait-posture	2	4	2	2	2	3	2	2	1	1	2
Bradykinesia	2	4	2	3	2	2	3	2	1	2	3
Rigidity Left	0	3	2	4	0	4	1	4	1	1	2
Right	2	4	3	5	1	4	1	2	1	1	3
% improvement BPRS	8	75	8	85	0	48*	43	79	30		
Clinical advice	0	+	0	+	0	+	±	+	±		

*Marked improvement on schizophrenic symptoms but increase in insomnia and anxiety
Nº 10 Prescribed another neuroleptic
Nº 11 Ran away from hospital

Table 6 : *DA stimulants in schizophrenia*

L-DOPA	╱Positive S.	╲Negative S.
Amphetamine	╱Positive S.	╲Negative S.
Apomorphine		
—high doses	╱Positive S.	?
—low doses	╲Positives S.	?

ing opposed DA states in these two groups. So, if DA blocking agents are useful in patients with positive symptomatology, implying an overactivity in at least some DA structures, impressive data indicate that patients presenting purely negative symptoms could, on the contrary, exhibit hypoactivity in some (other ?) DA structures. This is in agreement with the hypothesis of Chouinard (1978) and the results of Alpert et al. (1978) though limited to only some of the patients. The effectiveness of some neuroleptics at low doses, those shown to enhance DA activity (Puech et al., 1978) and those called « disinhibitory » by clinicians are therefore an important and an interesting field of research in schizophrenia.

The explanation for this effect of some neuroleptics at low doses is still controversial. The main alternatives are :

1) They preferentially block pre-synaptic DA receptors thus enhancing DA transmission (Lehmann and Langer, submitted). This effect does not occur in structures without pre- and post-synaptic receptors (hypothalamus).

2) They preferentially block structures controlling other DA structures as shown by Le Moal et al. (1977). The suppression of a negative feed-back could enhance DA transmission.

3) They block a subclass of DA receptors as proposed by Sokoloff et al. (1980) which control other DA receptors and DA structures.

4) They block inhibitory DA receptors at low doses and excitatory DA receptors at higher doses (Cools et al., 1980).

5) Many other possibilities remain, like an easier access of some neuroleptics to certain structures as proposed by Bartholini (1976), or an indirect effect of prolactin which is enhanced with very low doses (no blood brain barrier) and could facilitate DA transmission (Hruska et al., 1982).

Whatever the explanations, the clinical and pharmacological findings remain and when clarified, could form the basis for fundamental research.

It is just as difficult to explain why DA transmission should be enhanced or decreased in patients.

— The hypersensitivity of DA receptors found in schizophrenic patients, assuming that this is not due to neuroleptic treatment, could be a primary phenomenon or could reflect a decrease in DA transmission.

— The ability of schizophrenics to enhance their DA turnover when necessary, could be an explanation. Although some studies (Rüther et al., 1976 ; Van Praag et al., 1976) support this possibility, very little is known about this functional problem.

— The same can be said of the hypothesis of Ashcroft et al. (1981), the nearest to our own hypothesis, which supposes a constriction of the tolerated range of dopamine activity in schizophrenic patients. The reasons we had hypothesized a similar explanation is that normal ranges of DA metabolites are possible in this case and that the existence of both positive and negative symptoms in patients is not contradictory with such a mechanism of action.

The consequences of this hypothesis are both theoretical and practical. Theoretically, if DA modulates schizophrenic syptomatology in two opposite ways it follows that the basis of the disease process is necessarily upstream DA. Thought disorders may be expressed vigorously or poorly depending on variations in DA function (naturally or due to therapy), DA impairment does not explain their existence.

Practically, the hypothesis clarifies the use of neuroleptics in patients with negative symptoms :

— Low posologies of some neuroleptics like sulpiride or pimozide should be given in monotherapy, keeping in mind that a decrease in dosage is as logical as an increase when the treatment is not statisfactory.

— No improvement can be obtained on one side of the symptomatology without running the risk of an exacerbation on the other.

— If DA modulates the expression of the symptoms, the dosage of the neuroleptics should follow the symptoms should they change.

— The association of classical neuroleptics, often prescribed for their sedative (alpha blocking ?) properties, is probably able to antagonize to some extent the effects of « disinhibitory » neuroleptics by a mutual antagonism at the DA level.

As for biological investigations, the mean of the two opposite subgroups is likely to be similar to a normal population, although with a wider variance. Therefore such investigations should be made in clearly opposed clinical subgroups until more is known about the fundamental disease process.

REFERENCES

Alpert, M., Diamond, F., Weisenfreund, J., Taleporos, E., Friedhoff, A.J. *1978* — The neuroleptic hypothesis : study of the covariation of extrapyramidal and therapeutic drug effects. *Br. J. Psychiat. 133* : 169-175.

Angrist, B. Sathananthan, G., Gershon, S. *1973* — Behavioral effects of L-DOPA in schizophrenic patients. *Psychopharmacologia, 31* : 1-12.

Angrist, B., Rotrosen, J., Gershon, J. *1980* — Response to apomorphine, amphetamine and neuroleptics in schizophrenic subjects. *Psychopharmacology, 67* : 31-38.

Ashcroft, G. W., Blackwood, G. W., Besson, J.A.O., Palomo, T., Waring, H.L. *1981* — Positive and negative schizophrenic symptoms and the role of dopamine. *Br. J. Psychiat., 138* : 268-272.

Baro, F., Dom, R. *1976* — The interaction between neuroleptic treatment and sociotherapeutic approach in chronic schizophrenics. Investigations with haloperidol, penfluridol and pimozide. *Acta Psychiatr. Belg., 76* : 735-758.

Bartholini, G. *1976* — Differential effect of neuroleptic drugs on dopamine turnover in the extrapyramidal and limbic system. *J. Pharm. Pharmacol., 28* : 429.

Bleuler, E. *1911* — *Dementia praecox or the group of schizophrenia.* New York, International University Press.

Bobon, J., Pinchard, A., Collard, J., Bobon, D.P. *1972* — Clinical classification of neuroleptics with special reference to their antimanic, antiautistic and ataraxic properties. *Compreh. Psychiat. 13,* : 123-127.

Carlsson, A. , Lindquist, M. *1963* — Effect of chlorpromazine on formation of 3-methoxytyramine and normetanephrine in mouse brain. *Acta Pharmacol. Toxicol., 20* : 140-144.

Chase, T.N., Schnur, J.A., Gordon, E.K. *1970* — Cerebrospinal fluid monoamine catabolites in drug induced extrapyramidal disorders. *Neuropharmacology, 9* : 265-268.

Chouinard, G., Jones, B.D. *1978* — Schizophrenia as a dopamine-deficiency disease. *Lancet, 2* : 99-100.

Cools, A.R., Van Rossum, J.M. *1980* — Multiple receptors for brain dopamine in behavior regulation : concept of dopamine-E and dopamine-I receptors. *Life Sci., 27* : 1237-1253.

Crowley, T.J., Rutledge, C.O., Hoehn M.M. et al. *1976* — Low urinary dopamine and prediction of phenothiazine - induced Parkinsonism. *Am. J. Psychiat., 133* : 703-706.

Delay J., Deniker P. *1957* — Caracteristiques psychophysiologiques des médicaments neuroleptiques. *In : Psychotropic drugs,* pp. 485-501. Amsterdam, Elsevier.

Deniker, P., Ginestet, D. *1973* — Neuroleptiques. *Encycl. Méd.-Chir.* Psychiatrie, 37860 B20.

Falloon, I, Watt, D. C., Shepherd, M., *1978* — The social outcome of patients in a trial of long-term continuation therapy in schizophrenia : pimozide v.s. fluphenazine. *Psycholog. Med. 8* : 265-274.

Gerlach, J., Luhdorf, K. *1975* — The effect of L-DOPA on young patients with simple schizophrenia treated with neuroleptic drugs. *Psychopharmacologia, 44* : 105-110.

Hruska, R.E., Pitman, K.T., Silbergeld, E.K., Ludmer, L.M. *1982* — Prolactin increases the density of striatal dopamine receptors in normal and hypophysectomized male rats. *Life Sci., 30* : 547-553.

Inanaga, K., Nakazawa, Y., Inone, K. et al. *1975* — Double blind controlled study of L-Dopa therapy in schizophrenia. *Folia Psychiatr. Neurol. Jpn, 29* : 123-143.

Justin-Besançon, L., Thominet, N., Laville, Cl., Margarit, J. *1967* — Constitution chimique et propriétés biologiques du sulpiride. *C.R. Acad. Sci. (Paris), 265* : 1253-1254.

Kraepelin, E. *1913* — *Dementia praecox and paraphrenia 1913.*, p. 163. New York, Krieger.

Lecrubier, Y., Puech, A., Simon, P., Widlocher, D. *1980a* — Schizophrénie : hyper ou hypofonctionnement du système dopaminergique ? Une hypothèse bipolaire. *Psychologie Méd., 12* : 2431-2441.

Lecrubier, Y., Puech, A., Widlocher, D., Simon, P. *1980b* — Schizophrenia : a bipolar dopaminergic hypothesis. Abstract n° 390. Proceedings of the 12 th CINP Congress. Göteborg 1980. *Progress in Neuropsychopharmacology, supplement.*

Lehmann, J., Langer S.Z. — The pharmacological distinction between central pre and postsynaptic dopamine receptors : implications for the pathology and therapy of schizophrenia. (submitted)

Le Moal, M., Stinus, L., Simon, H., Tassin, J.P., Thierry, A.M., Blanc, G., Glowinski, J., Cardo, B. *1977* — Behavioral effects of a lesion in the ventral mesencephalic teg. Evidence for involvement of A_{10} dopaminergic neurons. *In : Adv. in Bioch. Psychopharmacol. Vol. 16*, Costa E., Gessa GL. (ed.) pp. 237-245. New York, Raven Press.

Marshall, W. K. *1971* — Pimozide (Orap) : a multicenter study. *Clin. Trials J., 8*, suppl. II : 49-54.

Puech, A.J., Simon, P., Boissier, J.R. *1978* — Benzamides and classical neuroleptics : comparison of their actions using apomorphine induced effects. *Eur. J. Pharmacol., 50* : 291-300.

Riviera Calimlim, L., Nasrallah, H., Strauss, J., Lasagna, L. *1976* — Clinical response and plasma levels : effect of dose, dosage schedules, and drug interactions on plasma chlorpromazine levels. *Am. J. Psychiat., 133* : 646-652.

Rüther, E., Schilkrut, R., Ackenheil, M., Eben, E., Hippius, H. *1976* — Clinical and biochemical parameters during neuroleptic treatment. I. Investigations with haloperidol. *Pharmakopsychiatr., 9* : 33-36.

Sutter, J.M. *1971* — Controlled trial of sulpiride in psychiatry. *Sem. Hôp. Paris, 47* : 446-455.

Sokoloff, P., Martres, M.P., Schwartz, J.C. *1980* — Three classes of dopamine receptors (D_2, D_3, D_4) identified by binding studies with ^{3}H-apomorphine and ^{3}H-domperidone. *Naunyn Schmiedebergs Arch. Pharmacol., 315* : 89-102.

Van Praag, H.M., Korf, J. *1976* — Importance of dopamine metabolism for the clinical effects and side effects of neuroleptics. *Am. J. Psychiat., 133* : 1171-1177.

Yaryura-Tobias J.A., Diamond B., Merlis S. *1970* — The action of L-Dopa on schizophrenic patients (a preliminary report). *Curr. Ther. Res., 12* : 528-531.

DISCUSSION

J.S. Kim
I have just practical questions. What is your best effective dose of sulpiride on negative symptoms ?

Y. Lecrubier
I would say between 100 and 300 mg/day.

J.S. Kim
For chronic patients ?

382

Y. Lecrubier
Yes, something like this.

J.S. Kim
According to the literature, this is just an antidepressant effect.

Y. Lecrubier
In a lot of these chronic patients depression has been described, I think, nearly as a part of the negative syndrome, so this raises another problem. The second point is that in chronic patients, sometimes the negative symptoms are the same as you have, for example, at the onset of the illness. I would not say that it is the same thing, if we are speaking about only chronic patients.

M. Ackenheil
I find it very important that you are looking for new ways of treatment of the different forms of schizophrenia and I agree with you in this sense. In our opinion, one should not consider the different schizophrenias as a uniform illness. However, there is one point which should be mentioned, that the different forms of different symptomatology, of plus and minus symptomatology, could occur in the same patient at the same time, therefore, I cannot agree with your explanation that the dopaminergic system alone should be responsible. If under- and over-function occur at the same time, then either another neuronal system is involved or there must be another localization of the disorder. The other point is that sometimes there is a shift in symptomatology and it is known, that very often at the beginning of the illness there are depressive symptoms, as described by Conrad. Later on, these patients were paranoid-hallucinatoric schizophrenics, thus bearing this in mind it is very difficult to explain this alone by an over-function of the dopamine system. I would believe that there must be an involvement of another system, for instance, the alpha-adrenergic system.

Y. Lecrubier
We do not know what sort of dysregulation in dopamine could exist in schizophrenics, but I would like to mention 2 things : One is, you have several illnesses where opposite symptoms are found (maybe from a single system). If you look for example at bipolar patients you have mixed states, where in both there are affective problems in one way and agitation and hypermotility in the other. You find this also in Parkinsonian patients with DOPA and so on, so it is difficult to stress that argument. Ashcroft, for example, proposed that the range of behavioral tolerance to the variations of dopamine activity in patients was restricted and that in this case, with a normal range of dopamine levels which should be the same in normal subjects, there is a very great difference of tolerance in the schizophrenic patients.

Ch. Eggers
I fully agree with Prof. Ackenheil and I would like to ask if you have paid attention to other factors, not only to the metabolism of dopaminergic systems. For example, we have to consider the age of the patients. You stated already that young patients have a tendency to have more negative symptoms than adults. If a child becomes schizophrenic before 10 years of age, the negative, unproductive symptoms occur more often than the productive, hallucinatoric or delusionary symptoms. Surely the age and stage of the development of the cerebrum and the cognitive functions play a very important role with regard to phenomenology and course of schizophrenic psychoses. Another statement : You surely know the work of Gruzelier and Venables, who have found nearly a bi-modal distribution of schizophrenics in such as responders and non-responders with respect to their psychogalvanic skin responses. Stimulation tests and psychogalvanic investigations in animals with experimentally-induced lesions of the amygdala and the hippocampus revealed distinct relations between these brain structures and information processing in schizophrenics. There are fascinating correlations between neurophysiological, psychophysiological, neuropsychological and psychopathological findings in schizophrenic adults and high risk for schizophrenic children on the one side and animal studies on the other. These correlations point out the importance of the mentioned limbic structures for the etiology as well as for the clinical phenomenology of schizophrenic psychoses (Eggers, 1982). Therefore, we have to take into consideration not only metabolic, but also anatomical, neurophysiological, neuropsychological and developmental aspects when discussing the causes of varying psychopathology and symptomatology of schizophrenic psychoses.

Y. Lecrubier
You are speaking of the reason why perhaps some schizophrenic processes develop in these children and I agree completely with what you are saying. What I say, is that dopamine is just modulating symptomatology and that neuroleptics antagonize this modulation. This even could happen spontaneously and thus dopamine is not implicated in the disease process, dopamine is probably the end of the process, the last thing that modulates some behavior, no more.

N. Matussek
The basic pattern of the dopamine hypothesis of schizophrenia, the amphetamine psychosis, is also characterized by a paranoid hallucinatory syndrome. So far, neither a hebephrenic, nor a catatonic syndrome, nor a schizophrenia simplex have been described after amphetamine. There is probably no hyperactivity of dopaminergic neurons present in these forms of schizophrenia. Whereas, on the other hand, there are a number of hints that in mania, too, a hyperactive dopamine system is involved. What is then the difference between schizophrenia and mania ?

Y. Lecrubier
I agree with what you say, there are of course probably other things than dopamine and I would not say there are no other biological disturbances. I was just stressing what behavioral position we should give it, perhaps irrespectively to schizophrenia. This is, I think, the more important thing in this investigation. As for manic states, dopaminergic blocking agents are naturally useful, but also agents which decrease noradrenaline. We tried clonidine and had good results in manic states. The best results are certainly achieved in associating low doses of neuroleptics (classical ones) and clonidine and I think this was replicated in the United States recently.

R.M. Post
The hypothesis you are proposing is very interesting. It also seems to be quite consistent with the most consistent findings in schizophrenia and that is the increased variance in almost any measure that is studied. Your hypothesis brings one back to the issue of dysregulation in the dopamine system with either hyper- or hypo-responsivity possibly accounting for differences in symptomatology. There is also an animal study that is interesting with regard to the idea that opposite behavior could be caused by the same pharmacological manipulation or the same biochemical change. Lesse and his collaborators gave cocaine to animals and observed that the same dose of cocaine, depending on the stimulus cues, either greatly increased their bar-pressing responding (when a light associated with previous reward was on), or decreased responding completely (when the light was off). So, in this case the context of the social stimulation and the animals' « interpretation of the experience » led to opposite behaviors to the same hyperdopaminergic stimulation. This phenomenon may also be an interesting additional concept for your model.

G.U. Corsini
While I agree with the finding that apomorphine in low doses is able to reduce the positive symptom of schizophrenia, I wonder how you could state that high doses of apomorphine worsen positive symptoms, because as far as I know, nobody has presented evidence for a worsening effect of high doses of apomorphine in schizophrenia ?

Y. Lecrubier
I think that what was published were psychotic reactions with high doses of apomorphine.

N. Matussek
With small doses of apomorphine Dr. Gershon's group in New York did not get a psychotic reaction in schizophrenics, but with higher doses and over a longer period a Hungarian group provoked a psychotic symptomatology with apomorphine.

B.E. Leonard
I think it is as well to remember that not all drugs that are supposedly neuroleptics seem to be modulating the dopaminergic system and conversely drugs which modulate the dopaminergic system are very often not neuroleptics, or antipsychotics. I am thinking particularly of two recent studies. One by Barchas and colleagues (Principles of Psychopharmacology, Academic Press, p. 105, 1978) on

thiethylperazine. This seemed to have a good neuroleptic profile according to the animal experiments, but it was found to be relatively ineffective as an antipsychotic in man. There was also a paper by Greenblatt and colleagues (Arch. Int. Pharmacodyn. 248, 105, 1980) on a new indoline derivative, which did not appear to modulate the dopaminergic system in any way and yet, in initial clinical trials it appeared to have antipsychotic properties. Thus, I think the point you are making is well taken ; we emphasize the dopaminergic system as being the key site of action of antipsychotics and tend to neglect other neurotransmitter systems, which could be effective in modulating the dopaminergic system, or even produce their antipsychotic effects by a mechanism not involving dopamine. The last point I want to make is that there is a growing literature supporting the view that the noradrenergic system may be derranged in schizophrenia. I am thinking particularly of Hornikewicz's work on post-mortem material, where he has shown clearly a dysfunction in the noradrenergic system in schizophrenic patients.

COMPOSITION : NORD COMPO,
VILLENEUVE D'ASCQ

ACHEVÉ D'IMPRIMER SUR LES
PRESSES DE L'IMPRIMERIE (istra) STRASBOURG
AVRIL 1983

N° ÉDITEUR : 1134